VIRAL CULTURES

VIRAL CULTURES

Activist Archiving in the Age of AIDS

MARIKA CIFOR

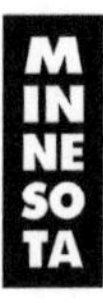

University of Minnesota Press

Minneapolis

London

Published by the University of Minnesota Press
111 Third Avenue South, Suite 290
Minneapolis, MN 55401-2520
http://www.upress.umn.edu

ISBN 978-1-5179-0935-2 (hc)
ISBN 978-1-5179-0936-9 (pb)

Library of Congress record available at https://lccn.loc.gov/2021061579

TO ALL THE ACTIVIST-ARCHIVISTS OF HIV/AIDS—
PAST, PRESENT, AND FUTURE

CONTENTS

INTRODUCTION

For the Record: AIDS, Archives, and Vital Nostalgia

if he were alive today he would be at this opening
if she were alive today you'd be texting her right now
if he were alive today he would be going gray
if they were alive today they could tell you about getting arrested at
    City Hall
if she were alive today you'd be so her type
if he were alive today you would have met him by now
if she were alive today she would have finished writing that book
if he were alive today he would have you on your knees
if he were alive today you'd still be arguing about that
if he were alive today he'd still be living with *AIDS*

"AIDS" STANDS APART in fierce pussy's *For the Record*. Printed in the retrovirus's signature bloodred hue,[1] "AIDS" breaks the singularity of the broadside's full-page, all-black text, a creative punctuation and punctum. Queer dyke art-action collective fierce pussy's text-based artwork reclaims language and public space for HIV/AIDS. With each iteration of "If he/she/they were alive today," the broadside intervenes in the strictures of AIDS time. Created in 2013 for arts organization Visual AIDS's twenty-fourth Day With(out) Art,[2] it is printed on cheap newsprint. With an intimate catechism of *ifs* repeating across the windows of New York City bookstore and gallery Printed Matter, fierce pussy transformed the site into a newsstand, taking their installation about the nature and meanings of the AIDS record to Chelsea's bustling sidewalks. *For the Record* also moved in posters distributed at museums, galleries, and nonprofits, on stickers and postcards, and in downloadable digital editions. Fierce pussy knew that passersby would only briefly scan the text, so they emphasized "AIDS" intentionally. HIV/AIDS, this project asserted, is still breaking news.

Fierce pussy is Nancy Brooks Brody, Joy Episalla, Zoe Leonard, and Carrie Yamaoka.[3] They met doing AIDS activism in 1991 and have collaborated on arts-based action ever since. These artists were acutely aware that in the twenty-first-century American popular imaginary, AIDS is static. The HIV/AIDS crisis in the United States is demarcated, when it surfaces at all in popular culture, as a past tragedy, a catalog of long-lost lives and decimated generations. AIDS is routinely marked as irrelevant to the unfolding crises and structural violences of our present. With each recurrent, yet distinct, utterance of "If he/she/they were alive today," fierce pussy speculated in conditional language about what might have happened differently in the epidemic's past, what could happen differently in its persistent present, and what could be different about HIV/AIDS's future.

For the Record in part is the expected AIDS record, an elegy for "dead friends, comrades and lovers."[4] Its textual performance mourns an accumulation of unbearable losses, utilizing the now-commonplace currency of imagining who could have been here and what work could have been accomplished if not for AIDS. Dominant AIDS narratives highlight treatment activism's political and aesthetic successes, driven by a heroic cast of now-departed AIDS activists—gay white middle-class men who died between 1981 and 1995 during their prime. Thus, aligned in structure and tone with other well-known AIDS artworks, the *if only*s in *For the Record* appear to focus on the valued lives of acclaimed gay cultural workers: artists, writers, designers, actors, directors, dancers, choreographers. "AIDS didn't just deprive us of millions of lives," Edmund White wrote, "it deprived of us of decades of potential masterpieces of fashion, art, design, theater and dance." For example, in "The Resurrected," White's 2018 *New York Times Style Magazine* article, Keith Haring (1958–91), who died from AIDS-related causes at thirty-one, is imagined and pictured as he would be at fifty-nine. Haring, a gay white cismale graffiti activist-artist who had already attained art world recognition, is one of four "geniuses, gone to the plague" whom White "resurrected."[5] In *For the Record,* too, there are traces of such conventional nostalgia, a potent longing for an earlier time shared with beloveds in the flesh. But significantly, fierce pussy refuses to us let stay comfortably in that space of uncritical, restorative yearning.

Conversely, fierce pussy conjures the dead not as martyrs but instead as wonderfully ordinary. The artists grant loved ones a mundane present in which they continue the everyday acts that constitute a life: texting, flirting, protesting, museum-going, fucking, talking, working. By making the present the focal point, fierce pussy pushes viewers to imagine and enact a different, more livable AIDS time—in which the past continues into the present in ongoing trivial tiffs, celebratory openings, and new relationships. Fierce pussy moreover asserts that mourning and loss are ongoing experiences that do not reside solely in the past. The artists deny cultural pressure to move on, to move past, to let go, to get over it in favor of embracing the future. The AIDS time rendered is neither linear nor progressive; rather, it is part of a vital nostalgia practice, an activist longing for a past time that interrogates, addresses, and repairs structural power inequities.

Through its unpunctuated litany, *For the Record* invokes a renewed urgency to curating and archiving as the care work needed to generate the AIDS record and to renew our commitment to HIV/AIDS awareness and action that can engender holistic cure. Fierce pussy created an AIDS record that requires viewers to reconsider our personal, social, political, and biomedical relationship to AIDS in the twenty-first century. Highlighting makes the final phrase pivotal: "If he were alive today, he'd still be living with AIDS." It repeats with only pronoun variations on the foldouts. Fierce pussy reminds us that even if the dead were animate, their histories and bodies would still be charged with HIV. Between an earlier epidemic era and our own AIDS time, so much, and yet so little, has changed. There are important advances in HIV treatment that prolong lives and improve their quality. However, even as biotechnology renders HIV a manageable chronic illness for some, it still requires arduous efforts to attain and sustain healthfulness. The virus still persists in infected bodies, living indefinitely in memory T cells containing integrated, transcriptionally silent HIV DNA.[6] Moreover, corporate, medical, and state apparatuses determine access, distribution, and production, rendering lifesaving antiretroviral medications inaccessible to many. Vulnerability and risk continue to be unevenly distributed by race, class, gender, sexuality, indigeneity, and carceral, housing, and immigration statuses; AIDS-related suffering and dying continue unabated in many minoritized communities; and an AIDS case plateau that is currently in progress makes a resurgence in new infections possible.[7] HIV/AIDS is still here, and it is still incurable in every sense—biomedical, political, cultural. A holistic AIDS cure demands dismantling the structural injustices that minoritize and marginalize HIV-positive people. Amid the ongoing AIDS pandemic, it remains urgent to use archives and records to raise awareness not only that people who died from AIDS-related causes were once here but also that people living with HIV continue to be here, and that those stories must be told and retold. The American HIV/AIDS crisis, John Petrus argues, needs "to be remembered not only as part of the past but also continuing in a different form into our present."[8] *For the Record* aims to ensure the everyday realities of AIDS time are documented, preserved, and accessible now and for posterity. In their creation and curatorial mobilization of the record through vital nostalgia, fierce pussy demonstrates the high stakes of documenting AIDS in America—then, now, becoming.

Viral Cultures: Activist Archiving in the Age of AIDS is about how we reckon with the AIDS past in this pandemic present. Archives are becoming as important to understanding AIDS as the biomedical event of HIV/AIDS itself. AIDS archives matter at this conjuncture for three primary reasons. First, archiving, the practices and acts of creating, collecting, preserving, and making accessible political, cultural, and medical knowledge, is a vital component of what Douglas Crimp terms "AIDS cultural activism."[9] Knowledge about HIV/AIDS would otherwise be marginalized, suppressed, or forgotten altogether.[10] Curatorial care work, the selection, organization, and maintenance of archives and records, enables them to be activated through creative works and events. Archiving and curation make possible the challenge and transformation of contemporary neglectful public understandings of the epidemic's persistence and lived experiences of HIV/AIDS. This book is an account of the people—activists, artists, curators, and archivists—and ideologies—temporal, political, technological, cultural, and biomedical—that shape AIDS archives and the cultural productions that animate these records.

Second, AIDS archives are produced by and reproduce the conditions of AIDS time. There is a continued urgency to AIDS cultural activism, and AIDS archives have a timely, evolving role to play in meeting and addressing it. In the accelerated registers of "epidemic time"[11] during the 1980s and early 1990s, AIDS activists responded by enacting the care work that Ben Alexander and Andrew Flinn call "activist archiving" at a furious pace, creating documentation, and collecting, preserving, curating, and making these records accessible. They accumulated rich, extensive archives that they mobilized for contemporaneous social change and that now shape the representation and conditions of HIV/AIDS with meaningful idiosyncrasies, erasures, redactions, and highlights. Almost immediately in the wake of 1996's biomedical breakthroughs, the advent of a more effective combination therapy of antiretrovirals for HIV and AIDS treatment, there was a shift in AIDS time. We entered and remain in an age of presumed HIV survivability and of ubiquitous end-of-AIDS declarations. The perceived urgency and relevance of documenting, collecting, and responding to HIV/AIDS was quickly evacuated. It is the records of a pre-1996 AIDS time that have been created, collected, and preserved for posterity by archives. Reckoning with twenty-first-century AIDS culture requires examining AIDS archives. We need to critically engage with "activist archiving," the archival care activists do as part of their efforts to engender social change, and with "archiving activism," public and private archival institutions' collecting, maintenance, use, and mediations of records created by AIDS activists.[12] Curation and archiving are practices of care enacted in activist archiving and archiving activism.

Finally, we are in a cultural moment that, amplified by the Covid-19 pandemic, is revisiting AIDS activism with a kind of nostalgia, but not the vital nostalgia that is going to be generative for AIDS cultural activism. From the 2010s onward, we have witnessed a proliferation of popular and scholarly AIDS crisis revisitations that are fundamentally grounded in the archival. These works are constructing what is known and knowable about HIV/AIDS through progressive narratives. Routinely, such narratives recenter gay, white, middle-class men as representative of AIDS activists and their treatment activism as a stand-in for AIDS activism as a whole. AIDS archives are positioned by such cultural productions as the location of the end of AIDS. Framing AIDS and its archives as relics of a distant past defangs contemporary AIDS crises in the United States, marking them as satisfyingly and safely over in the popular imaginary. Thus, simplistic historicization of AIDS can result in its depoliticization. However, there persists a deep, generationally inflected longing for the radical queer politics, coalitional community, and provocative aesthetics of pre-1996 AIDS activism. AIDS archival records, the people and systems that generate, collect, and care for them, and the ways that they are activated by activists, artists, curators, and archivists clearly merit a critical examination now. Despite the wave of scholarship, popular media, exhibitions, memorials, and other cultural productions on American AIDS activism during the 1980s and 1990s, the archives of AIDS on which such projects are built have not received proper attention. *Viral Cultures* examines the creation of AIDS records then and the activation of AIDS archival records now. How we engage with AIDS archives in the twenty-first century dictates more than HIV/AIDS's past. AIDS archives shape possible presents and futures and the distribution of life chances. Records, when harnessed through vital nostalgia, hold the power to be mobilized as forces that repoliticize AIDS and reinvest AIDS time with palpable urgency.

Viral Cultures demonstrates how nostalgia shapes the ways we record and remember in, with, and through AIDS archives. Nostalgia has long been dismissed and derided by scholars and popular commentators as a politically conservative, self-indulgent wallowing in the past that stands in the way of present and future social change. Using case studies from my ethnographic data, I center the vital potential of nostalgia as recorded and produced by archives documenting 1980s' and 1990s' AIDS activism in the United States. Vital nostalgia, the analytic inaugurated in this book, is a generative practice for interrogating, addressing, and repairing structural power inequities grounded in the bittersweet longing for a past time or space. This is the nostalgia we need amid crises and their aftermaths. Vital nostalgia enables a more complicated understanding of archives as both the site of AIDS's historicization and as the most powerful bulwark against dangerous end-of-AIDS narratives. Vital nostalgia names the critical examination of the present through an ongoing relation to the past. When activated within processes of vital nostalgia, AIDS archives showcase how activists and people living with HIV/AIDS are coping, struggling, and thriving with AIDS—not as the epidemic ends, but as it continues to unfold. Archives have powerful roles to play in developing a holistic, complex cultural cure for HIV's harms, to stem further suffering and death, and to improve life chances and quality for those continually marginalized. The temporal and affective drag of holding onto the past in such a vital nostalgic practice is about its political potentiality for feeling, imagining, and enacting a different, more just present and future. Ultimately, ethical scholarly, curatorial, and activist archiving practices must harness vital nostalgia in order to actively engage and serve diverse AIDS archival constituencies past, present, and future.

AIDS and Its Temporal Orders

"Tell the story of my life from zero hour to 12:00 a.m., from the good to the bad, tell the tale, save my life, a life I could have had just like Scheherazade," sings youthful, white, queer, well-muscled, leotard-clad Zero.[13] He croons while contact-juggling a disco ball and performing acrobatic feats to the accompaniment of synchronized swimmers. In the weird, wonderful opening number of *Zero Patience: A Movie Musical about AIDS*, we witness the melodic plight of a posthumous protagonist, the ghost of patient zero. Activist and filmmaker John Greyson's 1993 New Queer Cinema masterpiece was inspired by the true story of Gaëtan Dugas (1953–84). Dugas, a French Canadian flight attendant, was damningly misidentified in a 1984 epidemiological visualization as patient zero for the North American AIDS epidemic's contagion. In Randy Shilts's 1987 *And the Band Played On*, Dugas appeared as a sociopath who intentionally infected, or at minimum recklessly endangered, a promiscuous gay sexual network in coastal urban meccas.[14] "We were boys who loved our bodies, playing hard . . . boys who thought they'd live forever," Zero sings, reflecting the much-nostalgized, fleeting 1970s era of gay white sexual liberation. He marks that era's abrupt terminus with the advent of AIDS: "We didn't know we were playing for keeps." It is Zero's mission to find someone to, he repeats in the chorus, "tell the story, clear my name, why do they need someone to blame?" Dugas was not cleared of his alleged crimes until 2016.[15] As the musical number closes, the chorus of swimmers repeats the refrain: "Tell the story, tell the story, tell the story."

In my AIDS activism origin story, we are in early 1990s' San Francisco on the precipice of a dot-com boom. My grandmother has ventured out from her midwestern suburb to visit us—my father, mother, and preschooler me. We are walking through Union Square. Looking down, my grandma pauses, shocked, then asks, "What happened?" On the ground around us are chalk outlines of bodies piled upon bodies. It looks as if we stumbled onto a crime scene. We stand there in what appears to be the aftermath of a massacre carried out amid the high-end department stores, posh hotels, and holiday ice rink. My mother explains that, no, there had not been a crime—at least, not in the conventional sense. This was the remains of an AIDS Coalition to Unleash Power (ACT UP) die-in, an iconic "choreography of protest"[16] performed by activists who mimic corpses. By mirroring in their embodied acts the mass death of the AIDS epidemic, activists draw attention to the willful malfeasance perpetuated by the state, media, and public. The chalk outlines of bodies on the sidewalk likely faded quickly under the continuous assault of passing feet, but this memory of AIDS encounter has stuck with me.

Human immunodeficiency virus (HIV) and acquired immunodeficiency syndrome (AIDS) biomedically describe a broad spectrum of conditions caused by the body's acquisition of the HIV virion through the exchange of certain bodily fluids. While its circulation in the United States dates back to the late 1960s,[17] the medical community first clinically observed what would become known as AIDS in 1981. Its earliest recognized manifestations were in Los Angeles, San Francisco, and New York City among "clusters" of "homosexual men" who were diagnosed with previously rare opportunistic infections. These infections, Kaposi sarcoma and pneumocystis pneumonia, generally affect only those with severely compromised immune systems. That men with expectations of good health and access to health care were affected led to recognition of a more momentous epidemiological event.[18] Later that year, as word of a deadly new disease spread through gay communities, the *New York Times* first reported to the general public the possibility of an emergent epidemic under the headline "Rare Cancer Seen in 41 Homosexuals."[19] While the U.S. Centers for Disease Control and Prevention (CDC) recognized AIDS in 1981, its cause, means of infection, and scale remained unknown for the next few years. A toxic mixture of paranoia and scientific ignorance created widespread panic. Politicians and the media amplified these characteristics, leading to a popular hysteria, an embrace of fear-driven suspicions, and the shunning of entire groups.[20] In its early years, AIDS was frequently identified in the press as gay-related immune deficiency, or GRID. While it was not then and is not now a virus affecting only men who have sex with men, the symbolic and material association of HIV/ AIDS with sex, homosexuality, and the LGBTQ community was and remains important.

Materially, many of the best-known early HIV/AIDS responses came from gay and lesbian communities. In the early 1980s, facing widespread and far-reaching neglect, stigma, and discrimination from the state, mainstream media, pharmaceutical companies, health care and insurance providers, families, and religious organizations, and as the death counts rapidly rose, gays and lesbians organized. Many gay and lesbian communities were starkly segregated. Disparate resource distribution meant that early AIDS service organizations often arose from within gay white men's social networks and that they were staffed by white volunteers, supported by white donors, and oriented around a gay white cismale clientele's needs.[21] In turn, as they cared for people with HIV/AIDS and held public vigils to honor the dead, these early organizations' visibility reinforced the popular misconception that AIDS was a disease of gay white men, even as physicians found that the virus did not discriminate.[22] Framing epidemic commemoration now around only this first fifteen years constricts its subjects again to largely white, middle-class, gay American men.[23] The privileges these men held meant that they expected political and medical establishments to respond; when they failed to do so, it ignited outrage that fueled some fierce AIDS activism. The involvement of some in the arts, publishing, and media aided in securing selective attention within visible venues,[24] popular news coverage, and major museum shows. Meanwhile, the epidemic also raged in Black and brown communities, where it was less visible to the media and therefore to the straight white cisgender general public, policy makers, biomedical researchers, and, Dan Royles notes, in many cases to affected "communities themselves."[25]

By the mid-1980s, AIDS-related deaths surpassed twenty thousand nationally. Maddeningly slow progress in treatment, prevention, and care contributed to an escalating, unrelenting death toll and drove tactical shifts in AIDS activism.[26] In 1986 and 1987, groups emerged within gay and lesbian communities demanding confrontational direct action. Direct action was also provoked by a political climate with repressive tendencies, including the rise and entrenchment of neoliberalism under Ronald Reagan, growth of Christian fundamentalism, and institutionalization of novel biopolitical population governance forms.[27] ACT UP, the best-known oppositional group, formed in March 1987 in New York City and quickly expanded to over eighty chapters.[28] Building on the precedents of civil rights and Black power, gay liberation, and feminist health movements, activists mobilized a movement grounded in oppositional biopolitics.[29] They designated diverse intervention sites: mass media, pharmaceutical companies, the arts, medical schools, and government agencies. Activists became experts, educating themselves and others about pharmaceutical research and development, testing protocols, and developing alternative treatments.[30] They also contested policies restricting access to health care, housing, social services, and informal modes of discrimination and stigmatization. AIDS activists did more than work to save the lives of people made vulnerable; they changed culture, biomedical research, health care, and public policy—and in some instances, they made scathing critiques that situated HIV within the structural injustices constraining the life chances of people put at risk.

Activists did what they could to ensure the survival, thriving, and quality of life for people living with HIV and AIDS against impossible odds. Caring for those with AIDS involved daily and often extended labors, Crimp described, of "making innumerable hospital visits, providing emotional support, negotiating our wholly inadequate and inhuman human care and social welfare systems, keeping abreast of experimental treatment therapies."[31] This care work, which at its best is, as Marty Fink defines it, "a reciprocal process of mutual aid," engendered intimacies, familial connections, and bodily self-determination; it also facilitated forms of access not being met by institutions.[32] Activists' care was performed while coping with monumental loss, and in many cases the need to monitor and make treatment decisions about their own health.[33] Maintenance and care work, often unpaid and gendered labor, have not always been understood as activism; however, in the case of HIV/AIDS, touching and caring, whether for bodies or records, are political.

I picked up the copy of *For the Record* that hangs in my office from a tall stack near the entrance of the 2016 New York City edition of *Art AIDS America.* The exhibition was the first of such scale and national exposure to consider HIV/AIDS's powerful impact on contemporary art. Its curation reflected the racism, sexism, and classism that are routinely reproduced and reified in the veritable barrage since 2008 of retrospectively oriented HIV/AIDS cultural production. These works—films and documentaries, plays, popular and scholarly texts, performances, and exhibitions—draw on AIDS archives to advance a whitewashed narrative of AIDS creativity, care work, and impact. Of the more than a hundred artists *Art AIDS America* initially featured, only five were Black. Given that HIV/AIDS has always had and still has a disproportionate effect on Black, Indigenous, and people of color (BIPOC), this erasure was glaring. By the time I saw the show, its composition was amended in the wake of Tacoma Action Collective's die-in demanding that AIDS cultural production #StopErasingBlackPeople.[34] Curated omissions in progress-oriented AIDS narratives are far from exceptional. The willful disappearance of BIPOC, women, and trans and gender-nonconforming people is mirrored in productions that mine AIDS archives, from the Oscar-nominated 2012 documentary *How to Survive a Plague*[35] to the New York Historical Society's 2013 exhibition *AIDS in New York: The First Five Years* to 2016 debates over the New York City AIDS Memorial's form. The still-cresting wave of AIDS commemorations consistently begin their narratives with 1981 and end with the 1996 advent of antiretroviral drug therapy, marking a celebration of treatment activists' successes. Activism, reduced to the necessity of getting drugs into bodies, was marked as over. This telescoped temporal focus supports white supremacist patriarchy by acknowledging and celebrating only the efforts of gay, white, middle-class cismen, marking AIDS activism as past, ignoring failures and limitations of early responses to AIDS, and neglecting the existence and needs of minoritized communities where crises continue unabated. The represented face of AIDS in America is almost invariably white, male, gay, middle-class, and dead. The privileges of the men represented did not and could not save them from AIDS; however, they did and do protect them from vanishing from the historical record.[36] Now, AIDS time is marked by both the repeated erasure of minoritized bodies, actions, and experiences in dominant AIDS narratives, and the total evacuation of HIV/AIDS from the American cultural present.

On January 20, 2017, Donald Trump's inauguration day, the website and Twitter account of the White House Office of National AIDS Policy, in operation since 1993, disappeared. A perfunctory placeholder page stood in its stead, reading, "Sorry, the page you're looking for can't be found." This familiar notice symbolizes a conspicuous absence, and one that proved to be emblematic of national and global HIV/AIDS policy.[37] In June 2017, six Presidential Advisory Council on HIV/AIDS members resigned, citing that the Trump administration "simply does not care" about HIV/AIDS, a statement that was troublingly accurate. Seemingly disparate events—the 2016 adoption by the U.N. General Assembly of UNAIDS's Fast Track Strategy to "End the AIDS Epidemic by 2030," the 2019 media blitzes about HIV cures and celebratory marketing of pre-exposure prophylaxis (PrEP) as pharmaceutical curative, the disappearance of the White House Office of AIDS Policy, and many more—signify a prevailing cultural understanding that ending AIDS is not only achievable but also imminent, even inevitable.

AIDS, Susan Sontag identified, is a temporal condition.[38] From the beginning, the HIV/AIDS epidemic ruptured and reordered vectors of human existence: place, identity, relation, time.[39] I demarcate, drawing on Jules Gill-Peterson, the normative registers of AIDS time into "epidemic" time and "endemic" time.[40] Epidemic time, 1981 to 1996, was a period of nearly categorical AIDS dying, during which more than 350,000 Americans perished. Before the 1996 arrival of combination highly active anti-retroviral therapy, a long, relatively healthy life for people living with HIV/AIDS was nearly impossible. During epidemic time, HIV/AIDS registered as having an immediacy that, with efforts of HIV-positive people, queers, and anti-AIDS activists, managed to selectively surface it in the popular imaginary. For these individuals and communities, AIDS sped up time,[41] with bodies aging and deteriorating in a definitive disruption of chrono-normative logics. Unremitting waves of devastation called for an "immediate, in the moment, on the street" response.[42]

Normative AIDS time relegates people living with HIV/AIDS to a position out of time. As Sarah Sharma concludes, "The temporal is about power. Temporality is experienced as a form of social difference (margins) and a type of privilege (centers)."[43] AIDS time now has profoundly distinct valences. After 1996, we live in a time of "endemic" AIDS,[44] with HIV/AIDS having a depleted perceived public immediacy. Endemic time has also transformed the lived experience of HIV for those with privilege. For many, HIV is now a chronic illness with a life-span measured in decades; with better treatment, the risk of transmissibility for those with undetectable virus loads is gone. In endemic time, Americans who share my white, middle-class, cisgender, able-bodied privilege encounter AIDS (if they encounter it at all) as now only manifest in its relics, archival records created during and talked about only in curated commemorations of "epidemic time" that have only become more commonplace amid the Covid-19 pandemic. For those marginalized in AIDS's time politics, HIV/AIDS in the 2020s has a distinctive persistence; it is a present, unfolding emergency, one marked by unremitting immediacy.

It is popularly assumed that medically enabled long-term HIV survivability has been achieved. Yet globally thirty-seven million people are living with HIV/AIDS, and thirty-six million have died. In the United States alone, as of 2016, approximately 1.2 million people are living with the virus, fifty thousand new infections take place annually, and since 1981, seven hundred thousand have lost their lives.[45] Access to treatment and the stability required to maintain healthfulness remains out of reach for many; globally, approximately 60 percent of people have access to treatment. In America, conditions are disparate: many, especially cis and trans women, Black, brown, Indigenous, and undocumented people, and those facing poverty, addiction, homelessness, or incarceration, do not have adequate access to care. HIV is at the axis of contemporary political, social, and health crises, including mass incarceration, immigration, and opioid abuse.

Women have been profoundly affected by HIV/AIDS since the beginning. They have been put at risk and encounter challenges in accessing prevention, care, and treatment. Before 1993, CDC definitions were based on AIDS's manifestations in white cisgender men's bodies. Artaction collective Gran Fury famously charged, "Women Don't Get AIDS, They Just Die from It." Ignoring opportunistic infections as they manifested in diverse bodies enacted great harm, excluding women from research, proper diagnosis and care, and access to state benefits and resources. Willful negligence contributed to women with HIV/AIDS's cultural invisibility. AIDS continues globally to be the leading cause of death for women aged between fifteen and forty-nine.[46] Many women put at risk belong to marginalized communities, including transgender women, women who inject drugs, sex workers, and incarcerated women. The CDC estimates that 44 percent of Black, 26 percent of Latinx, and 7 percent of white transgender women are living with HIV. Black women of cis and trans experiences continue to be particularly affected, accounting for over half of HIV diagnoses among women. The likelihood of an HIV diagnosis in the United States is significantly higher for Black women (1 in 54) and Latinas (1 in 256) than for white women (1 in 941). As of 2017, AIDS was the seventh leading cause of death for Black women aged twenty-five to forty-four.[47]

Even with grossly inadequate data, it is clear that the epidemic's impacts on women are especially stark as they intersect with global migration. Before 2010, federal immigration law prohibited people with HIV from entering the United States. HIV status is now a basis for asylum applications—if an immigrant can demonstrate persecution because of their serostatus.[48] Nevertheless, immigration detention facilities routinely deprive people living with HIV of essential health care. In May 2018, Roxsana Hernández Rodriguez, a thirty-three-year-old Honduran migrant and transgender woman seeking asylum, died of dehydration and AIDS-related complications while in the custody of the U.S. Immigration and Customs Enforcement. Her death resulted from being denied access to lifesaving antiretroviral drugs despite officials' knowledge of her serostatus.[49] Gender-based inequalities, stigma and discrimination, and violence continue to present challenges to accessing the services and information that women need, with such challenges including structural barriers from poverty, racism, transphobia, and intimate partner violence. Despite, or perhaps because of, the challenges they face, women are powerful agents of social change; they are also some of the most prodigious and powerful documenters and collectors of HIV/AIDS knowledge and experiences.

American structural racism puts people of color, especially Black people, at significant risk for HIV infection as well as for AIDS-related suffering and death. Gay and bisexual men in their twenties, for example, made up 81 percent of new infections in 2016, and nearly 80 percent of those diagnoses occurred among Black and Latinx men.[50] Current projections are that one in two Black gay men will become HIV positive in their lifetimes.[51] Of the over two million people incarcerated in the United States, people of color, particularly Black people, are disproportionately represented. HIV rates among those imprisoned are five to seven times higher than the general public.[52] Intravenous drug use, sex work, domestic abuse, mental illness, poverty, and inadequate access to health care and resources inform who is subjected to the criminal justice system and who is put at greatest risk for HIV/AIDS before and during incarceration. Despite the work of those who have organized against injustices facing incarcerated people, including those with HIV/AIDS, conditions in jails and prisons continue to perpetuate infection, illness, and death. Inadequate access to health care, including access to prevention resources, such as condoms, in correctional facilities has a direct impact not only on incarcerated persons but also on the health of the communities to which they return. What's more, under neoliberal logics, individuals are understood to be "self-managing," responsible for making calculative choices about health and risk.[53] New infections or treatment failures are frequently blamed on individual recklessness rather than structural violences. Marlon M. Bailey, writing of the 2005 death from complications of AIDS of his Black gay interlocutor, Noir Prestige, notes that a hospice nurse told Prestige's partner, "We don't die like this anymore."[54] Bailey powerfully showcases that even now, some do still die this way.

AIDS is still a crisis, and it should be one to you. Now, more than four decades into the AIDS pandemic, triumphant biomedical and political discourses about the end of AIDS have been adopted by diverse stakeholders, including governments, nongovernmental organizations, major donors, the medical community, and the pharmaceutical industry. AIDS continues, as Crimp wrote in 1988, "not [to] exist separately from the practices that conceptualize it, represent it and respond to it. We know AIDS only in and through these practices."[55] To be certain, end-of-AIDS rhetoric and activist commitments to resisting it are not novel, just increasingly ubiquitous. Just four years after the July 1996 announcement of HIV treatment success, David Román traced the subsequent proliferation of end-of-AIDS discourses: major publications shifted their AIDS discourse, transfiguring it into something no longer deadly over the course of mere months. After issuing stories about its end, the media moved on. Román charted a simultaneous rise in rhetoric about a "post-AIDS" era by leadership in white gay communities as a means of disassociation from other minoritized communities that reinforced racist, classist, ableist, and geographic boundaries. These discourses encourage us to believe that "the immediate concerns facing contemporary American culture, including queer culture, are not-about-AIDS."[56] End-of-AIDS narratives counter the realities of an ongoing emergency characterized by sustainability challenges—withdrawals of resources from governments and nongovernmental organizations, donor fatigue resulting in reductions in long-term funding, failures to create effective, socially responsive health systems for treatment and prevention, and an unwillingness to confront the epidemic's root causes that are embedded in colonialism, imperialism, racism, heteropatriarchy, and socioeconomic inequities.[57] The AIDS crisis, as Sarah Schulman has shown, expedited a "replacement of complex social realities with simplistic ones"[58] and nurtured processes of gentrification, displacement, homogenization, assimilation, and upward wealth redistribution that manufacture consent through systemic, material foreclosures of possibilities for dissent.[59] End-of-AIDS discourse breeds ignorance and complacency; it contributes to weakening resolve to address HIV/AIDS.

As a queer person, HIV/AIDS is my inheritance. Dominant narratives, however, often divide queers neatly into distinct AIDS generations with disparate media modalities and platforms. First are people who came of age during 1970s' gay liberation—those who, like many of my interlocutors, remember both a time before AIDS and of watching scores of friends, lovers, and acquaintances die of a mysterious illness while institutions failed to intervene. This generation's activism is imagined as resolutely analog, its platform the city streets. Second are people of my generation, children of the 1980s and 1990s, who have never known a world without AIDS and who grew up alongside it. AIDS has suffused our identities and desires, shaping our sense and practice of queerness. Our platforms of AIDS media engagement are hybrid, crossing the analog and digital. Third is the generation born after 1996, the year that marks a transition to a highly effective treatment; this generation was mostly told that they don't have to think about AIDS at all. If this generation of supposed digital natives were to be engaged, then it would be through the mediations of digital media platforms. Yet these generational frames, attached as they are to different activist media modalities, offer only partial truths, only imperfectly reflecting the complexities of accepted narratives and lived experiences.

This book is situated within twenty-first-century AIDS culture and is part of an emergent critical HIV studies. HIV/AIDS and its activism have long been the subject of sociocultural inquiry, both popular and scholarly. In the late 1980s and throughout the 1990s, a number of still-influential cultural critiques focusing on AIDS and analyzing its activism appeared. Early works were often written by people who were themselves AIDS activists as well as scholars.[60] Much of the early AIDS literature was addressed to audiences beyond the academy. These works were not historical; they were about HIV/AIDS as an immediate concern. With a few notable exceptions,[61] AIDS did not receive much scholarly attention outside of public health and medicine in the early 2000s. Somewhere in the mid-2000s,[62] a focus on AIDS and its activism was renewed within history, sociology, political science, cultural studies, performance studies, art history, and gender and sexuality studies from scholars of my generation and those before us.[63] Much of this research is conducted in and sourced from the AIDS archives I analyze. Yet little scholarship addresses the archives themselves and the politics of activist documentation that gave rise to them.[64] Emergent HIV scholarship often newly centers minoritized activists, cultural workers, and communities' stories, and it articulates the twenty-first-century stakes of these histories. However, this scholarship is largely historical, focusing on HIV/AIDS during the popularly perceived height of the crisis, and can thus still unwittingly inform the dominant narrativization of HIV/AIDS in America as past.

The ways AIDS archives are constructed and used urgently matters. It is abundantly clear that the responsibility to stand against the lethal effects of misrepresentation, forgetting, and neglect and to insist on the ongoing urgency of HIV/AIDS, to document its history and record and remember its legacies, to point out its sprawling net of casualties and to confront its persistent stigma, discrimination, and racist, sexist, homophobic, transphobic, and ableist erasures will fall—yet again—on the shoulders of persons living with HIV/AIDS, activists, artists, curators, and researchers. AIDS archives routinely extend normative AIDS time, readily providing the "overexposed"[65] images that read as elegiac reminders of a bygone era. Yet AIDS archives hold the promising potential, when mobilized through vital nostalgia, to realign AIDS time in ways that expose its uneven valences and reset its social rhythms.

AIDS Activist Archiving and Archiving AIDS Activism

A 1995 Visual AIDS broadside-cum-recruitment poster by William Cullum insists, in all caps, "LET'S KEEP A RECORD." Fierce pussy's *For the Record* in its title also invokes the significance of AIDS records. Records are the central objects of archival collection, care, and use and are a conceptual preoccupation of archival studies' praxis. As Geoffrey Yeo defines, archival records are "persistent representations" of activity and experiences with attributes of structure, content, and context regardless of medium that travel across the bounds of space and time.[66] Cullum was among the first ten artists to have his artwork documented and preserved by Visual AIDS's Archive Project. He issued a call to action to his fellow cultural workers living with HIV and AIDS. "We need your help," he demanded. "Document our work now so that when you die and your boyfriend throws it all out on the street. There will be a record." Mortality was not an if but a when. Cullum's broadside underscores the urgency, born of the fatality of AIDS as well as the climate of the disease's acceleration, that drove many activists to create documentation of their actions and lives from the 1980s to the mid-1990s and to collect, care for, and activate those archival records on a significant scale. Activists' efforts provoking social change in their own time and for enduring posterity resulted in a vast, yet selective, archival representation. *Viral Cultures* takes this AIDS archival milieu as its subject.

Archives are deeply concerned with time and are central in constructing temporality, including individual and collective experiences of what time is; how it is constituted, organized, and mediated; and what it means to exist in relation to it.[67] Archives, much like HIV/AIDS, are conceptualized in the popular imaginary as static, always about the past, and dead, over, or at least irrelevant. Their immediate linkage to the emergencies that characterize our present and dictate future conditions are routinely neglected. However, archives are vital and relevant forces, "time machines"[68] that let us bridge past, present, and future. Brien Brothman posits that archives elicit a sense of continuity for the self, figure meaningfully into how communities understand and organize their past, and "foster a society's imagination of its future," effectually "establishing the quality and tensile strength of a community's composite temporality."[69] Archives provoke, he continues, "proximity [to] and integration with past and future generations" in ways crucial to building and breaking down solidarities.[70]

In an HIV/AIDS context, I draw together disparate concepts of *the* archive and archive*s*. The archival turn in the humanities transformed *the* archive from mere source to rightful analytic subject—a position it occupies in this book. Ann Laura Stoler describes the archive as a veritable Shangri-La, "a metamorphic invocation for any corpus of selective collections and the longings that the acquisitive quests for primary, originary and untouched entail."[71] In archival studies, the information studies subfield in which I am situated, scholars and archivists understand archives in a distinctive register. Archives, as Michelle Caswell defines them, are "collections of records, material and immaterial, analog and digital (which, from an archival studies perspective, is just another form of the material), the institutions that steward them, the places where they are physically located, and the processes that designated them 'archival.'"[72] *Viral Cultures* investigates AIDS archives as site and subject, examining both activist archiving and archiving activism within archival environments—institutions, digital media, galleries, and homes—imbricated in HIV/AIDS activism. I examine how AIDS activist archiving—activists' practices of archiving activities as part of their activism—has been and is being done. Further, I interrogate archiving AIDS activism, the ways that archives, whether community or institutional, document, collect, process, preserve, use, and make accessible the records of anti-AIDS activist groups and campaigns.[73]

Viral Cultures uncovers the cultural life of a constellation of AIDS archives and the people and lives that are implicated in those records and their animations. The three repositories at the center of this story— the New York Public Library (NYPL), New York University's (NYU) Fales Library and Special Collections, and Visual AIDS—are devoted to HIV/ AIDS in their collection development as well as in the processes, policies, and practices that they use to appraise materials for acquisition and make them accessible. These archives hold some of the most significant collections in scale and scope on HIV/AIDS activism during the 1980s and early 1990s. I examine the ways that these records are activated by archivists, activists, artists, and curators to mobilize AIDS knowledge and information as evidence that these things really happened, memories to preserve and transmit, and tools for demanding accountability and action. These archives' ideologies are informed by AIDS activist documentation and archiving, community archives traditions, and radical shifts toward addressing power in archival theory and practice.

Minoritized subjects have long been denied the pleasure and privilege of entry to the archive and to archives. People of color as well as queers, trans people, and HIV-positive people are routinely deprived of both history and futurity through evacuation from mainstream archival representation, relegated to a vulnerable existence in the present. AIDS archives emerged as—and in cases such as that of Visual AIDS's Archive Project remain—part of a long tradition of activist archiving within independent archives created by, for, situated within, and controlled by their communities of origin. Even within institutional repositories, like the NYPL and Fales, community-based archiving practices have troubled and transformed dominant practice.[74] Flinn, Mary Stevens, and Elizabeth Shepherd define community as "people who come together and present themselves as such;" they define "community archives" as "attempts to document the history of their commonality."[75] The community archives movement exploded in the wake of upheaval prompted by 1960s' to 1970s' social movements. In the 1980s, a gay and lesbian archives movement began to flourish, offering a means to locate and remember queer lived experiences and to evade and contest social subordination. Archival communities materialize around cultural, ethnic, racial, or religious identities, gender and sexuality, socioeconomic status, geographic locations,[76] and, as AIDS shows, health status. Despite harsh living conditions, minoritized subjects have always surpassed temporal relegation by willfully using archives to ensure more than just our present survival. The acts of creating, collecting, and preserving records that affirm the existence of communities that have been historically oppressed is political,[77] and community AIDS archives are a manifestation of archival activism.[78]

AIDS archives, and my account of them, are the product of a turn toward interrogating power in archival praxis. Before the mid-1990s, a set of positivist formulations undergirded mainstream archival practices; they dictated that archives' meanings were static and uncontested, and that archives are the natural product of institutional processes, one beyond archivists themselves.[79] In these traditional conceptualizations, the archivist's role is to act as a "handmaiden of history," a passive custodian of the historical record.[80] Sir Hilary Jenkinson, a leading early to mid-twentieth-century archival theorist, described archivists as engaged in an "unbiased" and "objective" record administration of "official" state-sanctioned agencies and corporations, forming an "untainted" collection which guaranteed accountability through unbroken chains of custodianship.[81] Over the past two decades, archives have been reconceptualized as spaces that were never neutral, and archiving has come to be understood as a far-from-objective undertaking. Critical archival studies[82] scholarship builds from and critiques humanistic theorizations of the archive and its powers. Jacques Derrida famously stated in *Archive Fever,* "There is no political power without control of the archive, if not of memory."[83] Michel Foucault conceptualized the archive as the "first law of what can be said, the system that governs the appearance of statements as unique events."[84] Mobilizing critical cultural theory, feminist, Indigenous, and queer scholarship, archival thinkers have reconceptualized archives and archival practices as manifestations of and instruments in the exercise of power and domination. This work exposes the myriad ways that archives have authorized power and abetted those with it—for example, by showcasing how supposedly objective and neutral approaches to professionalism are steeped in whiteness, colonialism, ableism, and heteropatriarchy. The archival record is heavily biased toward those in power, in turn enacting substantive harm. The AIDS activist record is also biased. Verne Harris noted that "the archivist" must be "a memory activist either for or against the oppression system."[85] The activists, curators, and archivists in the AIDS archives I examine are all proactive agents in the record's creation, management, and representation.

Contextualizing the ways that AIDS archives are made, developed, and animated through activist archiving and archiving activism requires interrogating ideology and power. AIDS archives are expressions of the relations, biases, historical moments, and acts of the records' creators and subjects. They are also reflections of archivists' appraisal practices that decide, as Terry Cook writes, "which creators, functions, and activities generating records will be represented, by defining, identifying, then selecting which documents and which media become archives in the first place,"[86] often along subjective measures of cultural and institutional significance and historical and research value. These acts deem records to be archival and thus worthy of preservation and accessibility into perpetuity.[87] "As archivists appraise records," Cook asserts, "they are doing nothing less than determining what the future will know about its past: who will have a continuing voice and who will be silenced."[88] Archivists cocreate the archives. The AIDS archives examined hold what Harris calls "a sliver of a sliver of a sliver" of the record.[89] Activist archives hold temporal particularities; the collections themselves and the movements they document may be temporary and ephemeral.[90] Social movement records frequently present preservation challenges as a result of activists' use of mass production and cheap materials, or unstable audio, moving image, or digital formats.[91] AIDS archives are always, Robb Hernández writes, incomplete, "caught somewhere between completion and oblivion," riddled with "redactions, omissions, editorial revisions, and serendipitous rediscoveries."[92] This book tells the story of how, in creating AIDS archives, archivists, activists, artists, and curators, in Tonia Sutherland's words, "influence what narratives and stories can and cannot emerge from the archives."[93]

New York City remains the city most recognized in accounts of the devastation of the American AIDS crisis, the furious and fabulous activism born in response to it, and the beautiful bounty of artistic cultural production on AIDS. There are many reasons for this AIDS fame. New York was long the urban center with the highest HIV case instances. To date, more than a 110,000 New Yorkers have died from AIDS-related causes. The city is home to some of the most recognized AIDS activist groups and institutions: ACT UP, Gay Men's Health Crisis (GMHC), the American Foundation for AIDS Research. In 1984, St. Vincent Hospital opened the country's second AIDS ward. Knowledge from within New York's gay community was used to draft an early safer-sex guide, *How to Have Sex in an Epidemic: One Approach*. It is the landscape of many acclaimed plays, films, and books about AIDS: *The Normal Heart, Angels in America, Rent, How to Survive a Plague, United in Anger,* and *Close to the Knives*. It was also home to famed cultural workers felled by AIDS: Alvin Ailey, Gia Carangi, Perry Ellis, Keith Haring, Félix González-Torres, Robert Mapplethorpe, Ray Navarro, Willi Ninja, Vito Russo, David Wojnarowicz. The *New York Times,* the city's paper and the nation's newspaper of record, is cited as the first mainstream outlet to report HIV/AIDS. AIDS memory projects are also fixated on New York, including the ACT UP Oral History Project and the Smithsonian Archives of American Art's Visual Arts and the AIDS Epidemic. The city is the site of one of few AIDS memorials. Virtual memorials, like the Instagram account @TheAIDS-Memorial, also routinely geotag and name the city as the site of loss.[94] Scholarly production about HIV/AIDS too has devoted significant attention to New York.

Though New York was and is at the center of AIDS accounts from the cinematic to the scholarly, it is by no means the only or arguably even the most important place in telling the story of HIV/AIDS in America. It is also not the only site of powerful AIDS archives. Indeed, as a native of San Francisco and later a resident of Los Angeles, two cities with their own remarkable archives and collections about HIV/AIDS, I was resistant to doing yet another project about New York. Yet there is something undeniably distinct about the AIDS archival activations that have happened there, making it worth the risk of talking about New York once again. While doing exploratory research in the ACT UP New York Records at the NYPL, I encountered the NYPL's 2013–14 *Why We Fight: Remembering AIDS Activism* exhibition and programming. This series exposed the constellation of activist archives that are the subject of *Viral Cultures:* the NYPL's Manuscripts and Archives Division, the Downtown Collection at NYU's Fales Library and Special Collections, and Visual AIDS's Frank Moore Archive Project and Artist+ Registry.

While not alone in the city or beyond it in their AIDS archiving, each of the institutions I focus on by the early 1990s had developed an unusually intentional and intensive collection development focus on HIV/AIDS and its implications for art and activism. While each contains materials that document AIDS activism in other locales, they are focused significantly on AIDS in New York City. The NYPL's Manuscripts and Archives Division began collecting materials related to AIDS activism in the late 1980s under its mission of supporting research on New York's political, economic, social, and cultural history. The institution holds over one hundred collections that it identifies as "pertaining to the history and culture of gay men and lesbians, and to the history of the AIDS/HIV epidemic."[95] NYPL collections include prominent AIDS activist individuals and organizations: ACT UP/New York, GMHC, the Estate Project for Artists with AIDS, People with AIDS Coalition, and Gran Fury. The division also holds the largest collection of AIDS activist videos worldwide. NYU's Downtown Collection, founded in 1994, holds over one hundred collections documenting the art scene in SoHo and the Lower East Side from the 1970s through the 1990s. It preserves the legacies of artists whose work dealt with AIDS and of many with HIV. The collection includes personal papers of prominent artists, filmmakers, writers, and performers: Robert Blanchon, Dennis Cooper, Avram Finkelstein, Frank Moore, Jack Smith, David Wojnarowicz, and Martin Wong. It also holds the records of art galleries and organizations, theater groups, and art collectives engaged with HIV/AIDS: Artists Space, Creative Time, Franklin Furnace, Group Material, and MIX's New York Lesbian and Gay Experimental Film and Video Festival. Visual AIDS, founded in 1988, is a community-based arts organization committed to raising AIDS awareness through visual art, materially assisting HIV-positive artists, and preserving and activating artistic legacies. Its Archive Project began in 1994 as a slide and research library to collect and preserve the work of HIV-positive artists. In 2012, Visual AIDS launched the archives' digital counterpart, Artist+ Registry. It holds digitized versions of many of the project's original slides, alongside new work by artist members forming the "largest database and registry of works by visual artists with HIV/AIDS."[96] Together, these archives tell an important story about how AIDS has been documented and archived since the 1980s. What is unprecedented is how these AIDS archives and records are being animated through programming, activist interventions, and archival relations in the twenty-first century. Because of the scale and significance of their mobilizations of the AIDS record, I cull from these three prominent AIDS archives.

Public programming has reactivated AIDS records with critical creativity. These efforts are enmeshed in and enabled by the complex network of relationships between the three archival institutions. They hold collections and materials created by and about the same individuals, collectives, and organizations. For example, the personal papers of Avram Finkelstein, an artist, activist, and writer, are part of the Downtown Collection, and his work as a member of Gran Fury is held by the NYPL; painter Martin Wong has a page on Visual AIDS Artist+ Registry, and his papers are at Fales; AIDS Coalition to Unleash Power/New York's (ACT UP/NY) Records are part of the NYPL, and Fales holds Bill Bytsura's collection of ACT UP photographs. They also have a number of formal and informal collaborations and partnerships. Visual AIDS's noncurrent organizational records are held by Fales, and Visual AIDS has facilitated Fales's acquisition of artists' papers, including those of Robert Blanchon and Chloe Dzubilo. In 2013 and 2014 alone, in exhibitions and other public programming, the relations between these institutions around AIDS records shaped their events, the objects displayed, and artistic and activist interventions made. In collaboration with Visual AIDS, the Downtown Collection was central in a number of important exhibitions held on site at Fales as well as in galleries, museums, and community organizations across New York City. These collaborations include the exhibition *Not Only This, but "New Language Beckons Us,"* comprising AIDS archival materials from the Downtown Collection and newly commissioned texts from contemporary artists. Smaller events and acts of coproduction were also common. Fales loaned one of Wojnarowicz's journals to the NYPL for *Why We Fight.* For the programing series accompanying the exhibition, the NYPL in turn worked closely with Visual AIDS on events from art workshops for teens led by Visual AIDS's artist members to the panel about the *Your Nostalgia Is Killing Me!* poster to the coproduction of Finkelstein's Undetectable Flash Collective.

As prominent AIDS archives, each institution holds tremendous, rich collections on 1980s' and 1990s' AIDS activism and its cultural productions. Their materials promise to reproduce and disrupt the stability of AIDS time as well as produce and mediate vital nostalgia for AIDS activism. The AIDS archival discourse they are producing through their "classification schemes, processing rituals, and economic modes for assessing historical or literary value," as Fales director Marvin J. Taylor asserts, have become "the cultural system par excellence that reifies, legislates, represses, normalizes, and creates the possibility of what can be known, who can know it, and how it will be preserved" when it comes to HIV/AIDS in the United States.[97] With attention to the intersections of gender, sexuality, race, class, nationality, and ability in the identities of the archives' stakeholders, *Viral Cultures* traces the creation and development of these collections across media modalities. I also examine the complicated connections of AIDS activists and artists to their archival materials, and curators' and archivists' relationships to the communities implicated in their records and programming.

Theorizing Vital Nostalgia

"Sometimes I can't stop thinking about dying. As a young faggot I knew I was going to die of AIDS, because, you know, that's what faggots did when I was a teenager. But things are different now; now fags are dreaming of white weddings and military service. Meanwhile, I'm still trying to imagine what the genocide was like."[98] Thus begins Ryan Conrad's monologue in his 2012 video *Things Are Different Now* . . . Conrad is a gay white artist and academic of my AIDS generation: one too young to be immediately implicated in that epidemic era but too old not to feel its impact. He deploys archival footage of ACT UP's iconic political funerals as captured by activist video collectives; this footage is held in AIDS archives, including the NYPL's vast AIDS Activist Videotape Collection. Layered between and over these famed archival images are twenty contemporary portraits of men in Conrad's network—young, gay, white. With audible melancholy, he asks, "Could I ever understand what it was like to lose twenty, thirty, forty, fifty of my friends and lovers? Would I have had the strength to drag my friends' dead bodies through the streets in protest?" AIDS activism of the 1980s and early 1990s may now seem like a strange object for nostalgic yearnings, yet there is a palpable nostalgia for that moment and those places, people, images, and politics that does not belong to Conrad alone. This nostalgia for AIDS activism distinctly inhabits, and also transgresses, generations and activist positionalities. There is a desire to abide, at least in a certain sense, in the past; the past seems to offer more.

Nostalgia for AIDS activism does not mean that anyone actually wants to restore AIDS's early years. Roger Hallas notes that it is diminishment of AIDS cultural activism that "gay men and lesbians mourn when they lament the absence of [contemporary] discussion about AIDS—for instance the empowering mutuality of ACT UP demonstrations, the graphic art of collectives like Gran Fury and General Idea, the complex installations of Félix González-Torres, or the politicized performance art of Ron Athey and Tim Miller."[99] Nostalgia for that time—mostly for flashy, provocative direct-action AIDS activism, with its attendant radical politics and lived purposefulness—has become a common language, both on the part of those who participated and by those who wish they had, through which people articulate their disappointments and frustrations with the present and its politics. Writing on retroactivism, Lucas Hilderbrand acknowledges that his relationship to the AIDS activist past is "romanticized," yet despite its limitations, AIDS nostalgia deeply informs his political and sexual identities.[100] Looking back is about the shortcomings of attention paid to AIDS now and is also deeply rooted in a deep dissatisfaction with the assimilationist 2000s and 2010s LGBTQ politics and activism, which focused on gaining inclusion in dominant institutions, from marriage to military. Ultimately, AIDS archives hold the records that provoke our AIDS activist nostalgia. Archives thus both mediate and produce AIDS activist nostalgia in ways that can be vital in repoliticizing AIDS time. This book builds on the collective affects articulated by Hilderbrand, Hallas, and other queer people; it situates AIDS archives as source and site to experience and mobilize vital nostalgia.

Nostalgia has a complex history. It names the condition or feeling of bittersweet longing for a time or space that is past. It demarcates relations to time and space that are tied, Katharina Niemeyer writes, "to a way of living, imagining and sometimes exploiting or (re)inventing the past, present and future."[101] Svetlana Boym asserts, "Nostalgia is not always about the past; it can be retrospective but also prospective." In other words, the past is shaped by the present's needs. Moreover, the ways in which the past is desired now directly affects future realities. Nostalgia for the past, intimately linked with present conditions and future imaginings, may be public or private, individual or collective. Nostalgia often arises as companion to social, political, and technological change.[102] Vital nostalgia, the analytic I develop in this book, names a process of questioning, contending with, and redressing power inequities that continually subject minoritized people to harm and violence that is grounded in a critical activation of a yearning for a past time and the people who occupied it. This nostalgia is vital in multiple senses. It is a vigorous, energetic force that is animate and changeable; it is fundamentally concerned with maintenance and continuance of life and living beings; it pertains to the recording of pertinent data about human lives. Vital nostalgia encompasses the complicated process of critical interrogation of our present through ongoing relation to the past. This is a nostalgia that emphasizes the longing for the past while also attending to and illuminating the ambivalences, violences, and complexities of that past that continue to dictate life chances. The temporal and affective drag of holding tightly onto the past in such a vital nostalgic practice is about its generative political potentiality for feeling, imagining, and enacting a just and livable now, and a more vibrant future.

Nostalgia is a composite of two Greek roots: *nostos*, "to return home," and *algia,* "pain."[103] Coined by physician Johannes Hofer in 1688, it identified homesickness, which was at the time associated with exiles and soldiers, as a psychopathological disorder. Those afflicted were characterized as manic with longing. It was described as "melancholic," "debilitating," and even "fatal."[104] Nostalgia's symptoms included losing appetite, hearing voices, seeing ghosts.[105] By the mid-nineteenth century, there was medical consensus as to nostalgia's basic attributes. It struck without regard to age, gender, nationality, or profession. Its onset could be provoked by any number of things: an overly lenient education; "disappointed ambition;" mountainous homelands; masturbation; "unusual food;" and "happy love."[106] Nostalgia's triggers were memories manifested in sounds, tastes, smells, sights, and feelings that reminded individuals of departed homes.[107] Some theorized that nostalgia had a physiological origin, "a pathological bone;" however, investigations were to no avail.[108] From the seventeenth century until well into the nineteenth century, nostalgia was curable. Cures were attempted by inciting pain or fear; opium, leeches, warm emulsions, or journeys to the Swiss Alps might also be prescribed.[109] The most successful cures were in a return, or the promise of one, to that which was familiar and local to the patient. By the late nineteenth century, nostalgia evaded cure. Nostalgia's object of longing became more prodigious than personal history, transforming into a collective sense of loss.

Nostalgia emerged as a cultural and literary mode, the purview of poets and philosophers. David Lowenthal labels nostalgia's transformation a shift "from a geographical disease into a sociological complaint."[110] Though the absence or removal from home and homeland remains an often-studied manifestation of nostalgia, it also came to define an urgent longing for departed times.[111] Nostalgia metaphorized from a treatable ailment to an incurable state. It signifies absence and loss that can in effect never be made presence again, except through the imperfect tools of memory and the "creativity of reconstruction."[112] Boym classifies nostalgia as sentiment, "the mourning of displacement and temporal irreversibility," that is at "the very core of the modern condition."[113] As a "historical emotion," nostalgia's transformation was about the increasingly common experience of dislocation and a temporal shift to "the modern conception of unrepeatable and irreversible time."[114]

From the 1970s into the 2000s, historians and social critics widely interpreted nostalgia to be apolitical, regressive, and ahistorical.[115] In particular, Marxist theorists denounced nostalgia. Christopher Lasch, for example, conceptualized nostalgia as a "betrayal of history" and derided its adherents as "incurable sentimentalist[s]" who were "afraid" of the "future" and "to face the truth about the past."[116] Raymond Williams framed nostalgia as an opiate with far-reaching dysfunctional consequences. Nostalgia, he believed, enticed people to take refuge in an idealized version of the past as a means to avoid examining present problems. Nostalgia was thus understood as a force impeding social change by lulling people into a ready acceptance of the status quo.[117] Tenacious resistance to nostalgia also carried into feminist projects.[118] Some scholarly reactions were shaped by authors' position within the 1970s' and 1980s' American "nostalgia craze," a zeitgeist embedded in the reactionary response to 1960s' sociopolitical upheavals, and a rightward political shift.[119]

Negative coding of nostalgia popularly is also informed by imbrication in late capitalist ideologies. Capitalism foregrounds linear, teleological notions of time and enshrines progress; thus, nostalgia's unrelenting grip on the past is derided. Fredric Jameson, whose theorization of late capitalist postmodernity situates us in a culture characterized by the demise of historicity, posits that we have replaced history with an aesthetic "nostalgia mode." Given the cultural estrangement from the past, its actual viscerality is substituted for commodified glossy, but empty, stylized "pastiche." Nostalgia thus names for Jameson the profiteering, plundering, and reduction of the past to stereotype and style. Damningly, nostalgia is a force that is constitutive of commodification's overtake of life under late capitalism's logics.[120]

Since the mid-1990s, a still-growing nostalgia scholarship in an array of disciplines has reclaimed it as a force with potential for criticality. Nostalgia is reconceptualized as generative in identity and cultural heritage, and for advancing political and social change. Boym's articulation of nostalgia as simultaneously past and future oriented, and Maurice

Halbwachs's nostalgic memory are foundational to such theorizing. Halbwachs framed nostalgic memory as "escape from the present," its escapist tendencies a virtue[121] that liberated people from dominant temporal orders. Nostalgic memory is dialogic. Constructed as it is in the present through hindsight, it has a significant comparative and animating purpose, selectively deploying objects and feelings from the past as creative inspiration and for possible emulation.[122] In Kate Eichhorn's words, nostalgia's alternative temporality "opens the possibility for a radical [feminist] politic that appears committed to longing for both real and imagined versions of the past as it is to futurity."[123] Nostalgia is a temporal mode that recognizes that forward progression and a clean break with past losses are often impossible, and sometimes undesirable.

Critical work on nostalgia has further reclaimed it as formative to identity and social movement mobilizations. Nostalgia allows for "a negotiation between continuity and discontinuity: it insists on the bond between our present selves and a certain fragment of the past, but also on the force of our separation from what we have lost," Nadia Atia and Jeremy Davies insist.[124] Linkages between present and past self are significant in identity development, communal belonging, and social movement building.[125] Boym writes, "Nostalgia is about the relationship between individual biography and the biography of groups or nations, between personal and collective memory."[126] As an example of this phenomenon, nostalgia affords activist-scholar Alexandra Juhasz the opportunity, by video remix in her experimental AIDS documentary *Video Remains*, to refigure time and feeling. Nostalgia is what takes her personal response to her best friend's death and makes it a collective experience that can produce novel feelings and knowledge that might catalyze action.[127]

Vital nostalgia builds on theorizations of reflective and critical nostalgia. Boym classified two types of nostalgia. Nostalgia can problematically be "restorative," aspiring to the perfect "transhistorical reconstruction of a lost home," or other space. Alternatively, nostalgia can be "reflective," thriving in the ambivalence of longing itself.[128] Reflective nostalgias, those with critical potentiality, do not aspire to actually reconstruct or restore that which is past. Vital nostalgia reaches beyond reflective nostalgia to the extent in which it is both deeply political and socially engaged; it is a mode of coherent critique that demonstrates more self-consciousness in its awareness and holds more strategic potential for action than reflective nostalgia allowed for. In a breakdown of critical nostalgia, Ray Cashman identifies nostalgia as a critical analytic when deployed to produce evaluations of our present that contrast it intentionally with our past. It is also critical in importance when used as inspiration to build a "better future."[129] Nostalgia's critical capacity is structural.[130] Vital nostalgia is distinct in the formative focus of its longing not just for lost objects, times, or spaces but also for lost individuals and communities, particularly those whose lives are marginalized, and life chances diminished by structural violence. Significantly, this study also expands the critical potential of nostalgia to catalyze ethical and morally invested human actions.

For individuals and communities living with and amid HIV/AIDS, vital nostalgia is a means to unsettle temporal conditions. Vital nostalgia draws on the AIDS past, real or imagined, to conceptualize and to construct a different, more just present and future. It provides a means for self-aware, complex, selective, or strategic retrieval and uses the AIDS past for contemporary utility. The past becomes a space to identify and deploy sources of agency, identity, relation, affect, and satisfaction that are lost in the present. Vital nostalgia names then a shared language, feeling, or memory. In short, it is a political tool by which people conceptualize, express, and challenge the ways that they are disappointed, absented, frustrated, or continually threatened in the present. Disrupting the linear and chronological ordering of life and being in the present crucially engenders the possibility for alterative livable futures, especially for marginalized subjects. Blurring lines between past, present, and future, vital nostalgia generates multiple through lines. It explores how to live in multiple times and places at once; this simultaneously presents ethical and imaginative challenges. Critical reflection, the feeling of longing, and action for social change become, within vital nostalgia, allied approaches.

To my knowledge, neither archives nor the archive have been studied or theorized in relation to nostalgia. Yet addressing nostalgia in the archival field promises deeper critical and ethical engagement with archival stakeholders, memory, temporality, and affect. It offers possibilities for transforming theory and practice. Nostalgia is theorized in this book in all of its complexity and capacity as a means of building and sustaining cultural heritage and identities, and as a tool for social and political action. In the archives, the past is both present in its material traces and yet no longer fully accessible, which makes the archives a powerful trigger for personal and collective nostalgias. Archives are thus an important subject and site for studying nostalgia. Vital nostalgia is a productive practice at every juncture between HIV/AIDS archives and the AIDS activist communities they document and serve.

Archival Ethnography

My efforts to discern the practices central to the construction and mobilization of AIDS archives took me from artists' studios in Jersey City to a bakery in Brooklyn, from the bustling Chelsea office of an arts organization to a Harlem row house's cozy living room. What I discovered in fieldwork in New York City from 2015 to 2016, and in follow-up visits from 2018 to 2019, were record-keeping formulations that both align with and contest archival traditions in their documentation, description, preservation, and animation of a virus through entangled networks of objects, people, and institutions, carefully collected ephemera and fragments, and artifactual and visual surrogates for departed loved ones and activists still fighting. *Viral Cultures* is an archival ethnography that follows the cultural life of archival objects as they move into, within, and beyond the demarcation of AIDS archives, and that follows the connections and collaborations between activists, artists, archivists, and curators. An understanding of archiving and curation as care work is reflected not just in objects of analysis but in the method of doing archival ethnography, which extends activists' HIV care work into contemporary time and space.

Archival ethnography, a form of qualitative field research and iterative naturalistic inquiry, enabled me to study cultures of AIDS activism and documentation, the form and formats of records and collections and archival processes that shape them, and the ideologies and power relationships that are reflected in and reproduced by archival systems from appraisal to outreach to use.[131] I did interviews, archival research and document analysis, and observation within archival environments to gain an understanding of the perspectives—social, political, and cultural—of the people who create, collect, maintain, and use records. Archival ethnography is unique, Janet Ceja Alcalá argues, in the ways that it "takes the archival milieu, broadly envisioned, as the subject of study, rather than solely requiring that the materials gathered as data be studied as historical artifacts of a particular social group's past."[132] I followed the "documentary" trails contained within archival records themselves and archival apparatuses that order, classify,[133] and make them accessible by archival institutions. This methodology offers epistemological advantages by accounting for the complexities of documents and human behavior and feelings, providing thick description, offering multiple viewpoints, and facilitating inquiry into obtuse but vital areas of human experience, affect, emotion, and memory, thereby enabling inductive research. I consider both what is deemed archival and what is left out of the AIDS record, moving between remembering and forgetting. "Societies institutionalize their collective archives," Sue McKemmish, Anne J. Gilliland, and Eric Ketelaar argue, "according to their own evidence and memory paradigms. These paradigms influence what is remembered and what is forgotten, what is preserved and what is destroyed, how archival knowledge is defined, what forms archives take, [and] how archives are described and indexed."[134] Archival ethnography affords me the possibility of exposing what stories AIDS archives can and do tell.

The formalized AIDS archives in *Viral Cultures* are housed within the country's second-largest public library, an elite private university, and a community-based arts organization in New York City. Yet the archives I study are even more prodigious, encompassing spaces in which archival records creation, care work, or use is a significant focus of interest and activity.[135] These sites range from artists' Facebook walls, Tumblr pages, and studios to major museum exhibitions and gallery installations; it includes personal collections stored in closets, up in attics, and under beds. Archival ethnography opens for interrogation the records' social, cultural, political, and aesthetic dimensions, the processes and systems that produce and maintain them, and the ways that they are activated by archivists, activists, curators, and artists.

In-depth semistructured interviews with more than thirty interlocutors form a substantive component of the rich data corpus I draw on in this book. The archival practices I examine are always in relationship to the individuals and communities who created, collected, and preserved the documentary evidence in question.[136] I am immensely privileged to have become a part of these AIDS worlds. Each of my interlocutors had a meaningful relationship, whether in the long term or as a one-night stand, with one or more of my research sites. I spoke with archives founders and library directors; professionally trained and volunteer archivists, curators, artists, and writers; long-term and former employees of each institution; executive directors and nonprofit staff and administrators; archives users; and lifelong activists. I interviewed people in quiet offices and staff lounges, in loud downtown cafés, in intimate domestic spaces, in reading rooms after hours, in artists' studios surrounded by works in progress, on the subway, on a rooftop overlooking the Christopher Street Pier, over the phone, and via videoconference in rooms thousands of miles away. Some interlocutors I met only once; with others, conversations unfolded over the course of years. The number of interlocutors interviewed at research sites varied according to institutional scale, scope of programming, and number of people involved in the collections and programming analyzed.

I engaged with each research site as an archives user and participant observer. Conducting archival research afforded me deeper understanding of the collections, the archival policies and processes that shape these records' use and interpretation, how the descriptions of materials reflect (or not) the contents and lives of individuals and communities implicated in them, and the scope and scale of AIDS activists' documentation strategies and ongoing productions. I also gathered and analyzed exhibition documentation, contemporary artworks and activist ephemera, digital exhibitions, press releases, social media feeds, and news about these sites and their records of HIV/AIDS activism to identify and interpret patterns. This process required taking the document seriously as "ethnographic object," "analytical category," and "methodological orientation," in Annelise Riles's words.[137] I used documents to supplement, verify, or contest concerns that emerged in fieldwork. I also recognized that these documents—archival records, statistical data, oral histories, and scholarly and popular writing—also mediate the meaning and elements of their contents.[138] At the sites, I participated in events from openings and tours to social media conversations. This study resulted in a rich description of phenomena that is fundamental to the project of building theory around vital nostalgia. Deeply embedded in and canonized by archives, the forms of nostalgia I explore are at once political, aesthetic, social, and personal, shaping the experiences, understandings, and memories of HIV/AIDS and its activism.

Container List

Viral Cultures is structured into five chapters and an epilogue. Each chapter centers on a case (or intertwined cases) culled from my ethnographic data. Some chapters zoom in on a single archives, object, or event; others reach across archival institutions, collections, or decades. Cases were selected to illuminate practices and potentialities of vital nostalgia. Mirroring the disruptive temporalities of AIDS and inviting comparison, I move between past and present to illustrate the contributions of vital nostalgia to the study of HIV/AIDS and its archives. This book grapples and grows alongside the epidemic's evolution. It is intentional that it addresses but does not end with cure. We are still living a paradoxical moment of presumed HIV survivability, projected epidemic end points, and unrelenting crises. In its structure, the book highlights the enduring importance and presence of the AIDS past to and in its present and future.

At this juncture, nostalgia for ACT UP's direct action is pervasive. In chapter 1, through a close reading of the poster *Your Nostalgia Is Killing Me!*, I analyze archivally mediated ACT UP nostalgia. Nostalgia for AIDS activism, its community, politics, and aesthetics by its participants as well as younger generations has become a common language through which people express disappointment and frustration with the present shortcomings of AIDS and LGBTQ politics. *Your Nostalgia* illustrates how vital nostalgia as an intergenerational archiving and curation practice can generate a historical counternarrative. With the aid of creative works, we can ethically address and redress racialized, gendered, and classed inequities that continue to characterize the epidemic.

Chapter 2 analyzes the cultural life of the ACT UP/NY Records. ACT UP/NY's extensive activist archiving was an essential, if underacknowledged, facet of care work. It resulted in a vibrant collection that has been institutionalized by the NYPL's archiving activism. AIDS archives can provide refuge for records and activists. However, archives are not free of conflict or exclusion. Through the exhibition and programming series *Why We Fight: Remembering AIDS Activism*, I examine how this archives was remediated by activists' vital nostalgia practices that demanded institutional experimentation. Understanding how power operates through activist archiving and archiving activism in this AIDS archives matters because its records mediate the possibilities and omissions of contemporary HIV/AIDS memory.

Cure has been narrowly defined in mainstream AIDS discourse as a medical solution administered to individual bodies; however, as chapter 3 posits, a holistic HIV/AIDS cure is imperative. Care work, curation, and cure converge in Visual AIDS's Archive Project. AIDS archives' thorough vital nostalgic curation processes can engender a holistic project of cure because they can provide a remedy for some of the losses and marginalizations experienced by HIV-positive artists. The Archive Project demonstrates that cure can be transformed and that archives—creating, caring for, accessing, and curating them—can play a vital role in a holistic cure that dismantles structural oppressions to meet immediate needs and affords critical measures toward healing and long-term survival for people with HIV/AIDS and their communities.

Chapter 4 focuses on AIDS's biomedical and cultural undetectability. Undetectability's dual sociotechnical logics afford archivists and curators a vitally nostalgic practice for attending to the relations between AIDS past and present, and for reigniting an urgency to fight AIDS in the public. Through close readings of exhibition documentation and creative output from the NYPL exhibition *Why We Fight,* including the Undetectable Flash Collective coproduced with Visual AIDS, and *Not Only This, but "New Language Beckons Us,"* held between Fales and Visual AIDS, I expose how curatorial acts can make HIV/AIDS newly detectable. Undetectability needs to be taken into deliberate account in order to curate ethically through vital nostalgia with and about AIDS's archives.

I chart in chapter 5 the significance of AIDS archives within contemporary viral media. By digitally remediating and transmitting viral imagery, aesthetic practices, and political actions from AIDS archives online through vital nostalgia practices, contemporary artists Jess Mac, Kia LaBeija, and Demian DinéYazhi´ reckon with the whitewashed dominant narratives of the AIDS past. Each uses AIDS records as viral catalysts in art-activist mobilizations of virality that navigate the tensions between a longing to understand AIDS activist histories and the urgency of generating action to address the epidemic's ongoing injustices.

As we live in the 2020s through Covid-19, we need to grapple with multiple pandemics at once—multiple AIDS crises, as well as multiple coronavirus crises. The epilogue turns to vital nostalgia's potential for navigating the conjuncture of archiving, curating, and living amid the convergence of AIDS, Covid-19, and racism pandemics. In the ways they have documented and archived experiences and events of illness and illness politics, AIDS archives have much to offer us during this upheaval to understand what has come before, what might be going on now, and what will come in the wake of these changes.

Viral Cultures traverses the past, present, and future of AIDS archives to explore the potential impact of vital nostalgia. I do this work because, as fierce pussy asserts with *For the Record,* we are still living with HIV/AIDS. This book addresses the power of AIDS archives and the responsibilities of those who activate them, from archivists, curators, artists, and activists to those most affected by HIV and AIDS, then and now.

1

"YOUR NOSTALGIA IS KILLING ME!"

ACT UP Nostalgia and the Meaning of HIV/AIDS

> It is not the remembering and it is neither the history, nor the material cul-
> ture nor the valorization of the battles won and lost that impedes our
> movement forward, but rather the unpinning of our past from the circum-
> stances from which the fights were born.
>
> —**VINCENT CHEVALIER** AND **IAN BRADLEY-PERRIN** (2013)

"YOUR NOSTALGIA IS KILLING ME!" screams the text in activist-artists Vincent Chevalier and Ian Bradley-Perrin's 2013 poster.[1] Titled after its all-caps proclamation, the poster makes in its curation a critique of AIDS commodification in digital media. It became an overnight social media sensation. *Your Nostalgia Is Killing Me!* (Figure 1) remixes AIDS archival images with contemporary AIDS advertising and pop culture images. The poster was introduced to a New York audience at a panel as part of the "Mourning and Militancy" screening that featured AIDS activist videos culled from the stacks of the NYPL's Manuscripts and Archives Division. This event was within the programming for the NYPL's 2013–14 exhibition *Why We Fight: Remembering AIDS Activism*. AIDS activist and then–Visual AIDS staffer Ted Kerr recounted the story for me of how one of the evening's featured filmmakers, ACT UP/NY alum Debra Levine, remarked on stage how she took issue with *Your Nostalgia*'s contentions. Levine argued that the poster's use of nostalgia in relation to AIDS was dismissive of ACT UP and its contributions. From her perspective, one shared by many of her fellow activists who participated in AIDS activism during the 1980s and 1990s, nostalgia was a frame that threatened to trivialize ACT UP's living legacy in ways that dishonored both those who lost their lives and the still-grieving survivors. Kerr, whose AIDS activism began in the 2000s, felt Levine had "misrepresented" the poster's content and contentions.[2] At home that night, Kerr shared the link to *Your Nostalgia* in a post to the ACT UP/NY Alumni Facebook group. He tagged others in his network who had attended the screening. Taking Levine's critique head on, he pulled the poster out from the archives into digital media. Within a matter of hours, the thread on the ACT UP wall exploded; the posts continued to build there and across personal Facebook walls unabated over the next few days. The most active participants in these online discourses, as well as those with the most vitriol, were former ACT UP/NY members, generations of activists active during the late 1980s and early 1990s. A younger generation of AIDS activists, among them the poster's creators, also stepped into the fray that week, alternately defending, attacking, and mediating. The heated critical conversations *Your Nostalgia* sparked among multiple generations of AIDS activists extended from the halls of the NYPL to social media, only to end up right back where they began: at the NYPL, for a discussion convened around the poster and the impassioned responses to it. As I will show in this chapter, the poster and responses it generated foreground the fraught legacies of ACT UP/NY and of the broader AIDS crisis.

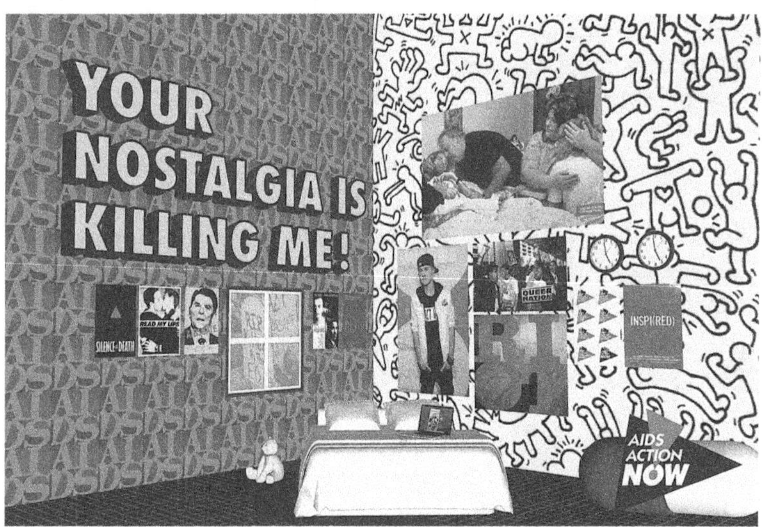

Figure 1. *Your Nostalgia Is Killing Me!* is a poster created by Vincent Chevalier with Ian Bradley-Perrin in 2013 for Toronto-based AIDS organization AIDS ACTION NOW!'s PosterVirus campaign. Courtesy of the artist.

Through a close reading of *Your Nostalgia,* the social media discourse and diatribes it sparked, and interviews with the poster's creators and interlocutors, I expose the operation and significance of contemporary ACT UP nostalgia. The poster's contentions and the intergenerational tensions over its meanings expose both possibilities and pitfalls of ACT UP nostalgia for the epidemic's present and future. This marked longing for ACT UP focuses on its affective enactment of community, queerly radical politics, and aesthetic sensibilities at the peak of its cultural currency. I will discuss how a vital nostalgia for ACT UP in service of interrogating, addressing, and repairing the structural power inequities that characterize AIDS then and now is grounded in AIDS archives and in their use and reuse.

The AIDS crisis may seem a queer object for nostalgia, as nobody wants to revive or relive the death, pain, loss, discrimination, and destruction that marked the early years of the American AIDS crisis. However, nostalgia for ACT UP's brand of direct-action AIDS activism, specifically for its community unity, radical politics, and aesthetics, both by the generations who participated and by younger generations who did not, has become a common language of dissent through which people express their disappointments and frustrations with the shortcomings of LGBTQ politics and the meager attention paid to AIDS in the twenty-first century. ACT UP was and is a nonhierarchical coalition of people taking nonviolent direct action to fight HIV/AIDS. In city-based chapters across the United States, beginning in New York City in 1987, ACT UP's actions utilized sharp wit and striking design. At its height in membership, activity, and media attention from the late 1980s through the early 1990s, activists came together to fight, march, educate, chant, fall in love, advocate, research, dance, mourn, build community, cruise, share meals, make art, testify, care, fuck, gossip, organize, debate, and document. It is precisely by considering how these quotidian acts were shaped by both HIV/AIDS and the activism created in response to it, alongside the present state of mainstream LGBTQ movement politics, that one can fully understand the powerful longing ACT UP nostalgia marks for a collectively imagined, more socially engaged, aesthetically alluring, and communal past. In the 2020s, there is dissatisfaction and despair among many queer people with the mainstream LGBTQ movement's assimilationist and neoliberal leanings over the last two decades, which have meant that already scarce resources and attention have been largely focused on obtaining entrance to two historically repressive conservative institutions: marriage and the military. Such narrow focus on issues pertaining largely to the lives of white middle-class gay men and lesbians has come at a steep price. The mainstream movement has frequently failed to address the daily struggles faced by LGBTQ people and people living with HIV/AIDS in housing, education, employment, health care, policing and incarceration, and immigration. ACT UP nostalgia is also fueled by an anxiety about the queer movement's failures or incapacities to tear down and remake civilization and its structures of power.

ACT UP is a major figure in scholarship and cultural production on AIDS and its activism.[3] That a great number of the accounts of AIDS activism have been produced and recorded by former ACT UP members figures into, but does not fully explain, the extent of the focus on ACT UP, and on ACT UP/NY specifically. The "affective conditions of political activism,"[4] as ACT UP/NY member and scholar Douglas Crimp puts it, were marked by the often contradictory but always intense coexistence of rage, mourning, pleasure, joy, love, and exhaustion; these were a profound component of what made ACT UP powerful. Sociologist and ACT UP/Chicago activist Deborah Gould argues that ACT UP created a transformative "emotional habitus" that profoundly remade queer life and politics.[5] It is not just the generations who actively participated in the group that remain in its thrall; Lucas Hilderbrand terms his nostalgic longing for ACT UP "retro activism." He, like me, grew up queer in the age of AIDS but was not of the right generation or in the right place to have been a part of such queer activist movements at their height. Hilderbrand acknowledges that his perspective on this activist past is "romanticized;" yet despite its limitations, ACT UP nostalgia deeply informs his political and sexual identities, as it does mine.[6] Those who were there have a meaningfully distinct longing for ACT UP marked alternately by yearning, grief, anger, and affection. It is in significant part the affective resonances of ACT UP, namely the feeling of queer community and artistically engaged political action across difference, that it make it subject and site for nostalgic feelings and memories.

The stakes of how, when, and where ACT UP is remembered are particularly acute in this moment, when a dominant narrative of the American AIDS crisis is solidifying through the activation of prominent AIDS archives. The epidemic's narrativization is still emergent and is therefore changeable. Popular scholarship on and cultural critiques of AIDS began to appear in the late 1980s, and a small but notable humanities and social sciences scholarship on AIDS flourished from the 1990s into the early 2000s. However, it is only after 2008, a period aptly labeled by Kerr and Alexandra Juhasz as the "AIDS Crisis Visitation,"[7] that AIDS has become a central subject of humanistic scholarly and popular inquiry. The late 2010s were characterized by heightened interest in AIDS and the activism and cultural production it spurred during the 1980s and early 1990s. This interest is evidenced by the proliferation of scholarship, documentaries, exhibitions, memorials, and other cultural production on that era. Kerr writes, "On screens, walls and in discourse, mass death and community responses are remembered through culled and curated video and film footage, photos and ephemera from personal collections as well as individual and institutional archives."[8] The archival records that are circulated through these works focus on a particular kind of AIDS activist—sexy, middle-class, young, white, and gay men—and AIDS activism—flashy "street-based, postmodern, confrontational" direct action.[9] AIDS history in these dominant accounts begins with 1981, when medical professionals first recognized a new illness affecting "homosexual" men in Los Angeles and New York City. Such neat, tidy progressive narrative arcs emphasize AIDS as a tragedy; audiences can be moved by graphically showing death and destruction wrought on beautiful protagonists. This tale is redemptively heroic, showcasing the passionate treatment activism of men fighting for their lives against the inevitable metronormative backdrop of New York City. As is to be expected, the heroes emerge victorious, the story ending as activists' successful push for the development of an effective AIDS treatment cocktail comes to fruition in 1996. AIDS activism, reduced to the curative necessity of getting drugs into bodies, is marked as over.

ACT UP is the superstar in these narratives, famous enough to stand in for all of AIDS activism, and through its acclaim reproduces anew gendered, racialized, and classed power inequities. Artist, writer, and ACT UP/NY activist Avram Finkelstein summed up for me: "So many of the things that suit the dominant narrative, [that] AIDS was an embattled community [who] fought for their lives and shook loose the pharmaceutical-industrial complex and now people no longer die. 'And look, they made really cool posters.' That storytelling around it really suits power structures."[10] He continued, "It's not to say that that story is wholly inaccurate, but as a narrative, as a cap to this story, it's ethically questionable."[11] Finkelstein's words demonstrate the dangers of historicizing AIDS activism in ways that support white supremacist patriarchy by acknowledging only white men, marking AIDS activism as past, and ignoring the failures and limitations of early AIDS activism, and thereby the existence and needs of marginalized communities, especially Black, brown, Indigenous, and trans, where the American AIDS epidemic continues unabated. Dominant narratives are a form of selective remembering practiced with archival documentation that conjures, to use Kerr's words, "memories and trauma for many who were there, as well as a possible displaced nostalgia for those who were not, and a desire for many to be able to return to such an engaged moment, yet without the loss."[12]

This chapter engages the question of why ACT UP figures so significantly into narratives about AIDS activism and into nostalgia for it. As I will discuss, ACT UP nostalgia names the desire for affectively unified community, radical politics, and powerful activist aesthetics. This matters because the ways in which the past of AIDS is desired in the present through ACT UP nostalgia has significant stakes in an ongoing pandemic. A close reading of Chevalier and Bradley-Perrin's poster and its provocations, creation, circulation, and responses provides a case study in the importance of negotiating intergenerational ACT UP nostalgia now. The poster exposes the operation of nostalgia in relation to AIDS archives and in the use and reuse of archival materials, as well as the generative potential of vital nostalgia for troubling and shifting dominant historical narratives in ways that address and redress injustice. Activists, scholars, archivists, curators, and artists have an ethical responsibility to interrogate and contest dominant historical narratives in order to intervene in the present. This requires us to engage critically with ACT UP nostalgia and its vital potential to challenge and transform historical narratives, and to mobilize for radical changes in present realities and future possibilities.

Looking at and Longing for ACT UP

"I had seen the footage like a million times and I had never seen myself in the footage," Jason Baumann, the NYPL's Susan and Douglas Dillon associate director for collection development and coordinator of Humanities and LGBT Collections, told me.[13] As a curator of the NYPL's archival exhibition *Why We Fight*, he had been watching on repeat the same few minutes of video documenting ACT UP's 1992 Ashes Action over the course of a year as part of the process of selecting and editing the footage for inclusion in the show. The two minutes he chose played in a loop along with short segments from other actions in *Why We Fight*'s main gallery. The

Ashes Action's climax was in the moments when ACT UP activists quite literally heaved their loved ones' cremains over the high fence, coating the green expanse of George H. W. Bush's White House lawn. It was an angry antidote to mournful forums like the NAMES Project AIDS Memorial Quilt, on display across the National Mall that same weekend, that perversely made from ACT UP's perspective "something beautiful out of this epidemic."[14] The Ashes Action was one event in a series of ACT UP "political funerals," actions deploying activists' bodies, living and dead, to make affectively potent political statements. Participant David Robinson described the action as "return[ing] people to the reality of AIDS. Hundreds of thousands of lives have been reduced to bone and ash, by the ignorance and apathy of the Reagan–Bush administrations. Today, we are depositing this reality on George Bush's doorstep."[15] Activists subjected invaluable objects to irreversible disposal, literalizing the devaluation of persons with HIV/AIDS as expendable. The Ashes Action was for Baumann "one of the most beautiful actions ACT UP ever did."[16]

The faceted meanings and lived experiences of ACT UP nostalgia—whether for its radical politics, communal orientation, and/or aesthetic sensibilities—are powerfully and profoundly shaped by generational position in relation to ACT UP and to the AIDS epidemic more broadly. Such nostalgia is also differently felt and experienced along the lines of one's membership positionality—whether someone was an activist only during ACT UP's perceived heyday, in the contemporary iterations of the group, continuously since the 1980s or early 1990s, or simply in spirit, wishing they had actually been on the street, in the march, or in the meeting room. For example, Baumann, "a rank and file" ACT UP/NY member in the early 1990s, described his experience viewing the show's Ashes Action footage. There is a "very clear moment" where he appears in the front of the line of activists as they advance toward the White House, a march dead quiet but for the beats of footsteps and funeral drums. However, it was not until the exhibition had been up for nearly four months that it hit him: "Oh, I'm right in this loop! Oh, there I am!" This late-breaking realization marked "a pivotal moment" in Baumann's contemporary relationship to ACT UP/NY. Baumann identified his initial inability to actually see himself in the archives as "trauma." From iconic moments of political direct action to the mundane daily tasks of AIDS activism, this work was "traumatizing. . . . It was just so much."[17] Baumann's failure of vision uncovers a larger concern of the continued generational immediacy of activist experiences for many who participated. The generational distinctions in experiencing the same AIDS archival records matter. The same archives can elicit distinct and mixed reactions, be they grief, vital nostalgia, or both held together.

The visceral investment of AIDS activists, especially former ACT UP members, in the formation of historical narratives about AIDS activism and in the archives used to create them is significant. Baumann's approach to curating *Why We Fight* and his larger engagement with the NYPL's AIDS archival content is informed by the knowledge that "a lot of the people who created them *are still here* and [that] a lot of the people who created them *aren't still here.*"[18] Holding those realities "colors" his curatorial decisions and the ways that they are interpreted by activist community stakeholders "both personally and politically." Talking about ACT UP activists' reactions to *Your Nostalgia,* Baumann noted that many people in Chevalier and Bradley-Perrin's generation, in their twenties and thirties in the 2010s, grossly underestimated how much firsthand participants continue to have invested in that time, and how many of them actually "sacrificed their entire lives to be members of ACT UP. . . . ACT UP was their entire life; they sacrificed careers, they gave up monetary gain, everything to devote themselves full time to being AIDS activists and whose lives, life trajectories suffered greatly as a result." Many participants in the early generations of AIDS activism dedicated "six to eight years of their lives to being full-time AIDS activists at a time when that wasn't a professionalized thing, and you didn't get grants, and you didn't get paid to do these things." Baumann identifies the magnitude of early activists' loss of lovers, friends, comrades, and acquaintances, often without space to mourn, as resulting in

> lingering feelings of failure [for these activists] of doing all of that work, and then not being able to save the people that you were trying to save. That [failure] sours everything. Even with the release of medications . . . whatever gains we had in ACT UP still doesn't save, it doesn't bring back to life the person that was the reason that you were fighting for all of these things, and even [knowing that many] . . . people's lives that may have been saved because of the things we did, right? It doesn't bring back the person who was the reason why you did this, or it doesn't fix your life if you're HIV positive and you've devoted your whole life to this. It doesn't necessarily save you or bring you back anything you've lost because of this.[19]

So many in ACT UP and its larger community died that the group's ranks rapidly dwindled in the first half of the 1990s.

For those who did survive the early years of AIDS, that activist experience and the ongoing mourning was and is profoundly draining. Prolific documentarians and former ACT UP activists including Juhasz and James Wentzy have noted that when they see or show footage from this period, they are waiting to see people they miss.[20] Similarly, Steven Kerry described carrying with him "the lingering remnants of the trauma, our numerous memories and ghosts, and our emotional scars with us every day," which means that viewing records was "a painful act of emotional masochism" that he and others would rather forgo.[21] The care for, connection with, and longing for those who have died continues to shape the feelings and practices of ACT UP nostalgia, as well as the frequent resistance to labeling some of those feelings and memory practices as nostalgia at all, among many in the generations of ACT UP survivors.

It is not just the persons who have been lost who are still longed for; nostalgia among many former ACT UP members extends to physical spaces. ACT UP occupied rooms each Monday night at the Gay and Lesbian Community Center and Cooper Union, and throughout the week at workspaces in Manhattan. These spaces are the object of a "yearning for home" among these former participants. In talking about a longtime colleague, an artist and ACT UP member, Kerr shared how he frequently "will say, 'I just want to go back to that room,' and when he says, 'I want to go back to that room,' he means the ACT UP room." Kerr, part of a younger generation who came to AIDS activism well after 1996, notes that in his contemporary labors he runs up against "the sanctity of that room." He acknowledged,

> Even in my most hardened heart, I know that that is devastating. . . . It's like their lives were robbed from them by illness and by a whole lot of shit, and so they were part of this thing that really mattered and changed the world for the better . . . so they can't handle even the slightest criticism. Because if you say, if you even hint, that ACT UP doesn't matter or ACT UP isn't as demigod as they need it to be, what you are saying is that *maybe even the most important thing in your life doesn't matter.*

Kerr identified these reactions as a powerful, generationally specific form of nostalgia that lives at intersections of "white fragility, male fragility, New York fragility."[22]

Yet the longing for ACT UP, though valid and meaningful, on such a scale contributes to the erasure of other significant AIDS activism from the collective imaginary. "When ACT UP is remembered—again and again and again—other places, people, and forms of AIDS activism are disremembered," Juhasz writes.[23] New York's Black and Latinx communities generated significant AIDS action, yet despite archival documentation, their stories and strategies remain marginalized. For example, Gay Men of African Descent (GMAD), founded in 1986, offered AIDS education and services by and for Black gay men. They strategically incorporated Black gay history into their weekly programming to promote empowerment through increased self-worth.[24] GMAD's archives have long been available at the NYPL's Schomburg Center for Research in Black Culture, yet only recently has there been any significant study of the group. Moreover, even longings for ACT UP's actions are partial and highly selective, especially as practiced by those who were not there. An unvital nostalgia ignores the full range of activities and practices—namely the insurance and medical research, needle exchanges, documentation, and administrative tasks engaged in by the group—favoring instead the theatrical, flashy public actions and noteworthy successes. Additionally, little work examines the local and transnational efforts of ACT UP/NY's Latino Caucus, which led a program collecting unused HIV medications and medical equipment in the United States and delivered them to nongovernmental organizations throughout Latin America.[25] The ACT UP desired and remembered is almost always populated and driven by dying, economically and educationally privileged, media-savvy gay white men in New York.[26] There were indeed plenty of such men in ACT UP; however, this narrow perspective dismisses without even considering it the labor and leadership of women, BIPOC, incarcerated persons, trans people, and intravenous drug users in AIDS activism within and beyond ACT UP. Nostalgia for ACT UP plays a powerful role in the development of dominant epidemic narratives now. The group's gendered, racialized, and classed documentation practices limit the collective imagination in ways that shape how artists, curators, and scholars enter and use AIDS archives. It is not a lack of archival evidence of the AIDS movement's diversity that drives erasures but rather the powerful assumption, informed by a limited AIDS imaginary, that they could not have possibly been there in the first place.

AIDS Archives and ACT UP Nostalgia

The profound vital nostalgic longing for ACT UP that is shaped by the group's archival representation reflects a desire to contest, disrupt, and refigure the political status quo. Nostalgia for ACT UP as practiced across generations is produced in significant part by a prevailing dissatisfaction with the intertwined politics of mainstream LGBTQ and AIDS movements. ACT UP nostalgia centers around three idealized facets of the group's practice and impacts: community unity, queer politics, and provocative aesthetics. Each of these facets is counter to the neoliberal assimilationist goals and practices that dominate mainstream LGBTQ politics and organizations, and the nonprofit-industrial complex that constitutes a contemporary AIDS response.

Since the 1970s, neoliberalism has become the pervasive ideology of American social, political, and economic practices and processes. Under neoliberal establishments, LGBTQ and AIDS work valorizes individual action and responsibilization, the professionalization and corporatization of activism, and the commodification of AIDS activism and cultural production. Neoliberalism, David Harvey describes, asserts that "human well-being can best be advanced by the maximization of entrepreneurial freedoms within an institutional framework characterized by private property rights, individual liberty, unencumbered markets and free trade."[27] Neoliberalism is a "governing rationality," Wendy Brown explains, "through which everything is 'economized.'" Most profoundly, she continues, neoliberalism renders people as "human capital who must constantly tend to their own present and future value."[28] Because neoliberalism favors private solutions, within its logics, the nuclear family is a primary provider of goods and services, including the provision of care and the stability of monogamy.[29] Aligning itself with this emphasis on the nuclear family, mainstream LGBTQ activism from the 1990s until its federal legalization in 2015 advocated for same-sex marriage. This activism routinely positioned gays and lesbians as perfect neoliberal subjects, deserving of rights by showing them to be responsible and worthy citizens. AIDS also played into these normative political aspirations; in the wake of so many deaths, marriage and its associated inherence and property rights were presented as a solution. AIDS also intensified mainstream gay community leaders' policing of sexuality and promotion of monogamy. Sex workers, people who have unprotected sex, and intravenous drug users are subjects positioned, René Esparza argues, by "neoliberal narratives as deviant, hedonistic, and, hence, as unworthy of care."[30] Under neoliberal logics in which individuals are "self-managing," responsible for making calculative choices about health and risk,[31] HIV infections or treatment failures are frequently blamed on individual recklessness rather than structural oppressions.

Neoliberalism espouses the value of privatizing social services that were once the state's purview, signaling an abdication of responsibility and care. In the context of AIDS, most early responses were community based. For example, Gay Men's Health Crisis (GMHC), founded in New York City in 1982, was the first organization devoted to providing HIV/AIDS care by and for the gay community. One of its earliest services, the buddy program, paired people living with HIV/AIDS with a volunteer who aided them in day-to-day tasks and served as a care advocate. By the late 1990s, several of the nation's largest AIDS service organizations transformed into large, professionalized organizations funded by major donors and state agencies and controlled by professional staff. While there is no question that they provide valuable services, such organizations work within market-driven corporatized models that often align with the neoliberal values of mainstream state and private agencies. In the 2000s, as professionally managed, nonprofit AIDS advocacy groups have proliferated, they have come to constitute in numbers and popular visibility the most significant contemporary response to HIV/AIDS. In the neoliberal frame, their care work is directed toward individual bodies rather than action aimed at the elimination of collective harms of racism, poverty, heteropatriarchy, and other injustices that structure the AIDS crisis. Contemporary nostalgia for ACT UP is a rejection of the neoliberal intrusion into LGBTQ and AIDS communities, cultures, and politics.

In contrast to neoliberalism's individualist logistics, ACT UP has long been portrayed as devoting substantive time and attention to building egalitarian community. That practice of community is understood as vital in their successes fighting damaging AIDS policies.[32] Mark Milano, who joined shortly after the group's founding and who has remained active in ACT UP/NY since, recounted how "it was extremely exciting back then to walk into that room" for ACT UP's Monday-night meetings. He continued, "Whenever you walk into a space like that and it's filled to the rafters, with almost no room for anybody else to get in, that's exciting. There is an energy that really is thrilling, and some people remember that energy."[33] When I watch archival footage of such meetings, the excited charge is palpable.

ACT UP activists did a remarkable and highly effective job of documenting their work as they were doing it in the late 1980s and early 1990s. Those records mediate ACT UP nostalgia now. Juhasz writes that ACT UP "got and gets most of the attention because it could and can and it wanted to." She continues, "It had the funds, time, and self-confidence. . . . Given that its participants were more photogenic, wealthier, more powerful, and simply sexier (in the eyes of dominant culture) than the ragtag group of feminists, lesbians, drug addicts, people of color, homeless people, poor people, immigrants, mothers, and Haitians who were also engaged in activism at this time, ACT UP activism is quite memorable."[34] The proliferation and mediation of video documentation now held in AIDS archives is particularly significant in nostalgia for ACT UP's community, politics, and aesthetics. Video is a media modality that crosses generational divides, presenting an immediate connection to this moment in AIDS activism. Analog, handheld footage, with its sun flares, static, and other technical glitches, allows viewers to viscerally experience some of the feelings of this activism, be it the threat of police advancing in riot gear, the drama and process of ACT UP's meetings, or activists crying, fighting, hugging, singing, and cheering.[35] The technological specificity of video recording technologies tied to particular moments, whether 1988 or 2018, moves the viewer to vividly imagine the production and reception of these videos in those moments.[36] The experience of unified community, queer politics, and provocative aesthetics in ACT UP is now distilled through the recollection of these intense moments, which seem to capture the energy of the group more than any comprehensive accounting of dates or facts ever could.[37]

Intimacy, especially "queer intimacy," has been widely cited by members as crucial to understanding the dynamics of the group in meetings and in actions.[38] Member Heidi Dorow recalls that ACT UP took on

> an urgency that made you want to do anything. I began to live in this world where you got to know people, and you got to love them, and you laughed with them and found out how beautiful they were, and they were going to die. . . . They like me and they love me, and they're there for me . . . and you're telling me they're going to be fucking dead in a few months, or a year, or two years? No way. That just made you enraged. That made you want to do anything.[39]

Being in ACT UP made activists feel, Milano told me, like they were "a part of something and we were a community working together."[40] The nostalgia for ACT UP among its former activist participants that Milano accounts for was born of that fraternal feeling, a collective affect "that's all gone [now], and I'm alone and that sense of brotherhood and sisterhood is gone. . . . The reality is that things were pretty depressing in the gay world before ACT UP, then they were pretty exciting during ACT UP, and then went back to being depressing again. The basic difference is isolation, community, isolation."[41] The longing for a queer community, real or perceived, constructed and practiced by ACT UP is not just the purview of former participants. Hilderbrand, from his white, gay, middle-class, cismale younger generational vantage point, mediated by his watching of AIDS activist videotapes, writes, "AIDS blurred the boundaries of class, race, and gender between previously disparate gay communities that united through activism" for a fleeting beautiful moment.[42]

The reality is that lines of difference—HIV serostatus, sexuality, race and ethnicity, gender, class, religion, citizenship and immigration status, education—were never simply or ever continuously transcended for all participants in ACT UP's community. Many AIDS activists did not want to or could not feel at home within ACT UP. Setting aside the different realities that inform one's perceptions about whether a beautiful moment of affective unity of existing together in community ever actually occurred, or at least whether it occurred in the same way for everyone, there is clearly a concerted longing for ACT UP's communal constructions now. It matters today that there is this acute longing for a kind of togetherness that can cross, diffuse, or make generative categorical differences and identity politics. Much of the contemporary response to AIDS comes from public health structures that focus on individual medicalized responsibility for maintaining health and halting contagion rather than on building community through shared experience among those most affected, thus serving to make living with HIV/AIDS an othered and sometimes isolating experience. The practices with which people engage in activism, including queer and AIDS activism, have also undergone notable technological shifts, moving into digital spaces and shifting the ways that community is lived and felt. Affective outlets of pleasure and sexual and physical intimacy are profoundly changed, tranforming the atmosphere of activism. The mainstream goals of the professionalized LGBTQ and AIDS advocacy organizations staffed by formally trained people, supported by grants, and with clear organizational hierarchies have turned to focus powerfully on individual entrance and benefits to be obtained from access to institutions such as marriage and the military. Such goals have failed to offer many young queers a compelling, urgent space to work for social transformation through communal practices. Community unity thus exists as a real, if distinct, object of nostalgic longing for both generations of ACT UP participants and for subsequent generations of queers. Bradley-Perrin noted of such nostalgia for ACT UP's unified community: "Don't forget that that was other people's demise, that moment was not only beautiful, it was painful and the painful part of that still exists; it's just the beautiful part that's gone."[43]

In addition to unified community, archivally mediated nostalgia for ACT UP now is fundamentally centered on the ways, real or imagined, that the LGBTQ community was not only unified but also politicized by AIDS activism. Those in ACT UP and its sister groups, such as Queer Nation, reclaimed "queer" as an identity, an antinormative politics, and an academic theory. My own relationship to ACT UP as a queer ciswoman who was too young to have participated in activism in the 1980s and 1990s is important here. ACT UP, from my earliest conscious encounter with it through archival records featured in a college course, epitomized what I wanted queer politics, community, and activism to be. It seemed from my perspective that there was a "radical past" at the heart of LGBTQ experience that I had missed out on. Lost persons as well as queer radical practices and politics are what is longed for. Many of the divisions within the political aims of LGBTQ community seem particular to the time of my queer adulthood, in which mainstream politics and activism has given priority to a relatively conservative homonormative agenda,[44] epitomized by the multidecade fight for marriage equality. It is not just in LGBTQ politics that normativity, institutional acceptance, and corporate interventions have become standard; AIDS politics has also now embraced pharmaceuticals and medical assistance as the most promising avenue, as epitomized in discourses around PrEP that emphasize the power of individual responses and responsibility. ACT UP's politics did not focus on assimilation or normative desires but centered a queer identity and antinormativity. For example, Esparza argues, Latinx ACT UP/NY activists' efforts in Puerto Rico and on the mainland were as queer and decolonial as they were "radical and international instead of reformist and domestic . . . favoring street protest and cultural production versus simply electoral politics and legal change."[45] He contends that activists' centering of devalued racialized subjects, including queers and intravenous drug users, demonstrates their "disavowal of heteronormative rubrics of social value as a precondition for personhood."[46] Many of ACT UP's direct-action tactics aspired to generate response beyond the queer community, but they did not shy away from anger and unpopular actions and messages. Theirs was not a politics grounded in likeability, relatability, responsibility, or mainstream acceptance.

"What I am nostalgic for is not ACT UP per se but for the way it mobilized a queer community," Hilderbrand wrote—a sentiment that I and many others of my generation share.[47] It will take a powerful queer response to create and sustain a queer politics that can address the pressing concerns of housing, education, employment, health care, policing, criminalization, incarceration, and immigration that affect and constrain the lives and life chances of those living with HIV/AIDS, especially those put most at risk. At a reunion of ACT UP/NY members in 2012, Milano attempted to get others in his generation of activists, now in their forties, fifties, sixties, and beyond, to rejoin the group he never left:

> I got up and said, "People, the reason you feel that way is because you left ACT UP. . . . If you want that sense of belonging, get involved again. The reason you felt great when you were in ACT UP was because your life had a sense of purpose . . . that is the greatest thing in life. You left that and now you obviously don't feel as good. So, come back! We need you—there are plenty of fights left to fight. We need you back." I got up and said that, and people got up after me, but nobody responded to what I said. They all just kept saying the same thing: "I'm so depressed now and it was so wonderful back then." They didn't come back.[48]

By clinging to ACT UP, its activists are working to maintain some semblance of subversiveness in a social milieu of LGBTQ life and politics increasingly shaped by the valorization of normativity. Nostalgia has thus become a shared language through which former participants and subsequent generations express their despair and continual disappointments with the lack of attention to AIDS, and with LGBTQ politics and activist energies and actions more generally.

Finally, today's nostalgia for ACT UP is about the group's aesthetics. Aesthetic nostalgia is particularly keen in this 2010s-to-2020s moment of 1990s' chic that is pervading fashion, art, film, and television as well as other modes of cultural production and commodity. The images of the AIDS art canon, captured in archives, circulate increasingly in high-culture spaces such as museums and galleries. These same images also now adorn T-shirts, tote bags, buttons, sneakers, Tumblrs, and baby carriers. ACT UP was image-driven and image-conscious activism. The group, with the support of art-action collectives like the Silence = Death and Gran Fury, strategically deployed graphics and other visually impactful tactics to enact its transformations of the public sphere during the 1980s and early 1990s. ACT UP positively courted media coverage.[49] Part of this visual work happened through street-based theatrical demonstrations, like die-ins, kiss-ins, and political funerals.[50] It also included video and film work, including public access television shows, documentaries, and video art. ACT UP was also hugely successful in creating and distributing AIDS cultural ephemera. These included cheaply produced posters, fliers, stickers, T-shirts, and buttons that were intended to inform diverse publics about HIV/AIDS, to gather support for their work, and to demanded necessary and continued attention to the AIDS crisis.[51] The graphic design of these materials captured in the group's archival records contributes to the appeal of such activism, particularly to those who were not participants in it. An earlier moment in AIDS activism is powerfully mediated by activist records including graphics and videotapes that feature witty, sexy slogans, and well-designed posters and videotapes.[52] So much of ACT UP's queer aesthetics has become mainstream, decontextualized and decoupled from AIDS, coopted for corporate profit and social media likes. The commodified and depoliticized appeal of images at the nexus of AIDS art and activism to younger generations of artists and LGBTQ persons is in large part what *Your Nostalgia* is responding to. The longing for ACT UP's authentically queer aesthetic sensibilities also marks a desire to repoliticize activist chic in service of a new form of radical LGBTQ and AIDS politics.

Reappropriating the AIDS Archives

Your Nostalgia Is Killing Me! contends with ACT UP nostalgia within the setting of a teenager's bedroom. Splashed across every inch of these bedroom walls are archival images, art, and advertisements that consciously translate and remix 1990s' digital aesthetics. The walls are papered in pieces by General Idea and Keith Haring. On them hang canonical artworks by activist-artists: Félix González-Torres, Gran Fury, and the Silence = Death Project. Artworks hang intimately near archival photographs of ACT UP and Queer Nation actions. Such iconic images of 1980s' and 1990s' AIDS activism and cultural production are paired with contemporary visuals, including advertisements for Product Red[53] and a photograph of pop star Justin Bieber sporting a classic ACT UP T-shirt on the red carpet at the 2011 Country Music Awards. *Your Nostalgia* moved across walls, both physical and digital, in 2013 and 2014.[54] Its creators, Vincent Chevalier and Ian Bradley-Perrin, are two young gay white Canadian HIV-positive men. They sought through creative response to address the complex roles that nostalgia, politics, affect, aesthetics, history, and digital media play in the ongoing AIDS crisis. *Your Nostalgia*'s sociopolitical context and creation process shapes its provocations, circulation, and interventions into vital ACT UP nostalgia.

Your Nostalgia confronts contemporary LGBTQ and AIDS politics that center whiteness, individual responsibility, corporatization, and ACT UP forward narratives. In this section, I analyze the conception, creation, and aims of the poster. The poster is the product of the artists' collaboration for the Toronto-based AIDS ACTION NOW!'s third annual PosterVirus project. Launched November 30, 2011, the thirtieth anniversary of AIDS's 1981 medical discovery, PosterVirus promotes contemporary dialogue and action on HIV/AIDS through public art with "complexity, depth, and an intersectional analysis."[55] Its curators, Alexander McClelland and Jessica Whitbread, bring together artists, community groups, and activists to create posters.[56] McClelland and Whitbread raised pressing questions for the project's 2013 iteration:

> How can we challenge the logic of the AIDS industry? What can art posters change? What do people care about in the AIDS response? In a movement divided by identity politics, how do we make sure that voices are being heard (and not only the ones with the privilege to shout the loudest)? Are we just talking to each other—what about all the people around the world who are not (or do not want to be) part of the mainstream HIV discourses?[57]

In their statement on Tumblr accompanying the posters' summer release, McClelland and Whitbread explicitly framed PosterVirus as counter to the popular revisitation of the 1980s' and 1990s' North American AIDS crisis, writing, "Hipsters across North America are flocking to get down with the AIDS movement and embracing some of our lost warriors. We are swimming in nostalgia."[58] They then raised further questions about AIDS nostalgia: "As we continue to romanticize the past, is the popular imaginary forgetting that AIDS still impacts us today? Has this created the false appearance that AIDS has made its way back on political agendas?"[59] Answering their own inquiries, McClelland and Whitbread concluded, "People are still dying. People still don't have access to treatment. People don't have housing. People are increasingly criminalized. People still spread ignorance and hate. And yet mainstream AIDS industry and media suggests that stopping all this is as simple as a 'cure.' A simple pill to make AIDS go away."[60]

The curators and artists contextualized their critique of normative AIDS discourse's dangers within discussions of PrEP. McClelland and

Whitbread's "simple" blue pill, Truvada, was approved by the U.S. Food and Drug Administration (FDA) in 2012, thus inaugurating the latest self-declared medical triumph over HIV/AIDS. When taken daily by HIV-negative persons, PrEP has been shown to significantly reduce the likelihood of HIV transmission through sexual intercourse.[61] In 2013, it was the hot topic in LGBTQ and AIDS communities. Gay men were and are the primary target for treatment-as-prevention models that require expensive pharmaceutical and medical intervention.[62] As marketed, PrEP reifies a neoliberal emphasis on individual responsibility for ending AIDS through prevention. Such framing sidesteps structural inequities that put at unequal risk certain lives: those of BIPOC, trans women, and intravenous drug users. As Bradley-Perrin noted, the promotion and adoption of PrEP as a magical AIDS "cure" in public health campaigns and casual conversation between gay men "perfectly described" what *Your Nostalgia* aimed to prevent.[63] He saw "young people getting sucked in by, like, the aesthetics of activism and action and, like, sex-positivity and all of those things without thinking through the deeper political implications."[64] There was a failure to ask in mainstream LGBTQ movement discourse, "What does it mean for a pharmaceutical company to say, 'I can just take this pill every day for the rest of my life and I'll be safe from everything and I never need to worry.' And how is this medication made? Who is getting tested? Who are the trials being done on? Who gets access to it? Where does that leave HIV-positive people?"[65] Leveling a critique of PrEP politics is evidence of a larger-scale dissatisfaction with the mainstream movement's promotion of neoliberal solutions to the AIDS crisis, emphasizing individual responsibility and relying on powerful institutions—the pharmaceutical-industrial complex, government, and health care—that have repeatedly failed to meet the needs of those put at greatest contemporary risk. Rounding up PrEP to "cure" ignores the needs of people living with HIV/AIDS, racialized structural inequities and institutionalized discrimination, and HIV fear and stigmatization. AIDS stigma makes PrEP as an easy "cure all," as Bradley-Perrin called it, deeply appealing to some young gay men—the same men who are Chevalier and Bradley-Perrin's intended audience.[66]

Bradley-Perrin, then a graduate student and AIDS activist in Montreal, told me in our interview how he coined the slogan "Your nostalgia is killing me!" in the midst of a discussion about AIDS and the art scene during a night out with a friend. That friend took to the phrase and began deploying it online. It was in a social media post of McClelland's that Chevalier, a video and digital media artist, first encountered Bradley-Perrin's slogan.[67] That post included an exchange between McClelland, Bradley-Perrin, and others about *Things Are Different Now . . .*, a video made by fellow Montreal-based artist Ryan Conrad and discussed in this book's introduction. The phrase "Your nostalgia is killing me!" was deployed in a post that was a takedown of Conrad's video for being uncritically nostalgic for the height of AIDS crisis in ways that its critics believed obscured the ongoing struggles for people living with HIV/AIDS with its aestheticizing lens.[68] In Conrad's video, archival footage of ACT UP political funerals is transposed with contemporary portraits in service of imagining the loss of these young queer subjects. In our interview, Chevalier noted that one commenter on McClelland's post directed a response to Conrad, suggesting, "Maybe art isn't your thing. There are many chapters of ACT UP reopening across America. Maybe you should join one of those and do something useful."[69] For Chevalier, this "Facebooking myopic bitchy thing to say"—that the artist should atone by joining ACT UP, a group that was then more than thirty years old and in his view "no longer [had] the same relevance"—was "the height of hypocrisy."[70] This moment of digital discourse was, in Chevalier's perspective, a perfect crystallization of "this nostalgic idea of ACT UP being the be-all and end-all of activism."[71] In subsequent work, Chevalier appropriated the phrase "Your nostalgia is killing me!," making it the core concept for his proposed PosterVirus contribution without Bradley-Perrin's knowledge. From its earliest conception, the poster thus aimed to disrupt a young queer generation's resortative nostalgic longings for ACT UP and its communal affects, politics, and asethetics.

Digital media circulations of AIDS images form and sustain ACT UP nostalgia for a younger generation of queers. *Your Nostalgia* began for Chevalier "from the Internet and my Internet brain."[72] It was a critical response to the ways that culture is mediated online through "aesthetic blogging." Aesthetic blogs are organized around stylistic themes like fashion or contemporary art, including numerous blogs valorizing the "white gay male body."[73] It was through the quotidian experience of surfing image-driven microblogging platform Tumblr that the sheer quantity of AIDS imagery consumed by the site's users became apparent. As Chevalier described it, here is "this amazing picture of Keith Haring and then you go to some contemporary porn, and just scroll through, scroll through, scroll through Félix González-Torres" and on and on.[74] In Chevalier's view, archival materials and artworks made during the AIDS crisis in the 1980s and 1990s were inserted in these blogs to be scrolled past quickly and uncritically, consumed along with vast quantities of other imagery. In their artists' statement, Chevalier and Bradley-Perrin evoked the iconic slogan made famous by ACT UP to illustrate the affective economy of AIDS digital circulation: "Silence = Death but the white noise humming from your latest post is keeping me up at night. Flying in two dimensions, scrolling through virtual space, virtual time, random access memories referencing deep memory held in those you find inaccessible."[75] For Chevalier and Bradley-Perrin, an endless cycle of blogging, liking, and reblogging threatened to flatten the context and meaning of AIDS archival images. Tumblr, with its largely youthful and often queer and trans user base, presented a potent venue for introducing a younger generation to past sexual cultures and politics. Chevalier noted a fascination and marked desire among younger gay men to connect with these archival images and objects, as well as with the queer community that they represent.[76] However, the actual practices engaged in remained in his view largely a missed opportunity to enact politicized consumption. Instead, Chevalier witnessed "a lot of revisionism," with users "ignoring the social, political, racial contexts" of these AIDS works.[77] Explicitly addressing aesthetic bloggers and their consumers in our interview, Chevalier said, "Fuck. What are you doing? Why do you get all this attention? You're not even HIV positive. How does your work circulate so much when you don't have a connection to the context that it was created [in]?"[78] In the digital economy, AIDS cultural productions come to "just exist without gravity," he continued.[79]

It was not until, in a recursive digital loop, Chevalier posted a draft of his PosterVirus entry on Facebook that Bradley-Perrin became aware of it. He commented that the poster's slogan "looked very familiar."[80] Chevalier responded, noting his strategy of appropriating material found on social media.[81] The two had a conversation that resulted in their collaboration. While each brought distinct skills, perspectives, and target audiences to the project, both creators sought to address people, especially young HIV-negative gay men, who were circulating and making work that was "capitalizing on the AIDS art of the past while ignoring the AIDS reality of the present," Chevalier said.[82] Bradley-Perrin was keen to reach multiple generations of queer men "who, through a focus on or over emphasis of the past, deprioritize the current lived experiences of people living with HIV." Many people living with HIV now have life stories that begin many years after the "accomplishments of ACT UP," which,

Bradley-Perrin argued, "made and brought about significant strides." Yet the problems that earlier generations of AIDS activists worked against continue, and moreover, there are significant new challenges faced by people with HIV and AIDS that still need our attention, "such as criminalization, and a lifelong dependency on the pharmaceutical industry."[83] What he was hoping the poster would say, Bradley-Perrin told me, was,

> Don't be bamboozled by, like, the look of the past; [AIDS is] the present, it's here; there is a clear line connecting the issues of that time to the issues of now; unresolved things still exist, and they are not being dealt with because people feel self-satisfied by being able to, like, play dress-up with the past, which is more sexy of course, the crisis period; the point is *it's still a crisis; it's just not a crisis to you anymore.*[84]

A narrow focus on AIDS in and as the past made the creators' own experiences as HIV-positive men culturally illegible.[85] Being young and seropositive is, more than four decades into the AIDS crisis, particularly stigmatized amid prevailing cultures of individual responsibility that moralizingly attribute an HIV diagnosis to individual failures to practice adequate responsibility despite knowing better. The artists called for, as Bradley-Perrin posted, a substantive revaluation of the present "as worthy of and in need of critical and subversive energy" in order to recognize "the ongoingness of the struggle that is continuing to be taken up by young people today with their own experiences of HIV and AIDS which are valid despite its distance from the canon of AIDS activism."[86] Through a set of emblematic signifiers, the poster asserts that a nostalgic focus on AIDS and its past activism too often results in neglecting the contemporary nature of the AIDS crisis, and thus prevents the initiation and implementation of lifesaving actions in the present.

A critique of digital appropriation, the poster is itself the product of digital reappropriation. The creation process was conversational and circular. Chevalier and Bradley-Perrin collaboratively determined the design, and appraised and selected images from digital media platforms. Chevalier and Bradley-Perrin's "methodology" for identifying images to be included within the poster as they circulated online is reflective of the ways that Tumblr curators collected, viewed, and shared images.[87] Unlike other image-driven social media platforms that emphasize amateur photography, the majority of images on any given Tumblr are reblogged from others in a feed, which are reblogged from others, and so on. Mirroring this seemingly endless cascade of images, Chevalier and Bradley-Perrin conducted Google image searches. The two often simply selected the top results for inclusion in *Your Nostalgia.* Yet this process was far from random; Chevalier and Bradley-Perrin drew on their own preconceived understandings of the AIDS cultural canon.

Both creators felt strongly about featuring iconic images from AIDS archives. The art-activism posters made by Gran Fury, for example, Chevalier said, "needed to be pretty much up front and center."[88] Chevalier had recently seen the 1988 General Idea wallpaper that appropriates Robert Indiana's iconic 1960s *LOVE* motif to read instead "AIDS" in bright red letters over and over again in its creation of what the art-action collective termed an "image virus" in a Museum of Modern Art show.[89] Describing his viewing experience, Chevalier said, "I always get overwhelmed because my nostalgia for something that I've never experienced comes in." He continued, "But I was standing there surrounded by this group of Uptown Manhattan girls on their cell phones. . . . For some reason they were all just drawn to the poster [of David Wojnarowicz's *One Day, This Kid*] at the same time as me, and we had maybe this three-second moment of silence where we read it, and then one of the girls just speaks up and says, 'Deep,' and everybody laughed." That gallery visit, nostalgic, superficial, and affectively engaged, "became my archetypal space for creating the nineties teenage bedroom."[90]

Digital affordances permit a complex layering of archival images within the poster. Chevalier built the bedroom in Google SketchUp. The 3-D modeling software's provisions include downloading and reusing objects created by other users. Chevalier appropriated the teddy bear, laptop, and bed on which it rests. Each design choice carried layers of AIDS referents. The bed's inclusion was requisite to the poster's bedroom setting. Moreover, though, its presence reflected the creators' conscious evoking of early AIDS portraits and mainstream media exposure. These images of AIDS, which come to constitute its meaning, almost inevitably depicted gay men in beds—as Chevalier remarked, "On their deathbeds, in the hospital bed, in their own beds." The men in these images were "surrounded by family, and friends, and stuff." Within the poster, Chevalier and Bradley-Perrin featured Therese Frare's portrait of bedridden, dying David Kirby held and surrounded by his distraught family, as reused in a newly colorized form by the United Colors of Benetton for a 1992 ad campaign. In the poster, the room, Chevalier noted, in contrast to such bedrooms, "is empty except for the flat signifier purpose surrounding that bed."[91]

Referring explicitly to its social media inspiration, *Your Nostalgia* visually cited Tumblr: a Tumblr page is featured on the laptop screen. The viewer can see a post circulating an image of Gaëtan Dugas, the French Canadian flight attendant only recently rehabilitated from his infamy as the North American patient zero.[92] Featuring Dugas, a man whose supposed promiscuity was to blame for an epidemic, rather than the structural inequities and oppressions that actually drove it, draws attention to social death through stigmatization and gross neglect of HIV-positive persons as that which is deadly, long-standing, ongoing.

The circulation of archival images and video footage plays an important role in contemporary nostalgia for ACT UP, particularly for those who were not participants. The bedroom window in *Your Nostalgia* looks out onto one such image. The zoomed-in still from video footage of an ACT UP die-in shows two activists, bodies flat against the pavement, holding headstone-shaped placards above their heads. The young blond man's headstone reads, "RIP killed by the FDA." On the right, rising above the dark brown curls of another young man's head, the text cannot be made out in full within the poster's cropped image, but "AZT" is visible.[93] This image documents a 1988 national ACT UP action against the U.S. Food and Drug Administration, where activists protested both the lack of AIDS-related medical research and development and the slowness of the agency's drug approval processes. My analysis of the full image revealed the second activist's headstone to read "AZT is not enough," his handwritten sign signaling the inadequate treatment options available to people living with HIV/AIDS. A close reading of the full-size image also showed that one of these men is clad in the same ACT UP shirt worn in reissued version by Bieber elsewhere within the poster.[94] I also examined related images taken by Associated Press photographer J. Scott Applewhite. These archival images of ACT UP have become so iconic and so frequently circulated online that it requires significant research to uncover which chapter and action the image documents, providing further evidence for Chevalier and Bradley-Perrin's argument about decontextualization. The intentionally superficial engagement of archival records and their juxtaposition with art and advertisements within the poster comments insightfully on how frequently AIDS records are disassociated from vital aspects of their gendered, racialized, and political context as they move out from archives into and within digital media. Chevalier and Bradley-Perrin wrote, "It is not the remembering and it is neither the history, nor the material culture nor the valorization of the battles won and lost that impedes our movement forward, but rather the unpinning of our past from the circumstances from which the fights were born."[95]

Intervening in AIDS Nostalgia

The poster's use of nostalgia as frame provoked the strongest and most polarizing responses from its interlocutors. In three-dimensional highlighter yellow, the text "YOUR NOSTALGIA IS KILLING ME!" eclipses in scale the poster's other elements. Chevalier and Bradley-Perrin's explicit use of nostalgia as core intervention is significant in identifying, acknowledging, and redressing the implications of the longing for AIDS's past. Nostalgia, in its unvital practice, favors the past at the expense of engaging the politics and realities of the epidemic's present. The title text could read as a call for the outright abandonment of the past of AIDS and present nostalgia for it. However, drawing on my interviews with its creators and a analysis of their "performatively academic" artists' statement,[96] I argue that the poster seeks to enable a more complicated, contextualized practice of vital ACT UP nostalgia. This vital nostalgia would necessarily recognize ambivalences, complexities, and intergenerational particularities and relations in order to mobilize contemporary audiences in the fight against HIV/AIDS. Vital nostalgia provoked by the poster and the dialogues it prompted addresses the possibilities and limitations of affective longings. These longings continue across temporal and spatial bounds for ACT UP's practices of communal relationality, queer politics, and aesthetic proclivities. As I will discuss, memories can serve, as Bradley-Perrin wrote, as a "powerful and productive force in activism."[97]

AIDS activism has not been widely acknowledged in scholarship or popular imaginaries as an object for nostalgia's longing relation. Nostalgia is often reductively conceptualized as rosy-hued longings for pleasant past personal experiences. AIDS is thus an uncanny object. Nostalgia is a valuation practice that establishes, as Chevalier described it, "certain narratives, and perspectives, and aesthetics" as ones that are positive, productive, and good, and others as their foil.[98] AIDS's affective spectrum is routinely understood within the confines of trauma, grief, pain, and loss, while representations of ACT UP are presented as only heroic, unifying, and ultimately successful. The juxtaposition of a desperate epidemic with a triumphant movement can be, as Bradley-Perrin highlighted, "used to construct a narrative of success in which certain key battles being won brought about a public understanding of AIDS as over."[99] He noted that nostalgia can "close space for conversation" and can "use important successes as end points rather than moments of reassessment."[100] However, ACT UP nostalgia, as reconceptualized here as a practice of vital nostalgia, opens possibilities for a generative relationship to earlier AIDS activism, both by its activist participants and by subsequent generations. *Your Nostalgia* then "reevaluates," Bradley-Perrin told me, "the way the past gets used in the present,"[101] and in doing so, it names ACT UP an object of nostalgic intergenerational longing. "I wanted it acknowledged," Chevalier noted, that AIDS is a "setting for nostalgia, and let's have a conversation around it through that."[102] It is only after its identification that ACT UP nostalgia's pressing contemporary power implications can be interrogated.

The current cultural relationship of the art world, fashion, and scholarship to the 1990s is important to nostalgia's operation in the poster. This was not only a decade that saw significant AIDS activism in terms of scale, attention, and impact, but 1996 was also a watershed year for HIV/AIDS in the United States. The advent of effective combinations of antiretroviral medications extended lives and improved life chances for those with sustained access. Biomedical innovation shifted public perceptions of AIDS at home. The year 1996 is when end-of-AIDS narratives first emerge, the nascent seeds of contemporary discourse. In 2013, when the poster was made, and now, in American popular culture, arts, and scholarship, we are caught up in a moment of 1990s chic, with fashion trends, major museum exhibitions, and a proliferation of historical texts revisiting the era. The contemporary allure of 1990s' digital aesthetics evidenced in the practices of Tumblr curators and corporate web designers also proves significant in the poster's design and impact. Its look and feel mirrors that of early web graphics, as well as the colors, fonts, and bold political graphic styles of early 1990s' AIDS cultural production.

Justin Bieber's image highlights the critique of aesthetic nostalgia made by *Your Nostalgia*. ACT UP is transformed by his wearing of its reproduced logo into just something cool, a T-shirt with words on it that does not require any political or historical connection to AIDS or its activism.[103] Bradley-Perrin described the frustration he felt attending small AIDS demonstrations in the mid-2000s while noting that "walking on the other side of the street everyone is wearing their ACT UP American Apparel T-shirt with their cut-off jeans."[104] ACT UP always had a self-consciously appealing aesthetic drive to its work and look, whether in fashion, graphics, or other media-grabbing actions. In the early 1990s, fashion writer

Guy Trebay noted "the street-side potency of ACT UP's graphics, which have defined a generation of activists through fashion presence."[105] The leather jackets, high-rise denim, and combat boots so popular among fashion-forward activists have made their comeback; many of my students in Seattle now wear outfits reproducing these sensibilities. Bradley-Perrin acerbically commented, "It bothered me that people were so ready to be obsessed with the ACT UP aesthetic, but so unwilling to engage with the issues that ACT UP actually had engaged with. . . . If you put half as much energy into doing the work that is needed today as you do in reproducing or resurrecting an aesthetic from the past, we might make some progress."[106] The poster grew in part from "an emotional response" to aesthetic nostalgia for ACT UP that circulates on street corners and Tumblr sites, Bradley-Perrin continued: "The people who *could have been in a movement,* but are *just choosing to dress up like they're in a movement.*"[107] The dangers of resurrecting aesthetics are in practices that engage only with "aesthetics of the past, rather than seeing the politics of the present," Chevalier said.[108] The poster created "a satirical space" that included "everything but the kitchen sink of AIDS, art, the AIDS canon in order to highlight when you're trapped in that space. You're not looking at the present realities of today."[109] There is also danger in the artists' own curatorial practice: by reappropriating only the AIDS archival canon in their view of what constitutes AIDS past, they in turn reproduce a white gay male–centered vision of AIDS activism and cultural production. Once again, artists and activists of color and women are excluded.

The High Stakes of the Conflict over the Poster

Your Nostalgia circulated as physical and digital posters. Evoking proliferation of confrontational posters in a pre-Giuliani-era New York City, including broadsides appropriated in *Your Nostalgia* by the ACT UP–associated collectives Gran Fury and the Silence = Death Project, *Your Nostalgia* was pasted to walls in North American cities throughout summer 2013.[110] It was, however, on Tumblr, Facebook, and other digital media platforms that most audiences encountered the poster. The format of its circulation shaped interlocutors' readings of it and their tones, sparking wildly disparate responses and tense conflict among AIDS activists of different generations that extended from NYPL's halls to social media walls.

After being cited by Levine at the *Why We Fight* film program, the account of which opened this chapter, the poster was also engaged within the AIDS archives. ACT UP alum and filmmaker Jim Hubbard curated that film series for the NYPL, with each evening devoted to a particular line of inquiry providing attendees an entry point, showcasing the NYPL's extensive AIDS activist video collections, and offering an analog discussion platform. Hubbard sought to display the breadth of short film and video made in the AIDS activist milieu during the late 1980s and early 1990s as a challenge to dominant HIV/AIDS narratives, which focus only on certain actions and actors.[111] His selections included rarely viewed clips, primary footage of historic ACT UP actions, and "once ubiquitous images that have been divorced from context."[112] After each screening, there was an informal discussion between the audience, Hubbard, and the filmmakers. On the night of January 8, 2014, the screening's theme was "Mourning and Militancy." It included Levine and Catherine (Saalfield) Gund's 1991 short film, *Katrina Haslip Memorial*, documenting through collaboration with their subject her life and work as an HIV-positive activist in prisons and a formerly incarcerated person. It was Levine's mention of *Your Nostalgia* that in turn prompted Visual AIDS programs manager Kerr's sharing of the poster to the ACT UP/NY Alumni Facebook group.

On social media, discourse erupted as it often does: at breakneck speed, with little civility and lots of fervor. "I really thought that Vincent and Ian's poster was going to be heralded by old ACT UP activists as something that they saw in their lineage, because what I saw Ian and Vincent doing was speaking truth to power by creating a counterpublic to the dominant narrative," Kerr told me.[113] He continued, "I really saw them in the same vein as Gran Fury and all these amazing examples of art being able to articulate the movement against the powers that be. But that's not what happened."[114] In the early morning hours and over the course of the next few days, the thread on ACT UP/NY Alumni's wall blew up. Responses also moved onto separate threads, posted as comments on Chevalier and Bradley-Perrin's personal Facebook walls. The most active participants were former members of ACT UP/NY, not exclusively but primarily from generations who had been active during the late 1980s and early 1990s. Early on, Chevalier and Bradley-Perrin attempted to respond directly to all of the comments and questions posted. As those comments grew more inflammatory and personal, both artists largely stepped back from the fray. Some younger activists also stepped in to voice their perspectives, largely but not entirely in the poster's defense. PosterVirus curator McClelland and Kerr also jumped in. Kerr said, "I just saw it as my job. . . . Ian and Vincent shouldn't have to absorb that criticism on their own. Alex and

Jessica commissioned the poster, and Visual AIDS really put it out in the world in a way, and I personally put it out in the world, so it was my job to absorb some of that, like, I think really violent rhetoric [directed] at them."[115] A few of the ACT UP activists on the thread took up roles as mediators or made measured defenses of the poster.

It was not the assertion that uncritical acts of nostalgia were detracting much-needed attention and diverting action on AIDS now that chaffed some interlocutors. Many veteran ACT UP activists took specific afront to the poster's choice to label anything related to ACT UP or AIDS as nostalgia. One activist posted,

> I deny the idea that "AIDS Nostalgia" even exists: It's a figment of imagination by people who weren't there. The definition of nostalgia is to look back at the past and see ONLY the good stuff! The definition of regret is to look back at the past and see only the bad stuff! I have never met an AIDS activist who looks back and remembers only the good times. Not a single one. But, yeah, there were good times & bad times, and we who were there remember it all. The question of seeing AIDS as a problem that was somehow "solved" years ago has nothing to do with anyone's warm & fuzzy nostalgic view of a rose-colored past that didn't exist.[116]

Of reading this and many of his ACT UP contemporaries' negative responses, Finkelstein shared with me, "You don't have to read very deep to see the responses . . . were surrounding that question, of whether it was a good time, and people were remembering it in a positive way, or whether it was a terrible time and we are the walking wounded and fuck you for not knowing that. That's what that thread is about. It's a class conflict about a conversation about the cultural meaning of history."[117] Among veteran comrades, he saw little desire to engage critically with the story of the early years of AIDS. He had followed the online dialogue but refrained from entering the "social media mosh pit" where there was "nothing I could do in this context that would be in any way useful."[118] Also following along with the heated conversation online was *Why We Fight* curator Jason Baumann, who could see where his fellow ACT UP activists' overarching critiques of the poster came from.[119] They saw it "as accusatory towards people who were from that time period, that we were nostalgic about that time period and unable to engage with the realities of HIV and AIDS today."[120] Some took the poster's frame of nostalgia as a personal attack. One activist went so far as to describe Chevalier and Bradley-Perrin as "an ACT UP hate group."[121]

It is worth noting that while the creators and some interlocutors were unprepared for such defensive responses, ACT UP, which aspired to "turn grief into anger," was always a space in which conflict, both between activists and with outside forces, played a pivotal role. However, within ACT UP, there were shared physical spaces, mediated practices for debate, and opportunities for resolution through consensus-based decision making. The scale of the breakdown of communication across generational lines online was also reflected in many other comments, like this one: "Rather than sneering at the supposedly oppressive 'nostalgia' surrounding them, Chevalier & Ian might simply show a bit of gratitude and move on."[122] The tone of the social media conversations moved between conversational, catty, cruel, defensive, patronizing, and reflective. Kerr concluded that the conversation's tone and its intergenerational conflicts were in part "a failure of a Facebook feed" that read the poster "in a silo."[123]

For their part, Chevalier and Bradley-Perrin grew increasingly frustrated by ACT UP's response. At the end of a long few days, Bradley-Perrin posted a reply on his Facebook page along with a link to the poster:

> This poster was not made about ACT UP, or older activists or "AIDS Art" of the past but rather the appropriation and uses of it in the present in a declawed and depoliticized way, turned into an aesthetic and deployed for the purposes of obscuring and rewriting history. . . . I consider myself to be a historian and activist as well as a member of a community that includes the ACT UP folks but this is BULLSHIT . . . to assume that all AIDS must be processed through ACT UP New York and their tired cronies and must pass the test of white male ACT UP supremacy bullshit under the guise of conversation is actually the most depressing assertion of the central message of "Chevalier and Ian's" poster ever. Your Nostalgia is Killing Me! UGH.[124]

Both Chevalier and Bradley-Perrin recalled being surprised by the strong reaction of these activists—an audience they had, perhaps naively, not considered as one of their primary interlocutors. Generational disparities were of crucial importance to all interlocutors' responses to ACT UP nostalgia. Kerr noted, "There is a phenomenon happening across activist communities in which emerging and younger generations of activists are feeling silenced or boxed in by previous generations. In turn, this makes the established and older generation of activists also feel silenced and can put them on the defensive."[125] It is clear from an analysis of the Facebook threads that many ACT UP activists felt attacked or confused. They, as Kerr saw it, "wondered if they did not have a right to broadcast their past, which relates to their life chances. Many felt that they were being silenced or attempts were being made to render them and their work irrelevant."[126] For many who fought the death and devastation caused by AIDS in face of violent institutional neglect, this history was hallowed ground that they did not wish to see trodden upon. Clinging hard to the sanctity of the real accomplishments they made, the lives they saved, is an important survival strategy to contend with the many lives that were lost, and the personal, financial, and professional repercussions of past sacrifices these activists made.

Despite *Your Nostalgia*'s having been created by two people living with HIV, there was a widespread misperception perpetuated in the on-line debates that its creators were HIV negative and thus could afford could to take an aestheticized view of HIV/AIDS, because they "didn't have skin in the game," Finkelstein said.[127] The "viral divide" between those living with HIV/AIDS and those who are not, while in this case imagined, matters.[128] The serodivide shapes the tone of each Facebook thread, where many of those involved were HIV positive. A "natural affinity" between the creators, themselves highly educated white gay HIV-positive men, and many of the older generation of activists, who share those identifications, Finkelstein believed, should have been possible.[129] However, stark divides meant that "HIV-positive gay men or people living with HIV were *not able to find any affinity across generations.*"[130]

The social media conversation's intense contentiousness prompted Visual AIDS to organize a public follow-up event at the NYPL around *Your Nostalgia*.[131] The event aspired to create a physical space that mirrored the ACT UP room at its best, a space open to conflict and configurations of empathy, inviting participants to bring their "confusion, criticism, anger, joy, will, and love" in order to "to work through and share" in collectivity.[132] Aspiring to work toward vital nostalgia in which the AIDS activist past is held onto critically and with intention, the event used it as a means to envision and enact a different AIDS present and future. For Baumann, including this panel, the last in the *Why We Fight* series, made perfect sense because the goal of the programming was to make the AIDS activist community "at home at the library."[133] He also noted that this conversation began at the NYPL and got heated there, so they "owed it" to the community to "continue" and to "help that community have that conversation."[134] Finkelstein, along with fellow early ACT UP member John Weir, joined Bradley-Perrin and Chevalier as panelists.

The first and only recorded portion of the event posted on the NYPL's website and on YouTube shows that each panelist briefly presented on the poster.[135] Bradley-Perrin and Chevalier's presentations aimed to clarify their poster's message and to personalize it by articulating their personal stakes in these debates. Weir had served alternately as peacemaker and instigator in the online threads; he called in his comments at the event for activists of all generations to engage with critical generosity with the poster and the issues it raised within an ACT UP context. Finkelstein was in firm agreement with the poster's contentions about AIDS history and "felt as the person who did half the work that is depicted as nostalgic in that poster that [he had] this distinct ability to and responsibility to speak critically about the meaning of that cultural production."[136] The event also included breakout small group discussions intended to offer space for all stakeholders within social media conversations to dialogue in shared physical space. Such dialogue is an essential component of how activists, as well as archivists and artists, might use vital nostalgia as they create and curate the records of AIDS's history.

The event represented an effort toward building a more vital nostalgia in the AIDS archives. However, none of "the people who screamed loudest" online attended.[137] For his part, Bradley-Perrin found it an "unsatisfying" conclusion.[138] The event's overarching tone was markedly different from that of the online discourse; as Baumann described it, "It was much more amicable in public than over the internet, as most things are."[139] Even while key participants found the event inadequate and the community did not come together in full to work through a conflict, it was still a pivotal moment. That this conversation began at all, where previously there was little more than silence, matters more than outcome. Moreover, that the poster used archival images of AIDS activism and cultural production, some of which are held within the NYPL's collections, and that its interlocutors returned to that archival context to engage are significant. By opening itself as a space for debate, albeit one with real limitations, this AIDS archives is ensuring through vital nostalgic practice its central place as an active participant in the ongoing conversations about the documentation and historicization of AIDS and nostalgia for its activism.

Moving AIDS Archives toward Vital Nostalgia

In sum, vital nostalgia for ACT UP is grounded and circulated through access, both digital and analog, to archival images, video footage, ephemera, and other records and provides just one case study into new and important considerations for the archival field. *Your Nostalgia* illustrates how digital media has created affective economies where archival materials documenting early AIDS activism and cultural productions frequently circulate and are appropriated in ways divorced from the context of their production. Archival images are disseminated across social media in ways that shape and are shaped by platform affordances as well as social, political, and cultural values. Activists have called for peers, scholars, and archivists to take seriously the contemporary reality that born-digital and digitized archival records are frequently circulating as objects without context across digital platforms. Such circulation can challenge their very status as archival records. Considering such objects will challenge and expand archival thinking about the nature of records. Is an archival record a record any longer when it circulates without metadata, other description, or even an acknowledgment of its archival origins? *Your Nostalgia* exposes clearly the dangers of digital decontextualization and related commodification.

Archives can and should be important players in these conversations about ACT UP, its records, and their circulation as well as the historicization of AIDS and nostalgia for its activism. Archives almost universally place significant emphasis on context for the creation, provenance, and culture of records in their work, whether it is through descriptions, maintaining original order in arrangement, or providing reference services. We in the archival field need to take such significant work and theorization of the importance of context into new and digital frontiers. Understanding AIDS images, including those featured within *Your Nostalgia*, anew as archival records resituates them within their full and meaningful AIDS context. Tracing nostalgia for ACT UP in the present is necessary to be able to continue to adequately contextualize archival materials documenting AIDS activism. Such contextualization is necessary so that these materials do not become the flattened signifiers that Chevalier and Bradley-Perrin critique with their poster. Moreover, complex contextualization is a part of the ethical responsibility of studying, archiving, and curating with AIDS activist materials. In order to make these records available to the greater community, including both activists and archivists, that may have deeply conflicted and conflicting affective connections in them, nostalgic relations require our deep interrogation.

David Lowenthal writes, "What pleases the nostalgist is not just the relic but his own recognition of it, not so much the past itself as its supposed aspirations, less the memory of what actually was than of what was once thought possible."[140] *Your Nostalgia* can be misread as antinostalgia, highlighting the pitfalls of dwelling in a romanticized version of the past that comes at the price of taking action in the ongoing HIV/AIDS crisis's present. However, the poster can be read more productively not as calling for the outright dismissal of nostalgia but instead as seeking a more vital practice of nostalgia. The nostalgic interest in and strong feelings for ACT UP, its community, politics, and aesthetics, both by those who participated in it in the 1980s and 1990s and those who wish they had, can be powerfully deployed with the aid of creative works like *Your Nostalgia* to bring attention to the contemporary nature of the crisis. Vital nostalgia can thus productively move contemporary scholarship, cultural production, and archival work toward a more complicated history and remembering of the AIDS activist movement.

Doing this work now is vital. As Finkelstein described to me, "We're in this pivotal moment because the solidification of an AIDS historiography didn't happen five years ago; it's happening now. The future is in our hands. We're in a potentially radicalizing moment. So the history of AIDS has nothing to do with the past. It has to do with now."[141] That *Your Nostalgia* was able to generate such intergenerational and heated conversations about the past, present, and future of AIDS is a sign of the power of vital nostalgia as an opening point for an ongoing discourse and a means of generating action. Finkelstein concluded, "Whether Ian and Vincent's poster was a success or a failure doesn't matter because it activated a whole generation of—two generations of people thinking about it," and maybe it inspired some of those people to act, something that is needed while "we're at war. You're either in resistance or you're in compliance."[142] *Your Nostalgia* aids in the development of a vital intergenerational nostalgia as a historical counternarrative that can address and redress racialized, gendered, and classed inequities in power in the present. Vital nostalgia for ACT UP crucially creates a much-needed space for imagining a different future, one in which queer politics can be radical, fashion can be fabulous, and activism can be cool again.

2

HOW TO ACT UP

AIDS Archival Temporalities and the (Anti-)Institutionalization

of the ACT UP/New York Records

AIDS is really a test of us, as a people. When future generations ask what we did in this crisis, we're going to have to tell them that we were out here today. And we have to leave the legacy to those generations of people who will come after us. Someday, the AIDS crisis will be over. Remember that. And when that day comes—when that day has come and gone, there will be people alive on this earth, gay people and straight people, men and women, black and white, who will hear the story that once there was a terrible disease in this country and all over the world, and that a brave group of people stood up and fought and, in some cases, gave their lives, so that other people might live and be free.

—**VITO RUSSO**, *WHY WE FIGHT* (1988)

"IF I'M DYING FROM ANYTHING—I'm dying from the fact that not enough rich, white, heterosexual men have gotten AIDS for anybody to give a shit," Vito Russo intoned. In Damned Interfering Video Activist Television's (DIVA TV) grainy video, Russo's voice and gestures, the tense grip on the loose pages and the shake of a fist, make his hurt and rage cutting and palpable. HIV/AIDS was actually happening to his audience, off screen until the final pan out but audible and visible in the camera's shakiness as the videographer jostled in the crowd. It was happening to him, a white, gay, middle-class man living with AIDS. They were constituents of the "disposable populations of fags and junkies who deserve what they get." The American public with its constitutive privileges (whiteness, middle-classness, heterosexuality, able-bodiedness, citizenship), he continued, "don't have to give a shit." By May 1988, Russo and fellow ACT UP/NY activists, including DIVA TV members, were bone weary. People living with HIV/AIDS and those who fought for them had borne the burdens of an epidemic more than seven years long, of discrimination and bigotry, of innumerable hospital visits and funerals. They had passed the breaking point. On a spring afternoon, activists gathered in Albany, refusing to do the expected: to "be home dying," or to be pitiable "helpless victims" exploited for human-interest stories. AIDS "is happening to us," they demonstrated in words and actions; moreover, "We do give a shit."[1]

As a concluding salvo, Russo envisioned aloud "Why We Fight." He emphasized a radical futurity in which AIDS would be holistically cured but not forgotten: "Someday, the AIDS crisis will be over. Remember that."[2] As he paused, an audible "Right on!" rung out. The certainty with which Russo claimed that there would actually be an end belied stark realities. With one phrase, "When that day has come and gone," he engendered a shift in AIDS time: from present crisis to past victory, from being "busy putting out fires and taking care of people on respirators" to a future thriving where "we're all going to be alive to kick the shit out of this system, so that this never happens again," from crisis to collective memory. He conjured a future in which there are survivors who "might live and be free." Russo's provocation, then and now, is a fantasy.[3] The forecasting he performed required that people "will hear" that "there once was a terrible disease."[4] Russo's future is one in which AIDS is not unremembered or misrepresented.

A future in which HIV/AIDS is widely acknowledged depends on "activist archiving" and "archiving activism."[5] Indeed, that digitized video of Russo's speech, with its sun flares, static, and technological glitches,[6] is itself an archival record, and one that afforded immediacy as I watched it. The demand Russo issued to generate AIDS memory work as activism is still provocative. It reflected the obsessive activist archiving efforts that were underway in ACT UP/NY between 1987 and 1995. In their performance of care work in the service of creating and sustaining social change in their own time and of shaping the enduring cultural record in posterity, ACT UP/NY produced a rich, vivid archives. Listening now, I hear Russo's call as evoking the need to interrogate the tensions and possibilities raised by archiving activism, the institutional stewardship of the records these activists created, collected, and cared for. Between their 1995 donation to the NYPL and 2016, the archives was transfigured. As I will show in this chapter, institutional experimentation was driven by activist interventions grounded in vital nostalgia, activist longings for a past time that interrogate, address, and repair structural power inequities. It matters urgently how this AIDS archives and the organization and people who made it came into being; it matters urgently how it has developed and whose lives are at stake in these records. The production of ACT UP/NY's archives mediates contemporary HIV/AIDS memory's possibilities and omissions. ACT UP's collection, housed at a prominent AIDS archives, steeped in matrices of power—race, gender, sexuality, class, ability, nationality, religion—shapes "the story,"[7] what is and can be known and felt about AIDS, who is visible, marginalized, or excluded, and how people and events are remembered, omitted, or forgotten. Records and the people and systems that create, collect, preserve, make accessible, and care for them, when mobilized through vital nostalgia, offer important possibilities for repoliticizing AIDS now among the future generations Russo dreamed of. AIDS archives enable us to benefit from the records of those whom Russo called "a brave group of people [who] stood up and fought and in some cases died," and to mobilize their archives to challenge AIDS's persistent and cruel injustices. More than four decades into the pandemic, giving a shit about AIDS is still required.[8]

This book is the first to showcase archivalization as central to ACT UP's organizing. ACT UP, a "diverse, non-partisan group of individuals united in anger and committed to direct action to end the AIDS crisis," took rage, mourning, and desperation and mobilized them into fierce action. ACT UP formed in March 1987 at New York City's Gay and Lesbian Community Center (now the LGBT Center, hereafter the Center). Its creation was part of a shift toward new modes of activism as death tolls and infection rates rose, and the fight grew increasingly desperate. Activists targeted indifference, neglect, and malfeasance. They demanded education, resources, and action in biomedical research, medical treatment, education, public policy, social services, and media and archival representation. They worked to end AIDS and improve the lives of people living with HIV/AIDS. Their actions were diverse in scale and approach—demonstrations, poster campaigns, research sessions, die-ins, kiss-ins, videos, workshops, occupations, political funerals, conferences, needle exchanges, zaps, and public access television shows.[9] Their disruptive acts, what Douglas Crimp called "cultural activism,"[10] were often image driven and theatrical, designed for late-twentieth-century televisual culture where transforming realities required changing representation.[11] ACT UP built affective ties between generations of activists who came together in fierce community. Scott

Wald described being there as engendering a "tsunami of feeling,"[12] simultaneously invigorating and exhausting, thrilling and devastating, hopeful and depressing, healing and painful. In the late 1980s and early 1990s, ACT UP/NY counted thousands within its loose network.[13] In New York City, General Meetings still convene on Monday nights, as they have for over thirty years, first at the Center, later at Cooper Union, and now back at the Center, just a few floors up from where they started.

Russo's measured words continue to be "right on." We are living in an AIDS time characterized by a prevailing cultural acceptance that HIV/AIDS in America is at, or at least near, its expiration.[14] Since 2008, there has been a flood of AIDS projects, popular and scholarly, that operate in retrospective register. The vastness and institutional situatedness of the archives that activists produced and sustained figure into the outsize role ACT UP/NY plays within the selective remembering practiced by these recent projects and as the queer object of contemporary cultural and political nostalgia. Many AIDS memory projects focus exclusively, or nearly so, on the crisis's anguishing first fifteen years during which 350,000 Americans died.[15] Standard accounts begin in 1981, when physicians observed and documented in print the first cases of what would become HIV among "homosexual men," a damning label of "risk" that soon expanded to people addicted to heroin, people with hemophilia, and Haitians. These accounts focus repeatedly on ACT UP's flashy treatment activism in New York City. They conclude with 1996, when the death counts slowed with the advent of antiretroviral drug cocktails that inhibited HIV, the development of which activists had driven, thus transforming the virus into a controllable chronic condition for those who can access and afford the medication regimens. Dominant discourses that focus on these medical advances appropriate Russo's freedom vision despite the vast contrary evidence that HIV/AIDS is and will continue to be for the foreseeable future a crisis locally and globally. The transformation of earlier crisis conditions into an age of selective HIV survivability opens space for end-of-AIDS discourse that perpetuates the delusion that AIDS is rendered harmless, and that suffering and dying are safely relegated to the past.

In addition to temporal limitations that foreclose urgency, the dominant AIDS discourse is also characterized by imaginative restraints in terms of affected communities. Early AIDS years were largely, and problematically, identified with white, gay, economically privileged men—the epidemic's first recognized victims.[16] Focusing on this period, contemporary revisitations continuously frame white, gay, middle-class men in urban centers as representative of all AIDS activists and activism. Revisitation projects reflect in part the power dynamics in ACT UP/NY (masculinity, whiteness, class, citizenship) that shaped who did the documenting and who and what was documented, and in turn collected and preserved by AIDS archives. Privileges did not and could not save many men from the ravages of AIDS; however, these archives did and do protect them from having their memories fade.[17] Yet the ways that these representations sideline activism by men of color, cis and trans women, incarcerated persons, intravenous drug users, and immigrants exceeds the archives' material constraints. It is not simply that the records of multiply marginalized subjects do not exist; it is that users enter the archives with a preconceived narrative about who AIDS affected. Through dominant racist and sexist practices of selective remembering, archives are situated as the site of the end of AIDS. Ultimately, perpetuating a narrow periodization and vision of AIDS as past impedes and defangs contemporary responses to the ongoing epidemic.

Archives also hold the promise of countering the lethal constraints of current AIDS memory projects. To capture how AIDS archives operate both as the site of AIDS's historicization, with all of this emergent history's attendant problematics, and as the most powerful bulwark against dangerous end-of-AIDS narratives requires understanding how they came and continue to be. In this chapter, I trace the ACT UP/NY Records' cultural life. I draw on archival research and observations at the NYPL, and on interviews conducted in 2015 and 2016 with current and former ACT UP/NY members and NYPL staff. First, I examine ACT UP's activist archiving. The extensive scale and efficacy of its documentation and collection emerged from and was shaped by activists' identities and experiences, technological affordances, and the group's politics and strategy. Second, I analyze activists' conflicts over the records' disposition and the collection's archival institutionalization. ACT UP's anti-institutional politics and intragroup differences figured significantly into the organization's decision making and its lingering affective resonances and political consequences. Finally, I turn to watershed relational shifts provoked by *Why We Fight: Remembering AIDS Activism*, the NYPL's major 2013–14 exhibition and public programming series. In donating its records, ACT UP did not cede control over the meaning of its archives; activists maintain complicated ongoing connections to their records and to the institution that houses them. In charting their relations, I focus on two events organized by ACT UP/NY within the archives, demonstrating that contemporary activist interventions grounded in vital nostalgia are shifting the contours of power through institutional experimentation. Like any other home, AIDS archives can provide refuge, a space of belonging for records and their creators, subjects, and communities. However, these archives are not homes free of conflict or exclusion.

Embracing the "Impulse to Archive"

"The impulse to archive,"[18] Debra Levine explained, struck her and many ACT UP/NY compatriots. Along with more widely recognized activist labors, such as demonstrations and petitions, activist archiving was a crucial part of some ACT UPers' practices and the organization's political strategy. ACT UPer and avid collector Maxine Wolfe, a seasoned activist in leftist causes since the 1960s, shared with me that "ACT UP was the first time that, in any activism that I was a part of, the people in the group itself were very aware [that] they should document their own history."[19] Unlike most earlier activist archiving, and in a prelude to the social media age, the impulse to archive in ACT UP/NY coincided with the peak of the group's activities. Yet like much of ACT UP's politics and tactics, its activist archiving built on civil rights, gay and lesbian liberation, and feminist movement legacies of direct action, civil disobedience, and organizing.[20] These earlier movements had taught activists the importance of documentation as a means of self-definition and representation, identity building, and empowerment[21] that bolstered efforts toward justice and healing, and that acted as an instrument for conceptualizing the past to shape the present and future.[22]

Archiving became and remains a vital component of AIDS cultural activism.[23] The ubiquity of ACT UP's video documentation in particular was simultaneously an archival act aimed at posterity and an element of activists' efforts to effect change in their own time to challenge the media narrative, advocate for better treatments, support community education, and create alternative television programming. Records were collected and preserved within the group's workspaces and a distributed network of private homes. Attention to activist archiving, evidenced both in self-documentation and later in the contentious debates over the archival institutionalization of its materials and ongoing relations to the NYPL, demonstrates that ACT UP saw archives as a site of political power and knowledge production demanding intervention. By creating, collecting, and caring for the materials that constitute the ACT UP/NY Records between 1987 and 1995, AIDS activists built an enduring home for themselves and their comrades. In this section, I cover the primary contributing factors in ACT UP/NY's activist archiving: urgency wrought by imminent mortality; members' backgrounds in media, arts, and the academy; innovations in video technologies; the group's affective communal orientation; key collectors' marginalized positionalities; and administrative practices.

AIDS's accelerated temporal rhythms before 1996[24] produced an urgency that led some activists to nurture documentation practices. David Román credits "the archival impulse" to shifts in AIDS time, arguing that it emerged in the mid- to late 1980s, when "it became clear that AIDS was not going to be resolved any time soon."[25] This period correlates with ACT UP's emergence. "The kind of temporality that we lived at that moment was a very kind of intense temporality," within which dying was nearly categorical and there was no treatment.[26] Activists did more "over the course of one day," Levine continued, than "in a normal life, where you really didn't have this sense of mortality that you lived with, among the people you lived with."[27] A heightened sense of mortality characterized the distinctive temporal immediacy of activist archiving in the heat of the emergency. Alexis Danzig highlighted the temporal aspects of video early on in DIVA TV. They were "deliberately documenting what [they] were doing" for the future, "creating something for posterity" and for the present, creating something "for safety" and for "being able to tell the story now."[28] Danzig described knowing "we were the news that we were making."[29] Through documentation, activists asserted that "our lives are in fact worth something, our lives are worth saving, our lives are worth documenting."[30] She concluded, "We did save our own lives."[31]

ACT UP was aware of the power in garnering and controlling media representation. The concern with representation is exemplified by DIVA TV's mission: "We are committed to making media which directly counters and interferes with dominant media assumptions about AIDS and governmental negligence in dealing with the AIDS crisis."[32] Many activists had professional media savvy. Media scholar and DIVA TV and ACT UP alum Alexandra Juhasz has noted that because HIV/AIDS in its first and still most recognized manifestation infected white gay American men's bodies, this community took to video and television for their material, educational, and artistic responses.[33] White, middle-class, college-educated professionals in media outlets, artists, and critics, some ACT UP activists, were a cultural elite who were situated within privilege so as to be outraged when their illnesses and deaths were met by mainstream media with indifference or blame.[34]

Privilege was also formative to activists' confidence that theirs was history worth documenting and that it held enduring archival value. Because they were already familiar with it, many activists used video and broadcast television as mediums of response, this time representing people living with AIDS. Such depictions countered mainstream phobic representations of those with AIDS as dying and alone. According to Ron Goldberg, ACT UP was always "extremely conscious of the media" as well as "extremely, extremely conscious" about timing its actions so as to best capture popular attention.[35] He emphasized that media awareness generated new records: "We did our own media. . . . When no one was covering us, we could still create coverage."[36] During our interview, Wolfe described those leading documentation efforts as "mostly the younger people," noting that "a lot of them were people who were in media."[37] Activists had disparate relationships to mainstream academic and media institutions by generation, which would later inform tensions around selecting an archival repository. In considering ACT UP's prioritization of activist archiving, Levine observed a predisposition toward documentation among artists: they were already "very attuned to making sure that their work is preserved in some way that can get seen later on."[38] Similarly, Danzig cited artistic influence: "These were mostly people who had come out of art school with a rich awareness of how you need to control images to be able to control what version of reality wins."[39]

It was not only rapid changes in politics, theory, and activism that aligned to make ACT UP's documentation extensive and effective; innovations in video technologies in the mid- to late 1980s[40] informed the format and tremendous scale and distribution of records. Activists brought video cameras "everywhere. Any action we went to someone was documenting it," Wolfe said.[41] She laughed, noting that she was doing the same thing with paper.[42] Video collectives, affinity groups of ACT UP "from the get-go,"[43] devoted to "direct, immediate, product-oriented activism,"[44] played an important role in video's ubiquity. "There was a joke, you know —they'd take pictures of us going to the bathroom. It was everywhere— we were always on video," Goldberg emphasized.[45] Video technologies' affordances distributed "responsibility" for documentation[46] and democratized possibilities for who, and what, were and could be captured in ways reflective of ACT UP's queer politics. Hubbard had "been filming the gay community since 1978 and often [in the early 1980s] I would be the only person with a camera" at an action.[47] Hubbard witnessed a profound shift "starting in '87, and even more so in '88 and '89, [with] the introduction of Video8 and HI8; suddenly there is this profusion of cameras; all of a sudden there is this small, easily portable, relatively high-quality video camera that was affordable."[48] Similarly, Danzig described shooting with DIVA TV: "You bought a camera for $1,000 and you put in a little tape and you filmed things. . . . And you bought a monopod and held it up at a demonstration and you filmed stuff. And if you were lucky, you caught some interesting stuff."[49] Additionally, innovations in satellite, the VCR, and computer editing made video technologies affordable and mobile. This enabled individuals and communities who had never had the option of mastering them to do so. Juhasz summarized, "The politics of AIDS—demands for a better quality of life for the people affected by this epidemic—are well matched by the potentials and politics of video."[50] ACT UP's video usage also has roots in 1970s' "guerilla television," which demonstrated the format's strategic accessibility, cost-effectiveness, and distribution potential.[51] At actions, the camera served an additional purpose: its presence could deter police brutality and provide activists with opportunities to review their strategies and performances.[52] ACT UP was one of the first activist groups to extensively use home video for documentary, educational, and legal purposes.[53]

Activists' impetuses to collect and preserve, their care work, were shaped by their feelings for one another. The powerful potency of affective intragroup connections, and the ways in which emotion figured into actions and informs ACT UP's historical significance, are widely noted.[54] Loss and a need for community alongside action led many to the group and kept them coming back. The ways ACT UP created and sustained community across difference have been greatly romanticized. Although in actuality decidedly more complicated, the connections that activists made with one another are still important in understanding the scale and practices of their documentation and archiving. Affect is both a motivation and result of activist archiving.[55] Hubbard emphasized, "AIDS was a public and political crisis, but it was also a personal crisis. So everyone who was working on AIDS in a political way had a personal reason for doing so."[56] Political commitments to memory work were a form of resistance to forgetting AIDS and reflected a sense of responsibility to the AIDS community. The work was personal; pain and memory are interconnected. Many activists cared deeply and literally for people who had been deemed expendable, their pain and experiences unrecognized. Connections, often with those who were sick, dying, or deceased, drove some members to collect materials on those whom they cared deeply about, holding them, storing them, keeping them as precious.[57] Describing the myriad ACT UP collections that are still in private homes rather than institutional archives, Levine told me: "I know who has what because I know who loved whom."[58] She continued: "That is literally how collections happened. Some people collected everything, but some people collected or kept things of the people in their affinity groups, the people that they loved."[59] Levine cited Aldo Hernández, who collected and still holds artist and fellow ACT UPer Ray Navarro's records. Hernández had dutifully cared for the records since Navarro's 1990 death; however, he had not actually looked at them before Levine's mid-2000s visit, when he had to break the lock of the filing cabinet where he had closed them away for safekeeping. AIDS archives are "very personal endeavours," Topher Campbell explained. "People have died, or been killed, or been forgotten or ignored. Some very fascinating, interesting people in a culture which, for lots of different reasons—not just racism, but class and poverty—has denied their existence."[60] Activist archiving offered for some a means to deal with pain, mourning, and trauma, and to make public the acknowledgment of suffering, love, and critical caring done in ACT UP in order to build the resilience required to face HIV/AIDS.

Activists' minoritarian identities and experiences of intragroup marginalization informed their commitment to documentation. Many people most active in ACT UP/NY's self-documentation and collecting hold minoritized identities, such as religion or gender, and frequently occupied marginalized positions even within ACT UP. Disinclined to trust that their voices would be captured or heard in the record, they took activist archiving into their own hands. Wolfe, a white Jewish lesbian, "picked up every piece of paper there was on the back table [at the General Meeting] every week."[61] She also "kept anything that I organized, I kept papers, including arrest records and lists of people who showed, who attended, people who went to actions."[62] Similarly, writer, artist, and former ACT UPer Avram Finkelstein, who is white, gay, and Jewish, described to me how he "realized it might make sense to grab copies of everything"[63] at ACT UP meetings and actions. The back literature table at Monday meetings that Wolfe and Finkelstein collected from offered an "incredible cornucopia of news."[64] These guides to the New York AIDS community included clinical trial updates, ads for New Age lectures, and personal testimonies.[65] Activists described picking up whatever looked appealing and circulating tidbits through their networks around the country.[66] Finkelstein recalled being aware that this print material was "fugitive," by which he meant it could easily disappear.[67] For him, creating "an archive under my bed" was motivated by this knowledge as well as his history.[68] Of this need to archive, he told me, "Part of it is a Jewish response I think as well. Nobody in my entire family knew the name of the village my grandmother fled during the pogroms in Russia, including my grandmother. And so I feel this Jewish compulsion towards history. . . . It was just like a personal impulse for me to save this material."[69] ACT UPer Stephen Shapiro made the same connection. In a note following up after our second interview, he wrote, "One reason why ACT UP was so self-consciously archival (on the individual level) is that it had a very large Jewish membership. And this is a cultural-ethnic group with a fundamental dedication to textual preservation, especially in the aftermath of the Holocaust (a primary metaphor for the crisis)."[70]

ACT UP is often portrayed in scholarly and popular accounts as constituted by white, gay, middle-class men, yet women shaped ACT UP/NY's activist archiving. Women have always been marginalized in American cultural understandings of AIDS and its lived experiences, in access to resources, and as activists who made vital contributions to anti-AIDS activism. ACT UP's women were driven to documentation to represent and to preserve women and other marginalized persons' stories. With histories in feminist health activism, many women activists understood HIV/AIDS not as exception but rather as part of a long history of health crises affecting marginalized persons for which the only remedy was to take these concerns into their own hands.[71] Women, many more of whom had long been activists, brought tactical expertise to ACT UP. They also did much of the documentation labor, especially in video collectives. Yet women are rarely represented either as subjects living with AIDS or as leading activists in the fight against it. Some activists argued that women's marginalization in current crisis narratives was due in part to the focus of their footage; many women filming, like Levine, were not "really looking at ourselves as the center of documentation."[72] Women activists, many of whom were white, middle class, and HIV negative, often "had less reason to think our life and death survival at that historical moment was the primary subject."[73] Levine recalled that she and her counterparts recognized that creating documentation had "political benefits for us as women."[74] Others, like Juhasz, argued that gender informed their video content.[75] For example, video collectives created extensive educational media explicitly for and about the needs of women with HIV/AIDS, who were often ignored by clinicians, researchers, and politicians as well as absent from mainstream representations. It was always clear that for women's epidemic experiences to be centered or captured, women would need to do the documentation.

Like much activist knowledge in ACT UP/NY, activist archiving expertise was gendered. Many women in ACT UP had long-term prior and simultaneous involvement with the Lesbian Herstory Archives (LHA), a grassroots feminist lesbian community archives founded in 1972 that by the mid-1980s was part of a full-fledged LGBTQ archival movement. Experiences as LHA "archivettes" informed some women activists' keen awareness of the need to document, collect, preserve, and make accessible for posterity records of their activism. Polly Thistlethwaite credited the LHA with her understanding of "how archives are constructed and who gets to be in the archive and . . . what parts are going to be available to the public, what parts are going to be excised."[76] Moreover, the LHA's training afforded the skills and experience required to archive. Wolfe, an LHA volunteer since 1984 who joined ACT UP just after its founding, drew others into AIDS activism. Wolfe, Danzig, Thistlethwaite, and other lesbian members of the ACT UP Women's Caucus were part of ACT UP and the LHA throughout the late 1980s and early 1990s. The LHA was even the direct material beneficiary of ACT UP.[77] Prior to ACT UP, Thistlethwaite's social world, like that of many lesbians, had not included many gay men. The personal connections she and others formed in the group in turn led some activist men to aid in the LHA's efforts.[78] Wolfe, Thistlethwaite, and Danzig all credit the LHA with shaping their strategies and heightened awareness of the significance of self-documentation and value of archival access for activists. ACT UP and the LHA, Danzig concluded, were both "very much about ownership and about community."[79] The feminist community archiving backgrounds of many women activists also informed their perspectives about where the ACT UP records should be located.

Navigating sexism and its nexus with racism, classism, or marginalization as lesbians within ACT UP/NY motivated some women activists to document. Levine, a white woman, aimed with the videos she created to produce an understanding of "the parameters of the work you were doing." She primarily filmed "people whose lives we knew were fairly precarious," given their positive serostatus and minoritized racial and class identities. Levine was involved in collaborations with incarcerated activists, most of whom were women of color from economically disadvantaged backgrounds. These activists did not garner much attention within ACT UP or from the general public. Documenting incarcerated lives and activist work within prisons required, from Levine's perspective, determining "platforms" that attached these activists' work to those of more dominant art and activist practices in ACT UP. Video was a medium capable of "refiguring" representation by showcasing the breadth of activist community. Levine noted that "AIDS was this crazy nexus, where like people who had extraordinary privilege were in a moment denied those privileges and actually depended on people who had never had the privileges, who really understood the way to organize themselves in order to demand or to claim the things that they needed."[80] Significant conflicts over movement priorities, which became especially fraught in the early 1990s, were informed by experiences of sexism and racism in ACT UP. For some ACT UPers, these tensions and their experiences of marginalization produced their desire to document.

Yet creating, collecting, and preserving records about women's AIDS activism within the ACT UP/NY Records and associated collections has not proved sufficient to obtain recognition of women's contributions. Ann Cvetkovich noted, "Lesbians, many of whom came to ACT UP with considerable political experience, seem to be some of the first to disappear from ACT UP's history."[81] Wolfe, reflecting on that sexist erasure, told me: "One of the things that people don't get about ACT UP, when they always call it a gay male organization, was that most of the leadership was female."[82] Thistlethwaite concurred: "We—many of the political leaders in ACT UP were based in the Women's Caucus. . . . Lesbian political sensibilities were driving a certain part of the organization."[83] According to Wolfe, women "did the marshal trainings, we did the CD [civil disobedience] trainings, we did the logistics for organizations, we did a lot of organizing of actions, et cetera. We were the facilitators at meetings, and we also had a Women's Committee besides that, and we made the Women's Committee be national, so we knew women in all these ACT UP groups all over the world."[84] Regardless of the archival record they produced, cis and trans women and people of color continue to be widely marginalized in memory projects that activate AIDS archives. Levine noted, for example, that despite her efforts to ensure the presence of their records in AIDS archives, "incarcerated activists' contributions to the movement are not central to most of the recent historical narratives."[85] Standard narratives operate through the lens of their creators' preconceived gendered, racialized, and classed notions of who was in the room or on the street, reflecting and replicating ACT UP's presumed whiteness, maleness, gayness, and middle-classness. Such representational realities do not dismiss the value of marginalized activists' valiant efforts that shaped the ACT UP/NY Records.

Activist archiving was a core organizational function. ACT UP/NY's administrative practices fashioned its archives. ACT UP/NY collected records within its administrative spaces. This effort was without a systematic or formally articulated process or mandate. I found no direct mention of the archives or archiving procedures within the group's meeting minutes. However, that the "workspace collection" existed at all and its tremendous scale provide evidence of ACT UP's organizational active, if haphazard, commitment to archiving. "Workspace" was, in Shapiro's words, "1980s activist slang; we never would have called it the office—that was too bourgeois."[86] By the early 1990s, the workspace was in Midtown West.[87] The upper-floor industrial loft space was neighbored by cheap clothing manufacturers. Activists erected their own drywall to construct small rooms. In the drawing he made me (Figure 2), Shapiro noted the locations of filing cabinets used for storing posters next to the group's Xerox machine; another cabinet he labels enthusiastically the "ACT UP archive!"

Individual activists determined what was collected and preserved in, and what is absent from, ACT UP's organizational records. ACT UP/NY never had paid staff, but it had a workspace manager.[88] Jason Baumann,

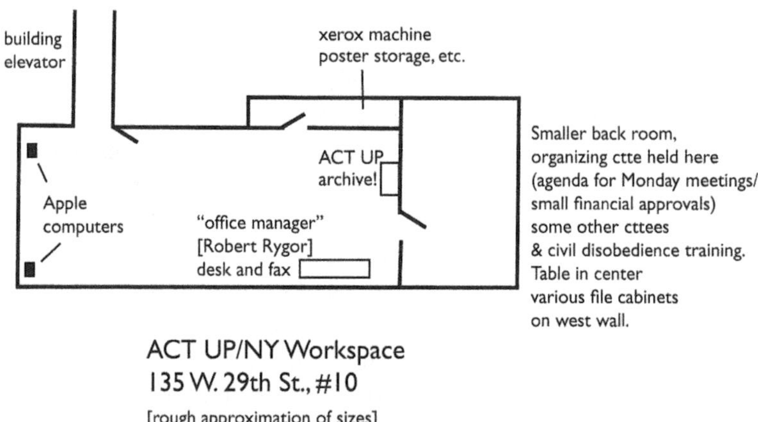

Figure 2. ACT UP/NY's organizational records had a prominent place in the group's Midtown workspace in the early 1990s. Drawing by Stephen Shapiro. Courtesy of the artist.

Susan and Douglas Dillon associate director for collection development and coordinator of Humanities and LGBT Collections at the NYPL and former ACT UP/NY member, shared with me that he often "think[s] about how much of what we have is because of . . . what Robert Rygor filed."[89] Rygor was manager throughout the early 1990s.[90] His effort points to how "even organizational and institutional archives are traces of people's decisions of what they decided was worth keeping."[91] It is difficult to draw neat distinctions between the records of individuals and those of the organization. As a result of personal and idiosyncratic collection development, Shapiro identified the contents as "really random."[92] Wolfe noted particular limitations, reporting that the workspace collection "didn't have any of the women's stuff, practically, and nothing about the actions themselves. What was there basically were the media materials, the media coverage, and the Treatment and Data books," efforts often led by white men, whose singular focus on "getting drugs into bodies" sometimes excluded contending with the structural inequities that characterize AIDS.[93] Shapiro contested this perspective, arguing that more network materials were incorporated, including some he obtained though research undertaken to allay the group's financial issues.[94] The workspace collection, with all its particularities, forms the core of the ACT UP/NY Records.

ACT UP/NY's archive is a product of the group's internal context and epidemic conditions. ACT UP's activism engendered fierce clashes over issues, agendas, and priorities that shaped their archival project. Conflict was a crucial communication practice reflective of a queer politics that rejected identity norms, hierarchies, and political coherence.[95] Power disparities were at times reenergized by such conflicts. ACT UP/NY's precarious coalitional politics eventually proved unable to provide a home spacious enough to contain its constituencies. Significant divisions that routinely broke down by generation, serostatus, gender, and race emerged by 1992. By 1995, internal factionalization over tactics and priorities, experiences of racism, classism, and sexism, and their relationship to both the AIDS movement and the lesbian, gay, and queer movements had become serious. Along with mounting death tolls and widespread burnout, divides depleted ACT UP's ranks by 1994–95. These factors interfered with its activist archiving; the bulk of ACT UP's documentation stops in 1995. The end of 1995 into 1996 also marks the advent of a new crisis era, when new treatments and greater access to them made it possible for some to live with HIV in the long term for the first time. That shift has contributed significantly to the misperception that the crisis is diminished and activist response superfluous. Tumult and the group's dwindling ranks are reflected not only in the ACT UP/NY Records' contents but also in ACT UP's heated decision making about their disposition.

Seeking an Archival Home

In the early 1990s, ACT UP/NY had financial crises from which it had difficulty recovering. One result was that ACT UP needed in 1995 to "leave the workspace extremely precipitately."[96] This event prompted the donation of its records to the NYPL. Activists did not cede responsibility after their records' creation or collection. On a Monday night in 1995, the ACT UP/NY membership gathered for a General Meeting. That night's agenda included a deliberation about where the organization's records belonged. It quickly became a contentious debate on the floor about the politics of who, where, and how archiving AIDS activism—within communities of origin versus major institutions—is done. This event demonstrated activists' deep care and commitment to their communities, politics, and legacy. It also reflected the positions of power held by many members that produced these activists' assurance of their records' enduring value. Debate waged on the floor was a characteristic ACT UP communication form. This debate was "extremely compressed," given the imminent workspace closure. Shapiro summarized: "If we did not have a decision within literally a period of 10 days, the papers would have been completely lost. . . . Everything ACT UP had would be on the street."[97] Their decision was also informed by internal factionalization, including tensions over some activists' chummy relationships with mainstream institutions. Regardless of position as to the most suitable archival home, the central ACT UP members in this debate—whose whiteness, middle-classness, and educational privileges enabled them to focus on the future and more than basic daily survival—each framed an argument around belonging as an ethical concern requiring balance between facilitating access and use and securing preservation. All sought to ensure that people living with AIDS would have ready access to the records while also making sure that the collection was going to survive in the long term.

ACT UP's democratic organizational structure encouraged individual initiative, so fittingly, Shapiro, a gay white man with a graduate degree, made it his mission to find the records a permanent home.[98] He approached Mimi Bowling, then the director of the NYPL's Manuscripts and Archives Division. He remembered: "I just walked into Mimi's office" and "said, 'Look, we want to give the archives to the NYPL.'"[99] This was not the first time this possibility had arisen; an NYPL employee had attempted a few years earlier to acquire ACT UP's noncurrent records. However, that arrangement had disintegrated when a dissenting voice stalled discussion at a General Meeting. Shapiro was met with some skepticism from Bowling. Whatever her hesitations, the "interest on the part of the library was still there, and so, it was just a matter of handling the logistics," Bowling insisted during our interview.[100] Like its feminist predecessors, city-based ACT UP chapters were organized horizontally. Volatile coalitions included caucuses, bodies set up by communities to create space for their needs, and affinity groups—that is, groups loosely organized around specific advocacy issues and personal connections. ACT UP's coalitional ethos at its peak in membership and activity during the late 1980s and early 1990s was powerful. At General Meetings, participants shared announcements, provided action information, and made operational requests. Actions were generally brought to a committee and then to the floor for a vote, but radical democracy meant anyone could bring a motion to a vote. It was not unusual for activists like Shapiro to initiate a project or action and then return to the General Meeting to present it for debate and a vote. This was "a very effective and powerful system," Shapiro asserted, and one that enabled nimble action while providing "accountability."[101]

Activists on the floor that night took up two major positions on archival institutionalization and its outcomes for security, access, and preservation. The first faction held that it was most important for the records to remain within the gay and lesbian community at a community-based archives. This position, Shapiro said, was predicated on the idea that "heterosexuals, or straight society, wouldn't understand the materials, and wouldn't protect them, and that we should build up community organizations."[102] He recalled that some active members, including Wolfe, Danzig, and Bill Dobbs, wanted the records to go the Center,[103] where ACT UP/NY held its weekly meetings. Wolfe asserted that the NYPL's lesbian and gay collections were limited in the mid-1990s, even if "stuff from our enemies" were counted.[104] She was concerned about the record's safety outside of the community. Those in favor of the NYPL donation kept saying, "'We want it to be protected,' and I said, 'Well, here is why again you should give it to a grassroots archives because I'll tell you something: if there's a fire at the New York Public Library, the ACT UP collection is gonna be the last thing they save,'" Wolfe recounted.[105] In contrast, from her LHA experiences, she believed at a grassroots community-based archives, the collection would "be the first thing they save."[106] Danzig also saw the Center as the "rightful place" to house the materials. She wanted the records to "remain in the community," where activists would have ready, culturally comfortable access.[107] Others, like Hubbard and Levine, were supportive in theory of donation to a community-based repository, but they did not think that there was a viable candidate that had the capacity to process, preserve, and make ACT UP's materials accessible. Levine, despite her hesitations over its capacities, could see why some in the group saw the Center as the best choice; at least it "gave a framework" to the ACT UP/NY collection.[108]

ACT UPers of the second faction argued that the materials rightfully belonged at the NYPL. Shapiro saw his position as reflective of contemporaneous conditions in ACT UP/NY: "Where instead of three hundred people coming to an ACT UP meeting, as I recalled in '92, when we're at thirty people [in late 1995] . . . and you think, okay, in 2027, how many ACT UP members are there going to be?"[109] For those on this side of the debate, the decision was just as much about the limitations of community-based archives as about the possibilities the NYPL offered. Shapiro extended his concern about diminishing community resources to the alternative proposed archival home, the Center. The NYPL was a sure thing; they "might have budget cuts. But they're going to have a rare archive. . . . It was going to be there," he told me.[110] The LGBT Community Center National History Archive opened in 1990.[111] In 1995, a major renovation promised to close the Center's West Thirteenth Street location, a historic former school building, for years.[112] This was an important consideration, Shapiro described, because "the archives would be inadmissible, and we were fighting the clock. Today in the postcocktail age, it's a very different thing; two years [in 1995] meant that people would not be there," and that simply "was not acceptable."[113] The activists' most pressing consideration was access, especially related to staffing. The Center archives had limited hours and was volunteer run. At the NYPL, there would be regularly scheduled reading room hours, and the NYPL "would make a financial commitment" to accessibility as well as preservation.[114] Despite heated debate, the vote on the floor was "overwhelmingly" in favor of donating to the NYPL.[115]

Activists' identities and experiences, as well as their politics, shaped their positions on selecting an archival home; they continue to inform their relationships to the ACT UP/NY Records and the institution that houses them. The potential legitimization offered by a mainstream archival institution is an important break. "ACT UP was New York history and American history. And that we had a right to be seen as such," Shapiro declared.[116] From the start, many activists were already considering the historical significance of their movement. Shapiro continued, "I also thought . . . that in fifty years, there's going to be an ACT UP [commemorative] stamp. . . . They're going to incorporate it into the mainstream narrative history, which will be bad and good. But . . . we deserve to be there."[117] Those in opposition to a mainstream archival institution take affront to such framings. Wolfe read the desire to belong at the NYPL as masculinist, with men being more invested in the "status of having your stuff at the New York Public Library."[118] Danzig too described with dismay the NYPL's institutional appeal.[119] At least in retrospect, it is many women who maintain the greatest distrust toward institutional archives. Thistlethwaite noted, "There was some evidence of personal collections being heavily edited by the New York Public Library to exclude the lesbian and the queer content in collections."[120]

The conflict about the archives' donation was also shaped by generational tensions. Shapiro noted that the "people who were for the Center were . . . of a slightly older generation, who wanted to build up autonomous institutions . . . [people] whose life experiences with the academy had been primarily negative."[121] That older generation of activists, many lesbians and gay men who came of age before and during the 1960s' to early 1980s' gay liberation and feminist movements, feared that the security, accessibility, and particularity of ACT UP materials "would be lost" in the NYPL move.[122] Shapiro was part of a younger generation of ACT UPers, in their twenties during the early 1990s. His was a constituency with close connections to and greater comfort with the academy; he had studied queer theory, and he saw academic and archival institutions as tools that could be utilized to their political ends.[123] Shapiro also highlighted to me the importance of the City University of New York's (CUNY) Lesbian and Gay Studies program, located just across the street from the NYPL. CUNY graduate students were offered research carrels in the NYPL, and ACT UP correctly anticipated that their materials would be part of meeting that group's research demand.[124] For others in this debate, academic researchers were secondary; they were most keen to make the archives accessible to activists, youth, artists, and others who might feel more welcome in an informal LGBTQ space. Danzig attributed the vote in favor of the NYPL as about "people get[ing] starry eyed about authority and about institutions," as well as a fundamental unwillingness to put in the hard work of creating and maintaining a community archives.[125] She continued: "I think that something has been lost by putting it in [the NYPL]; something will always be lost" by removing records from their community of origin.[126] After the vote, the donation was not discussed at length again. ACT UP/NY's furious pace meant, Shapiro said, that the matter of the archives "was done and then we moved on."[127]

Acquisition, Appraisal, and Access

Housed in the NYPL's Stephen A. Schwartzman Building in Midtown Manhattan, the Manuscripts and Archives Division holds over 5,500 collections of individuals, families, and organizations, with a focus on New York.[128] It began collecting lesbian and gay materials in the mid-1980s.[129] Bowling's interest "in documenting the AIDS crisis" predated her NYPL employment.[130] In the mid-1980s, Bowling attended an Archivists Roundtable of Metropolitan New York meeting at the GMHC. Activists were overcome with "an overwhelming sense of mortality," Bowling remembered; they knew "we may not be here that long, and we must leave a record behind. And somebody's gotta preserve it."[131] A representative from the GMHC stood up and addressed the archivists: "No one is dealing with this. No one is saving the records," she recalled him saying.[132] When she joined the NYPL in 1989, Bowling had the opportunity to prioritize collecting on HIV/AIDS. In this period, the NYPL was unique in its collection development, both in commitment level and in interest as an archives outside of the LGBTQ community in collecting AIDS activist materials. Bowling sought out and was approached by activist groups, individuals, and estates. My interlocutors remembered the institutional support and constraints for archiving AIDS activism quite differently. Bowling described the NYPL as being supportive, with the staff sharing an awareness of the significance and urgency of documenting AIDS.[133] Shapiro recalled a more mixed reaction: "Not everybody wanted them within the NYPL."[134] It was clear to him that Bowling was making every effort to ensure a smooth acquisition. In negotiating donation conditions, Shapiro described how "Mimi and I kind of played good cop, bad cop. . . . Occasionally I would throw tantrums strategically so Mimi could use that" to gain institutional support where needed.[135]

ACT UP largely entrusted to Shapiro the practical details of the donation. He asked Danzig to join him. Together they attended three meetings with Bowling, the director of the NYPL, and another staff member. After each meeting, Shapiro and Danzig reported back to the ACT UP floor, creating "a constant recursive loop between conversations" over the two-month acquisition process.[136] Shapiro and Danzig voiced their concerns and those of ACT UP writ large. Shapiro recounted at one early meeting sharing some ACT UPers' apprehensions that an organization outside of the lesbian and gay community wouldn't know how to handle their materials.[137] He remembered the NYPL staff laughing "because half of them were queer, as well. After all, it's a library!"[138] ACT UP brought to the table three major concerns reflective of their investment in immediate and enduring access, especially for nontraditional archives users, including fellow activists.

First, ACT UP was committed to ensuring public domain status for the records. Copyright was counter to the group's ethos. Activists intended their records and designs to circulate widely and to be reused by other activists, so ensuring that the materials were under no copyright restrictions was significant. Many activists were invested in rethinking intellectual property, given the widespread appropriation of images and symbols, especially in arts-based activism.[139] The NYPL had never acquired a collection with "a public domain grant," and it took a number of weeks for the lawyers to sort everything out.[140]

Second, ACT UP wanted to ensure that the records had neither time nor age restrictions. The NYPL was "stunned by the fact that we put no time restrictions on the material."[141] Conditions in 1994 and 1995 within the epidemic and in ACT UP, when despite years of activist toil there were no effective treatments, meant that many were ill and dying in a relentless, awful parade. Shapiro emphasized that he was thinking about lost comrades and friends, "all the people who can't be here to speak to this."[142] Referring to the standard archival practice of restricting access to records with sensitive information to protect third-party privacy, he couldn't help but imagine with horror what "adding twenty-five years" to that tally would mean.[143] After the negotiation wrapped, Bowling contacted Shapiro to notify ACT UP that "people's names and numbers are on these contact sheets."[144] Bowling was, in Shapiro's memory, "very nervous about it because there were no time limits. . . . 'We were like, 'Mimi, this is our point. . . . We're comfortable with it, and we want people to be able to contact people.'"[145] In an environment of inadequate information, treatment, and care, ACT UP knew the value of building networks that could quickly generate and share resources—like news stories, medical research, and community periodicals—to support services that might save, or at least improve the quality of life of, people living with HIV/AIDS. Danzig was also committed to there being no age-based access restrictions. The records included materials created by YELL (Youth Education Life Line of ACT UP/NY), "information that had been made by teenagers, non-researchers."[146] For Danzig, it was of the utmost importance that these young records' creators and their peers could and would use them. Though ultimately successful, it "took time to negotiate" such a policy with the NYPL.[147]

Finally, ACT UP wanted reassurance that the NYPL would prioritize the archival processing—that is, the arrangement and description—of ACT UP's records. Processing is essential in ensuring that a collection is open and accessible for diverse users. The group had reservations stemming from the composition of the NYPL's board of trustees. Cardinal John O'Connor, then the Catholic archbishop of New York, and who famously touted condoms' ineffectiveness and opposed their distribution as an AIDS-prevention measure, was a board member. ACT UP had already had a series of public confrontations with him, including an iconic 1989 die-in at Saint Patrick's Cathedral. As Shapiro succinctly summarized it, "There was not a lot of love between these two."[148] The activists were "freaked out that O'Connor could place restrictions" on their materials or delay their processing.[149] Shapiro noted this last access issue was settled to ACT UP's satisfaction "on a handshake deal; nothing was written in" the donor agreement.[150]

ACT UP's collection challenged the NYPL's definition of a record. It was in working with LGBTQ and AIDS collections that the institution developed an awareness of the need to collect nontraditional formats, "things like T-shirts that tell stories that don't exist anywhere else." In their hasty appraisal visit amid the impending workspace closure, archivists evaluated records for "research potential," something Bowling defined "very broadly." Appraisal criteria were informed by AIDS: "Everyone recognized that this was an epic horror that was affecting all of our lives, and colleagues at the library died, and my friends died, and whole fields of endeavor practically got wiped out. . . . We felt a very profound obligation to document that time in history." Bowling continued, "We tended to err on the side of inclusiveness." When it came to the ACT UP records, "essentially, if it was 8½ by 11, NYPL took it." Storage constraints limited the acquisitions. "There was this giant room full of all of those posters and placards and banners that you see in all of the now historic photographs of

ACT UP actions," Bowling recalled. "There was no way we could take . . . even most of them." Archivists did their best, she continued, to acquire graphics that they "recognized as iconic or that were particularly special and off the wall." A record's "exhibition potential" also figured into appraisal.[151] Subsequent digitization reflects a similar logic, with its prioritization of high-impact visual materials.

The NYPL March 1996 press release announcing the records' acquisition noted that it had "already begun the organization, preservation, and cataloging of the papers so that they can soon be used by researchers."[152] The ACT UP/NY Records are 97.4 linear feet of administrative and subject files, minutes, notes, correspondence, legal and financial documents, fliers, photographs, posters, placards, and ephemera.[153] Within six months of opening, it became "the most frequently asked for material in all of the NYPL catalog. We're not talking about the Shelley letters. We're not talking about the Wordsworth letters. ACT UP's material is the information which people want to see the most," Shapiro recalled.[154] The volume of public interest in and the accessibility of their materials are points of pride for activists on both sides of the donation debate. The records were processed initially in the late 1990s. In the same period, the collection was filmed through a partnership with Gale, a private educational publishing company. The microfilm was available at the NYPL and "to other organizations that wanted to purchase it."[155] It is these same microfilm reels to which I was granted access during my 2015 and 2016 NYPL visits. They are also the basis for the digital copy of the records held in a privately owned for-profit database. "A lot of people had personal stuff they had hung onto. . . . We hoped that once they were in the NYPL, that would magnetize them," Shapiro told me.[156] The group's donation informed the NYPL's acquisition of associated personal collections from ACT UP/NY members in the 1990s and early 2000s, including fierce pussy's records and Vito Russo's papers.

In addition to defying conventional logics of access and definitions of record, the ACT UP collection also proved complex in terms of its overarching categorization. The Manuscripts and Archives Division holds over one hundred collections pertaining to the history and culture of gay men and lesbians and to HIV/AIDS. "Gay and lesbian history and AIDS history are not a single subject," the digital reference guide for these collections noted; "however, because of their interrelationships, both types of collections are included."[157] The construction of this descriptive apparatus makes explicit the correlation of the LGBTQ community activism and history with HIV/AIDS. Such a linkage is a reason that some within ACT UP were ambivalent about the NYPL, fearing that ACT UP's materials would be secluded "in a gay and lesbian collection."[158] Supporting this point, the microfilm is produced and sold by Gale as part of a series on the "Gay Rights Movement," and its primary subject classification is "Gay and Lesbian Studies." Ironically, Shapiro favored the NYPL over the Center in part over this same correlation, "because a lot of people conflated the [gay and lesbian] community and AIDS activist community . . . just because there were a lot of gays and lesbians [involved] didn't mean that they had any better sense of what AIDS activism was than anyone else."[159] Shapiro believed that the NYPL would offer a broader context for the records within histories of activism in New York.

While the ACT UP/NY Records are part of a division with a broader collecting mandate, it is noteworthy that the problematically simplistic cultural linkage of gays and lesbians with AIDS is reproduced through its archival apparatuses. The finding aid, the description of the records that provides the archives with physical and intellectual control and that assists users in gaining access to and interpreting the records, again reifies this conflation. Writing the gay and lesbian community into the proper home of AIDS activism through archival description is complicated. It informs access to and the subsequent interpretations of these collections by archival users. If not done carefully, it powerfully recenters gay, white, middle-class men; it informs who and what is accounted for and who is excluded from dominant AIDS narratives; and it reproduces the historical belonging they enact.

Absences in the ACT UP/NY Records

Archives are defined as much by what is absent as what is present. The NYPL collection's boxes and folders contain only some of the memory, experience, and affect that constituted ACT UP. In the records, there are notably gendered and racialized absences that inform racist and sexist dominant narratives. A note on the ACT UP/NY web page publicizing the NYPL's 1996 press release, "ACT UP/NY Archives Donated to the New York Public Library," reads, "Other sources of comprehensive information about ACT UP can be found at the Lesbian Herstory Archives in Brooklyn."[160] It offers the LHA's phone and fax numbers, directing those interested to contact "Maxine Wolfe via her Voice Mail."[161] Wolfe, one of the most active creators and collectors, always "knew" her materials were going to the LHA. When she retired in 1996, she spent eighteen months arranging and describing her fifteen cartons of political papers.[162] Thistlethwaite also collected materials, including items from the Women's Caucus, and donated most of them to the LHA.[163] For Wolfe, the LHA's Park Slope brownstone was its rightful home "because I'm a lesbian, and because I want people to know . . . that the people who were in ACT UP weren't just the men that everybody thinks."[164] The LHA's contextualization centers women's voices, labor, and leadership in AIDS activism. Wolfe's decision was also the result of negative experiences in the move from ACT UP's first workspace. She recounted going to pack up, describing with a cynical laugh how "what the men were concerned about was packing up all the Treatment and Data Committee work. . . . They weren't interested in any of the other stuff that was up there."[165] Wolfe's biting comments reflected a consequential fissure, often by gender, over ACT UP priorities. Members of the Treatment and Data Committee and others, often gay white men, pushed for a narrow focus on pharmaceutical research and access, including working with government agencies and corporations. Other activists, including Wolfe and many in the Women's Caucus, favored a wide-ranging intersectional approach to ACT UP action that would take up structural oppressions like poverty or xenophobia. They correctly forecasted that even if better drugs became available, access and the care needed to sustain complex regimens would be inequitable. The workspace collection, Wolfe recalled, included "papers from eighty chapters of ACT UP, which they [the men] didn't think were important."[166] Wolfe proceeded to collect the materials that were being discarded. This experience confirmed that "nobody thought it was important to save the stuff on women, except the women."[167] Thistlethwaite's and Wolfe's collections offer the most substantive documentation on women, lesbians, feminist politics, sexism, and gender dynamics within ACT UP/NY. Therefore, Wolfe emphasized, the ACT UP Records at the NYPL have "very little on women."[168]

This institutional division has significant ramifications for who is accessing and using the ACT UP Records. Locating ACT UP materials at archival institutions that have focused on serving disparate constituencies shapes the stories they are used to tell. The LHA prioritizes serving lesbian and queer communities. They make it clear online that any time volunteers are there, the archives is open to all for browsing, socializing, or doing research in the open stacks.[169] Academics are also welcomed, but this population is not the archives' focus; its alternative access and use practices are more likely to surprise and inhibit those with more conventional archives experience. The NYPL, with its Midtown Manhattan location, is more likely to be the destination for academic researchers, especially those who are not members of the lesbian community, for a number of factors. These include its cultural prominence—it is widely acknowledged as a premier collection on New York City and its social movements—and the logistics of using the archives, with regular reading room hours, paid reference staff, and standardized provisions for copying, digitization, and so forth. These divides in collections and archival practices figure into the exclusion of women's lives and experiences in AIDS scholarship. In addition, that the ACT UP materials at both sites lack explicit descriptive links to related materials at the other archives means that users may remain unaware that there are other ACT UP materials, which powerfully shapes dominant accounts. Wolfe stood firmly behind her decision to donate to the LHA. Shapiro's response was more ambivalent: "On one hand, it's contextualized within lesbian history; on the other hand, it further exacerbates the split of the material, because it's not in the wider social context."[170]

The question of where the most suitable home is, of where and to whom the materials will be most accessible, for other ACT UP/NY materials remains open. "A lot of people have shit in their basement and still are conflicted about what to do with it. Basements, attics, little sections of their tiny, overstuffed apartments," Levine told me.[171] Even among those who have donated some of their records, where the remainder will end up is still being determined. Goldberg, for example, still holds papers in his apartment.[172] Similarly, Thistlethwaite kept records at home that were most "special" to her—letters to the Women's Caucus, documentation from particular actions, photographs.[173] There are also complex racialized as well as gendered power relations to these pending decisions. For example, Julián de Mayo described how in researching the Latino Caucus he learned that many of the relevant records are still in key participants' hands, held within private homes in the Latinx community.[174] Those who hold the Latino Caucus records were deeply concerned about their survival, but they remained unsure as to what archival institution, if any, those materials belong within—with ACT UP's records at the NYPL or in a Latinx-serving institution. Archival self-determination and community control are important, and these records are perhaps more accessible to the record creator's immediate community at a private home than they might be if donated to a major institution. However, the multiple barriers to access for those outside of the Latinx AIDS community makes it difficult to learn what materials even exist, and moreover, access to them even within the community is likely to be limited and individually mediated. In line with the academy's own structural barriers, such minoritized ACT UP records and stories are often excluded from dominant narratives.

Ultimately, while the NYPL does offer a central locus to link AIDS activist archives, some activists are still wary of the institution's provisions for access to their records. When Finkelstein was determining where to donate his papers, including ACT UP materials, his critiques of the NYPL's description of the ACT UP/NY Records in the finding aid and catalog record figured prominently. He cited as example the misattribution of two iconic AIDS activist posters he created in the NYPL's archival descriptions. ACT UP gave rise to and worked closely with art-action collectives whose designs provided the anti-AIDS activist movement its provocative aesthetics. Included in the accession of famed collective Gran Fury's records were two posters, "Silence = Death" and "AIDSGATE." The NYPL's finding aids marked the posters as Gran Fury productions. However, both posters were actually created by a different collective, the Silence = Death Project. In addition, Finkelstein saw marked differences between how Gran Fury's records and ACT UP/NY's records were described. The ACT UP/NY Records, in his opinion, had duplicates and ill-labeled files, which he argued is reflective of archivists' devotion "to the stuff that had some marquee value, the cultural production that had come out of Gran Fury." ACT UP's records, largely administrative and textual, did not receive the same care as the Gran Fury Collection; the finding aid has "holes" that perpetuate "inaccuracies [that will] make it harder after we're all gone for people to find their way through the material." Finkelstein concluded, "Those things matter."[175] He donated instead to NYU's Fales Library and Special Collections. While significant in scale and scope, it is clear that the ACT UP/NY Records also perpetuate—through their gendered, racialized, and classed contents, access, and use—archival silences and omissions that shape the dominant narrative of AIDS.

Activist Intervention and Institutional Experimentation

Refashioning the contours of archival power is critical in ensuring that the ACT UP records are animated to repoliticize AIDS. In the late 1990s to early 2000s, there was a perception within the AIDS activist community, especially among ACT UP activists, that their materials were inadequately processed, used, or exhibited. Danzig noted, "It becomes one of the million collections, and that's a problem."[176] Regardless of factual accuracy, that bad feelings were articulated is important in understanding the NYPL's strained relationships to records' creators, subjects, and the larger communities they represent.[177] By the early 2000s, the NYPL faced significant processing backlogs that encompassed many LGBTQ and AIDS collections. With access as many activists' top priority, word of delays with related collections fueled tensions. Moreover, even for those collections like ACT UP/NY's that were technically open to researchers, for many activists, "because they might not be interacting with it as users," Baumann noted, it looked like the materials were "closed."[178] "Community relations" had been sorely neglected.[179] The NYPL, like many archival institutions, had focused on serving traditional researchers: academics and students. Moreover, archiving activism within institutional repositories does not always emerge from "an affinity" in politics or care work between the archives and the activist group being collected.[180] Additionally, the process of archiving these materials "does not automatically signify that this collecting establishes a relationship between the archives and the community that it draws materials from."[181] Problematic relationships with activists can troublingly invoke or maintain legacies of oppression, colonization, and displacement. The relational shortcomings of these early years of the ACT UP archives' institutionalization shaped activists' troubled relationship to the AIDS archives. They also set the stage for activists' recent interventions at the NYPL that mobilize vital nostalgia to embolden activism and provoke institutional change.

The same excerpt of Russo's "Why We Fight" speech that is this chapter's epigraph, printed in ACT UP's signature hot pink, adorned the opening wall of the NYPL exhibition *Why We Fight: Remembering AIDS Activism* and its promotional materials. Titled in homage to Russo, the exhibition and programming series marked a watershed in the complex relations between the NYPL and activists. Running from October 4, 2013, to April 6, 2014, in a gallery off Astor Hall in the Schwartzman Building, the exhibition showcased archival records—posters, pamphlets, videos, and artifacts from the 1980s and 1990s drawn primarily from the NYPL's collections of organizations and individuals pivotal in their responses to HIV/AIDS. The show featured many items from the ACT UP/NY Records. It was curated by Baumann with Laura Karas, the archivist who had done the (re)processing of many AIDS activist collections, including substantively revising the ACT UP/NY Records finding aid in the mid-2000s. The events and programming shifted the NYPL's relationship to the AIDS community it documents and serves, as well as activists' connections to their archival home. The NYPL was ready and receptive, if slow, to enact such change. Baumann's position was created in 2008 to "interface with this community and this content," supporting the NYPL's LGBT initiative through community engagement, fund-raising, and collaborating with staff and the public to promote and facilitate their use. Improving relations with the activist community was a top priority with "these collections because they have, because there is a community," Baumann noted. "It's our history, and these people need to know that it's here, and there needs to be somebody to negotiate that nonprofessional access and relationship."[182]

"All the programming was about making this [AIDS activist] community *at home* at the library," Baumann told me.[183] *Why We Fight* programming was a pivotal political project in bringing the AIDS activist community to the archives and the AIDS archives to the community. It showcased diverse voices, testimonies, and activist actions. In collaboration with NYPL colleagues, Baumann planned some events. For example, the first panel, "We Were There, Too: Black Gay Activism and the Fight against AIDS," was developed with the Schomburg Center for Research in Black Culture's Steven G. Fullwood. Archival records on loan from the Schomburg also featured in the show. Programming was also done in collaboration with community-based organizations. Visual AIDS developed art-making workshops for teens led by their artist members. Baumann invited artists and activists to engage the show and wider collections it drew from. ACT UPer and documentarian Jim Hubbard curated a film series with selections from the NYPL's AIDS activist video collections, and Finkelstein blogged to contextualize the show and facilitated the Undetectable Flash Collective's arts-based intervention. The NYPL prioritized supporting programming initiated by the vibrant community of records' creators, subjects, and stakeholders. These programs featured many ACT UPers, including panels organized by activists and hosted by the NYPL on "Women of ACT/NY," *Your Nostalgia Is Killing Me!* (see chapter 1), and, detailed below, "How to ACT UP." This programming sparked institutional experimentation and greater engagement of the AIDS archives with contemporary social movements and politically involved artistic traditions. Activists' leadership thus activated vital nostalgia for an AIDS activist past as captured in the NYPL's archives as the means to call out and work toward redressing harms perpetuated by the epidemic's persistence.

Activists did not wait for institutional intervention or support. ACT UP mediated the meaning of its past, which dictates powerfully their presents and futures, as well as those of all people living with HIV/AIDS. The two instrumental events analyzed—the opening night die-in and how-to workshop—demonstrate the ways that activists' vital nostalgia informs their interventions that promise to remake often-troubled relationships between AIDS activists and the institutions that house their records. Through vital nostalgia, activists engaged in a substantive refiguring of AIDS's present through its ongoing relation to the AIDS activist past. These examples show how caring for ACT UP, as well as its records, requires critical engagement from both activists and archivists.

The Die-In

ACT UP/NY activists chanted, "Act up, fight back, fight AIDS!" Their voices reverberated through the NYPL's imposing Astor Hall. The activists, falling silent, staged a die-in, one of the group's most iconic protest practices. Their prostrate bodies spread, overlapping in a nongeometric configuration across the white marble. ACT UP intervened in public space and consciousness. Mathew Rodriguez then rose to his feet. He spoke, insisting that neither the AIDS pandemic nor AIDS activism is over, and he criticized New York City's cuts to HIV prevention funding, which put at unequal risk the lives of young queer men of color—men like him. This die-in happened on October 4, 2013, the opening night of the NYPL exhibition, *Why We Fight: Remembering AIDS Activism*. ACT UP/NY activists, some of whom created or were the subjects of the records on display, performed their die-in in their archival home to make the point that "AIDS IS NOT HISTORY" and that it is dangerous to memorialize it as if it were. For its curators, the show's title and frame of memory were political, a resistance to forgetting and to sensationalized misrepresentation of AIDS activism. However, activists read references to memory and the focus on the 1980s and early 1990s as dangerous distraction. Drawing on legacies of contesting misrepresentation, activists challenged the prevailing temporalization of AIDS as past. By intervening, activists made themselves into the structure that mediated between the archives and the public, generating a new cultural perception of the archives as a space of debate and critique. Activists contested the dominant perception of archives as fixed spaces devoted to preservation of the past. Hearing accounts of this die-in for the first time in summer 2015 crystallized my project's focus. Although I did not witness their protest firsthand, the activists' embodied action and their message still resonated powerfully with me. I interpret their mobilization of the AIDS past in service to the AIDS present as vital nostalgia practices.

ACT UP today is invested in activating its archives to repoliticize AIDS in the popular imaginary. The exhibition was organized around themes of "Changing Perceptions of People Living with HIV," "Safer Sex and Needle Exchanges," "Public Mourning," "Healthcare Activism," and, the final panel, "HIV Today." The brief acknowledgment that those who survived the epidemic's early years and AIDS are still here did not for these ACT UPers do enough to disrupt the show's curated emphasis on remembering. Mark Milano, continuously involved in ACT UP since 1987, noted that today, "*We're not remembering* AIDS activism, *we're living* AIDS activism."[184] Members of the current ACT UP iteration, along with the ACT UP/NY Alumni group, were invited to the exhibition preview. ACT UPers there notified Baumann, the curator and coordinator of Humanities and LGBT Collections, that they were going to stage a die-in on opening night both inside and outside the gallery. ACT UP was generally supportive of the NYPL's effort to honor the history of AIDS activism; however, the group justifiably feared that this history would continue to eclipse contemporary AIDS realities and ignore the activism that persists in the face of them. Controlling the narrative of their past was self- and community preservation. Activists that night wanted to make clear ACT UP's position in this fight: they had never disappeared or disbanded, despite myriad historical accounts that locate the group's demise in the mid-1990s, and they would never do so without the pandemic actually ending. In the video, Milano, staring down the camera, announced, "We're here today to make the point that this is not just something that was just going on in the '80s and '90s; *it's something going on right now.*"[185] Included in their ranks were many who have been active since the late 1980s and younger activists who came of age long after ACT UP/NY's height in membership and activity. A younger member, Bacilio Mendez II, chair of ACT UP/DAWG (Digital Activism Working Group), appeared next. He argued "that while we should be respecting the activists and the work that has come before us, AIDS by no means is over and should not be memorialized as if it is."[186] He went on to assert, "Teaching young people about the history of AIDS and LGBT activism allows them to connect with a tradition of empowerment that occurred before they were politically conscious." Mendez cautioned, though, that if we want such knowledge to do more than create a longing admiration for that past, "if we want new generations to repurpose these tools of activism and empowerment to fight HIV today, we have to start with the statement: 'AIDS is Not History!'"[187]

This was the first time that a demonstration had happened inside the NYPL. "There was some anxiety from our security about how to handle it," Baumann reported in our interview.[188] Despite their trepidations, the NYPL's public relations and security teams agreed that "the only right thing to do was to let them demonstrate . . . as long as nothing was harmed in the gallery" and no patrons were bothered.[189] These comments illustrate the importance of balancing the needs and relative power of different parties within archival relationships. Archivists' roles were to facilitate activists' vital nostalgia practices. The NYPL provides an example of how as archivists we can move toward accomplishing such support. The activists' agential acts challenged the institutional AIDS archives to overcome its conventional caution and to engage in present AIDS politics. They pushed the institution toward, forging new forms of alliance and asymmetrical collaboration between anti-institutional movements and the archives. Rather than social processes being given an aesthetic makeover or deactivated, the die-in helped to generate a collaboration in which the archives forms a part of social struggles.

Die-ins are a signature form of ACT UP protest and confrontational care work. This demonstration's form was itself a nostalgic referent; however, the activists refused to let such nostalgia remain about the past. Through the NYPL die-in, activists intervened in the narrativization of an earlier crisis era. They utilized nostalgia for the early AIDS era and its archival objects to garner focus and give rise to actions to ameliorate the current epidemic's harms. Embodying the acts of activist predecessors, these activists performed with their bodies the function of the action they were protesting. By moving their bodies from vertical to horizontal, they emulated dying and the body's stillness in death. The activists symbolized visually the many comrades, friends, and lovers who had died as well as the many socially precarious others whose lives are still being put at risk for HIV/AIDS. In these choreographies, activists' bodies aggregated in intimate proximity to one another, heads touching, sometimes even resting on the legs and arms of other bodies. This intimacy created part of the power of these clusters, which radiated outrage even in silence.[190] Breaking their stillness after Rodriguez's statement, the activists rose to their feet, lifting signs overhead while streaming through the hall, out the NYPL's doors, and down the steps toward Fifth Avenue. The building, which is a tourist attraction as much as a functioning library, provided the ideal site for activists to produce a self-consciously nostalgic visual spectacle. They embodied the multiplicity of publics engaged with AIDS. Between the famed lions, they staged a second die-in witnessed by reporters, NYPL staff, a crowd of onlookers, and, with video mediation, eventually by me. The activists evoked for their audience the earlier ACT UP takeovers of public spaces in New York City as a strategic intervention from the past for the present and future. Through vital nostalgia, they utilized the AIDS activist past to provoke awareness of and action against the epidemic's ongoing violences. Through activist intervention, the AIDS archives moves to become a generative touchpoint for contemporary reflection and action.

How to ACT UP

Like the die-in, the "How to ACT UP" workshop was motivated by activists' commitment to mediating both the archivally driven story of what transpired in AIDS's early years and how it is being told now; nostalgia for that past was mobilized to provoke attention and action addressing the contemporary epidemic. ACT UP's Milano recalled responding to Baumann's announcement of the upcoming exhibition at an ACT UP/NY alumni gathering by saying, "That's great. But you cannot talk about ACT UP in the past tense."[191] Alumni made "it very clear that we would not sign off on the exhibit unless they did something about ACT UP today."[192] The workshop emerged as an activist intervention from these early conversations. Milano summarized its goals: "(a) ACT UP is still going, and (b) we need you to get involved, and (c) here is how you do it.'"[193] The event focused on transmission of tactics and strategies for direct action—or, as Baumann framed it, around questions like "How you do this? How do you pull this off?"[194]

The workshop's activation of the archives included publicity: promotional materials featured ACT UP's signature hot pink triangle standing vividly against a black background and above stark white letters spelling out "Silence = Death." In 1986, the art-action collective Silence = Death Project created this design, made famous by ACT UP, appropriating the inverse pink triangle used by Nazis to brand homosexual men, marking their bodies for destruction. Activist-artists turned that triangle on its head. Their reclamation of the emblem reminded viewers of the suppressed history of gay men's oppression and annihilation in the Holocaust and, placed above "Silence = Death," materialized the reality that cycles of silence and inaction must be dismantled as a matter of survival. This image appeared on innumerable posters, stickers, placards, T-shirts, and buttons, including ones displayed in *Why We Fight.* Digitized, it became askew in its scanning, appropriately queer in orientation (Figure 3). The January 14, 2014, workshop, initiated by ACT UP/NY activists and hosted at the NYPL, invited participants to "learn the nuts and bolts of grassroots political activism from current and former members of the historic AIDS advocacy group."[195] Mediating the archives and exhibition, the activists began multiplying the publics involved and catalyzing action through training that crossed generational divides—if not those inflected by race, class, and gender.

Animating the event was an anxiety about whether knowledge about HIV/AIDS activism was actually being transmitted from one queer generation to another within queer sexual ecologies that lack the ready-made structure of reproductive generationality. In the context of AIDS's decimation of entire generations of minoritized persons—especially Black and brown queer and trans people—there are cultural and political knowledges and modes of resilience and survival that are in grave danger of loss. Older activists thus have a commitment to passing on queer heritage between generations and across time and space. Panelists, selected by ACT UP, included Jamie Bauer, Jay Blotcher, Danzig, Goldberg, Milano, and Rodriguez, with Andy Velez as moderator. With the exception of Rodriguez, with whom I share a millennial positionality, the panelists were at least in their fifties—old enough to have been in ACT UP during its most active period, between 1987 and 1994, and including survivors of the pre-1996 crisis. Half of the panelists were white, male, and identified as queer—factors that shaped responses to them, including their relative safety in performing civil disobedience. Imparting what they had endured in service of personalizing their activism and building affective connection with the audience, panelists addressed how concepts and practices from earlier organizing might inform present direct action. The event was open to the general public, but it specifically hailed younger queers. Educating others was an activist function for Milano. "As those of us involved in ACT UP are getting older," he said, we need "to make sure there is a new generation of people carrying the torch."[196] The how-to workshop drew people from the current ACT UP/NY and other relatively youthful activists, born in the 1980s and 1990s. Baumann recalled that they sought answers from the seasoned panelists to practical questions.[197] For example, attendees wondered

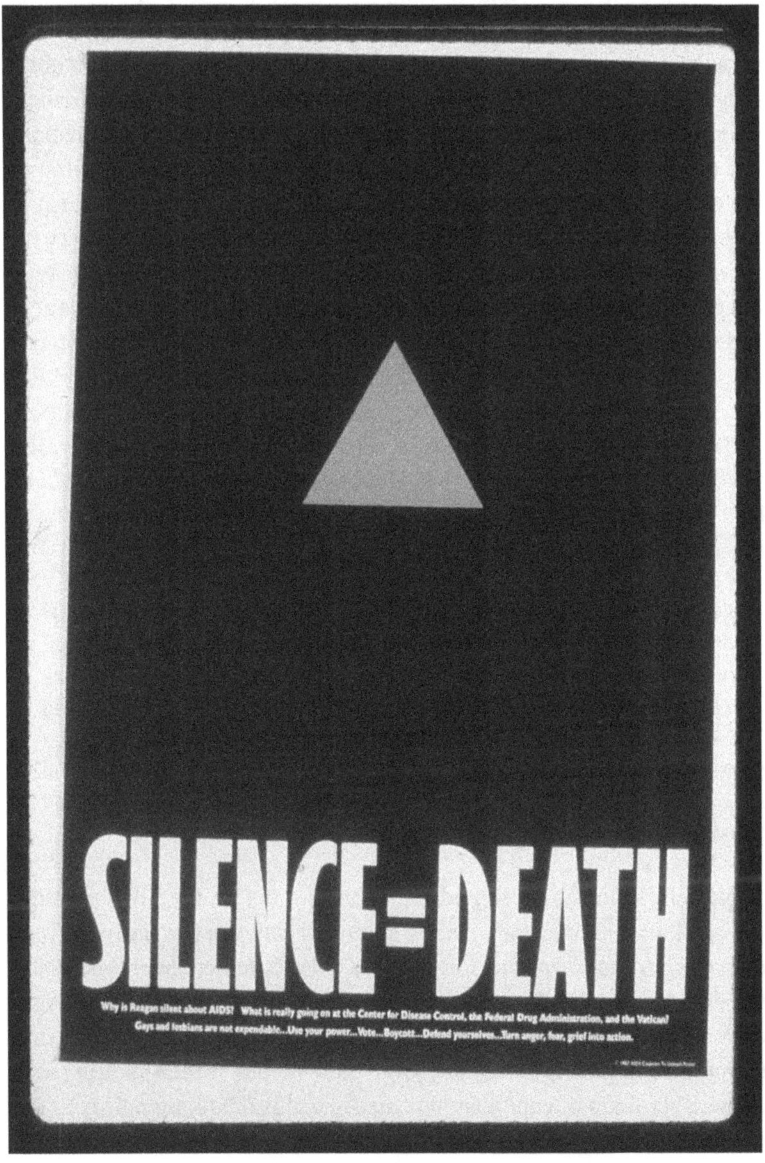

Figure 3. The "Silence = Death" poster was created by the Silence = Death Project (Avram Finkelstein, Brian Howard, Oliver Johnston, Charles Kreloff, Chris Lione, and Jorge Socarrás) in 1986. Made famous by ACT UP, the poster as digitized by the New York Public Library is appropriately queerly askew. Courtesy of Digital Collections, New York Public Library.

about the quotidian details of running a meeting: "Do you take names down and run down the list, or do you just keep calling on people?"[198] The panelists called out how HIV/AIDS, then and now, is a constituent component of structural violence—racism, transphobia, poverty, criminalization, and incarceration. Yet in its limited representation of the persons and communities most affected now, the panel could not hope to impart the diversity of knowledges and particular communal strategies, such as those created and enacted by Black, Latinx, and Indigenous activists, for survival and thriving. The panel was an important step toward activating the past for the present, but it stopped short of fully centering the voices and work of communities of color and trans folks—those often most starkly affected by the contemporary crisis. This step, current activists and critical AIDS scholars argue, is requisite to engendering meaningful AIDS action.

The workshop moved between celebratory narratives of ACT UP's actions and legacy and more critical engagement with the meaning of its history for present AIDS politics. The event's online description offered this brief history:

> Beginning in 1987 with an action calling out Wall Street profiteering on AIDS drugs, ACT UP . . . significantly improved HIV drug development, championed HIV prevention, cared for its members, and won laws helping people with AIDS and HIV. The AIDS activist group's unique form of fierce and fabulous direct action confronted the opponents of people with AIDS and stopped onerous laws targeting that population. With ACT UP's powerful messaging and political engagement, people with AIDS were transformed from "AIDS victims" into a movement that saved millions of lives.[199]

This event synopsis presented the expected, heroic narrative charting the inspirational successes of early treatment activism and flashy, fervent direct-action interventions for which ACT UP is famed. Such historicizing can support the dominant crisis narrative that emphasizes activist-driven transformative progress in legal reform and medical research that culminated in getting better drugs into more bodies.[200] Yet beginning with activists' critique of capitalist pharmaceutical profiteering points to the group's ongoing relevance, as corporate curtailment of drug access is a significant issue for contemporary AIDS activists globally. In person, the event largely embodied a nuanced, powerful set of radically queer political aspirations and contemporarily relevant critiques and strategies. The panelists mobilized personal accounts and archival records in line with contemporary cultural nostalgia for ACT UP, its affective enactments of community, its queer radical politics and irreverent actions, and its provocative aesthetics. These activists, some of whom were navigating their own nostalgic relations to an earlier AIDS activist moment, were aware that ACT UP nostalgia is experienced acutely by younger queer generations seeking a usable past of resistance and valor in AIDS activism—even as we still navigate HIV/AIDS realities.

Throughout preparations for and during the workshop, activists deployed the ACT UP brand's power to enable the conditions for production, rather than just consumption, of AIDS activism. Vital nostalgia requires such a critical relationship with the past. To do so, panelists deliberately leveraged the AIDS archives, drawing from records held in personal and institutional collections. Each speaker addressed distinct aspects of direct-action activism, ranging from conducting outreach and public relations activities to planning a message and staging civil disobedience under current technologically enhanced surveillance. Milano focused on how actions with small participant numbers could and can effect meaningful social change. His point is salient now when actions on HIV/AIDS are small and media and public attention difficult to garner. Milano was painfully aware of such difficulties as a member of the current ACT UP/NY, a small but active group.

Milano began by showing archival footage from his personal materials of a June 1999 ACT UP action with only twelve participants, including him, in Carthage, Tennessee. At this action, activists disrupted Al Gore's announcement of his presidential candidacy. By intervening at a key moment, a few ACT UPers brought due international media attention to the United States' racist profiteering policy on the importation of generic AIDS drugs to South Africa. While the most iconic ACT UP actions, on which nostalgic longings often center, drew thousands together, in this action, a few ACT UPers radically shifted the cultural conversation, and eventually policy, transnationally. Milano's presentation linked nostalgia for past victories to present work, the archives to the demonstration, in a way that challenged dominant narratives of AIDS activist history that focus solely on United States, and especially New York–centric 1980s' and early 1990s' demonstrations.

The panelists sought to empower attendees and subsequent viewers to apply knowledge gained about activist strategy and tactics to produce cultural resistance through direct action. The workshop was designed to culminate in a march on City Hall, generating democratic public space rather than just talking about one. However, the freezing temperatures and an unexpectedly favorable recent election outcome led activists to cancel the march. "Once they all got into a room, they were more interested in communicating with each other than they were in marching anywhere;" for Baumann, this shift in plans was "a great relief."[201] The NYPL, a public institution entrenched in political neutrality, would neither endorse nor oppose ACT UP's proposed action. Baumann had planned to step back after sharing with the crowd that "they are free when they leave the library to do whatever they want. . . . I can't tell you should, but the people on the stage can tell you that they think you should, and you all are free to go do what you wish."[202] Playing mediator at such moments was uncomfortable for him.[203] Even without actually activating imparted knowledge into immediate action, by holding a conversation within the space of the NYPL, the activists enacted the first steps in the radical activation of AIDS archives. They produced the groundwork of dialogue and skill sharing required for developing AIDS awareness that exposes power inequities in the epidemic and its narrativization in ways that can engender change.

As a workshop, this event issued a corrective to didactic, unidirectional practices of cultural transmission that are expected from institutional archives. Originating from the AIDS activist community, it demonstrated both activists' agency and deep commitment to vital nostalgic practice. Utilizing the skills earned from experience and long-term survival, as well as deploying cultural and political yearning for ACT UP and the radical politics it represents, activists intervened in the present. The organizers acknowledged the power of legacies of loss and queer persistence from the early AIDS years while opening up fruitful possibilities for filling in broken links in a queer cultural and political genealogy through dialogue. Reaching beyond geographic and temporal accessibility constraints, the panel was recorded and posted on YouTube and in the NYPL's digital collections, creating a new AIDS activist record and opening opportunities for people not in attendance to participate vicariously. By drawing from the AIDS archives, whether through the incorporation of archival records as teaching tools or in the transmission of embodied practices and political strategies, activists strategically activated the archives to build community resilience and generate action in response to the sociopolitical forces and gross inequities that have produced the AIDS pandemic. These archives aid in activists' developments of unconventional and resourceful practices. The activists moved the archival record from the dimension of consumption to production. Even on video, I see how they materialized the memory work of the exhibition to create the conditions and skill sets instrumental for radical social change.

The event was also pivotal in charting the development of more ethical care work in engagements of NYPL staff with the activist community that calls the archives home. Simply having an archivist be a member of that community is not enough to ensure responsible relationships. At the ACT UP alumni gathering and in the *Why We Fight* exhibition, I see Baumann's history as a member of ACT UP/NY in the early 1990s as informing his curation; he said it provided him with deeper "understanding of what the materials I was looking at were, and who people were."[204] It also informed community responses to him and the show. Baumann acknowledged to me that his activist past also created "a measure of comfort" for some in the community.[205] However, he refused that this is most significant; in his view, the fact that he "was willing to show up" is what made the difference in community engagement.[206] Baumann surmised, "I could have been a member of that community, but I could [still] be appropriating that history to my own commercial ends, to glorify myself."[207] It was part of his task to prove to the community that he was actually "creating a forum for a historical conversation that's crossing different kinds of generations."[208] Out of the entire exhibition and programming series, Baumann saw the "How to ACT UP" workshop as its most striking accomplishment. He remembers that it was "my moment, where I felt like I had really accomplished something with that show, was when that connection got to be made between present activists and veteran activists about real concrete questions."[209] Activists, with the NYPL's cautious support and through vitally nostalgic interventions, remade the archives, at least temporarily, into a generative space of belonging.

Legacies of Activist Archiving and Archiving Activism

The position of AIDS archives, simultaneously as the site of and source for AIDS's historicization and as the most powerful bulwark against the lethal threats posed by end-of-AIDS narratives that mark AIDS as past, requires understanding how AIDS archives and their collections came to be and persist. While acknowledging that it did not act alone, ACT UP/NY undoubtedly has played a significant role in the transformation, through bodies, words, and graphics, of AIDS's meanings, experiences, and temporalities.[210] The group led the push for development of and greater access to HIV/AIDS treatment and prevention, ensured that AIDS was understood as political and social, and reshaped the lived realities and representations of those with HIV/AIDS.[211] Archiving has also been too long unrecognized as vital to ACT UP's work and accomplishments. Activists' valuation of their efforts and lives through documentation and activist archiving provided a powerful counter to the ways that those most affected by HIV/AIDS were deemed expendable, subject to biological and social deaths. The answer to the temporal imperative Russo issued in 1988, that "we have to leave the legacy to those generations of people who will come after us," was one his fellow activists have heeded through activist archiving. Many ACT UPers' diverse acts of archiving during the late 1980s and early 1990s amounted to a transformative practice of critical care.

Tracing the ACT UP/NY Records' cultural life demonstrates that activists' deep sense of responsibility, care, and commitment to making their work accessible and actionable could not and did not end at documentation. On the floor of the General Meeting, pivotal conflicts over the proper disposition of their records, care, anti-institutional politics, and inter-group power dynamics and divisions shaped the questions of where and how they would belong in an archival institution. Though many records were moved to institutional AIDS archives, the affective resonances and political consequences of the conflict over archival belonging and what access means in this context linger. As many activists feared, archival institutionalization processes often focused only on the past; they failed to account for or meet the current needs of the AIDS activist community, whose lives are intimately tied up with the archives' fate. Activists' concern with how and when their materials would be made accessible and who would have access to them is clear from the analysis of their debates over donation, the terms they dictated during the NYPL acquisition, and their continued mediations of the archives, and with it their legacies.

The institution has taken steps to refashion its previously troubled relationship with the activist community, pointing toward an ethical archiving activism practice. The activists' ongoing archival intervention through vital nostalgia was strengthened by the institution's new hospitality. The NYPL shifted toward prioritizing the archives' potential to engender connection, manifest in actions including Baumann's appointment and the *Why We Fight* exhibition and programming. Baumann was formative to such shifts by immersing himself in the community, listening and engaging. It is the challenging work of building and sustaining human relationships that led to the successes of *Why We Fight* in drawing together the archives and the community and empowering past and present politics. Through activists and archivists' labors, the AIDS archives is beginning the transformation process into a home not just for the activist community's materials but also for their bodies, memories, identities, and actions.

I see the NYPL in the wake of *Why We Fight* attempting to continue to honor activist intent in broadening access to ACT UP's materials, especially for nontraditional archives users, including activists. However, current approaches have real limitations. The high stakes of ongoing activist intervention through acts of vital nostalgia become clear when considering the newest home for ACT UP's archival collections, the Archives of Human Sexuality and Identity, a proprietary Gale database of eighteen digitized archival collections that explore LGBTQ history from 1940 to the present. It holds a digital copy of the microfilmed portions of the ACT UP/NY Records. Arrangements with private corporations like Gale for digitization have become commonplace in an environment characterized by decreases in public funding and increases in users' expectations for digital access.[212] ACT UP's archival records are made digitally available primarily through this for-profit subscription database. On its surface, inclusion within the Archives of Human Sexuality and Identity offers the tantalizing opportunity to open access and broaden use in line with ACT UP's priorities. However, databases like this one reproduce and reify systematic power differentials. The digitized records are accessible only to users who have privileged access to them behind costly paywalls, putting in danger access, use, and intellectual freedom.[213] The NYPL offers free on- and off-site access to the database to users with NYPL library cards; however, for those who might wish to use the collection and who are located outside of New York, no free access is available, and obtaining a library card requires ties to New York State.[214] *Why We Fight*'s successes were grounded in human relationships—the creation of physical spaces to gather, to learn, to see one another, and even to die-in. To recreate these in a digital space would require a creative community-engaged platform. That Gale and similar corporations lack the mission-driven commitments of institutions like the NYPL to community engagement endangers future efforts. Access to and preservation of the ACT UP/NY Records remains contested. The institutional archival homes of the AIDS activist past, digital and analog, matter in the present and for the future because it is these records that lay the groundwork on which dominant retrospective whitewashed, gay middle-class male–centric narratives of the crisis are built and replicated.

Through temporal interventions aimed at interrogating and redressing structural power inequities through yearnings for a past time and space—vital nostalgic practices—activists and archivists are reshaping and repoliticizing the AIDS archives and its meanings. It is clear that archives can be a critical tool for remembering AIDS in ways that honor its legacies and losses and that challenge its ongoing devastations and the sociopolitical conditions that produce them. ACT UP's archives challenge us to reflect on the state of AIDS in America now, to reflect why we are where we are at this moment in time, having survived and persevered. "In many significant ways," Charles Morris wrote, "we are here because of ACT UP."[215] The issues, internal and external, that prompted ACT UP's factionalization in the late 1980s and early 1990s foreshadowed many of the racist, classist, sexist, ableist, transphobic, and xenophobic elisions, neglect, and violence that continue to plague HIV/AIDS activism, service work, and its representation. The visceral tensions that emerged between radical action and institutionalization, principles and access, and justice for all and survival for some, shape HIV/AIDS in the twenty-first century. Contending with ACT UP's legacies is an urgent material necessity while AIDS is often forgotten, marginalized, and misremembered. ACT UP archives, even while, Morris wrote, "partially assembled, widely circulating, fragmentary and fragile, grant-funded and stuck in some basement, in the public library and precariously pitched on a sidewalk awaiting the garbage collector,"[216] are powerful forces that can be harnessed with vital nostalgic practices in order to actively engage and serve diverse AIDS archival constituencies. Activists and archivists, by critically deploying the AIDS archives, can remake AIDS temporalities. Scholarly, curatorial, and archival practices demand reframing in order for us to demonstrate that we do indeed, as Russo insisted, "give a shit" about AIDS.[217]

3

AN ARCHIVAL CURE

Remedy, Care, and Curation with the Visual AIDS Archive Project

Decades into the epidemic we find ourselves between: between past battles, lost loves and a loss of what is next. Between ongoing trauma, trauma
anew and uncertain hope. For many, the urge to focus on the cure is a
cultural imperative for resolution—we have come so far, and we want
badly to feel the triumph of defeating HIV. But we are not there. Instead,
we are between a rock and hard place—a middle ground that is thick with
possibilities.

—**TED KERR**, "A ROCK AND A HARD PLACE:
BETWEEN HERE AND THE CURE" (2014)

ON MARCH 5, 2019, headlines went viral in a way that almost no HIV/
AIDS news does anymore. Posts topped my social media feeds, the chime
announcing e-mails dinged, and NPR reporters crisply enunciated the
details at the top of the hour. At every turn, I was inundated with cure.
News that the second ever person was "cured of HIV" was everywhere.
The so-called London patient's cure came just over a decade after the cure
of the "Berlin patient" had been announced at another international AIDS
conference. The latter subsequently outed himself as Timothy Brown, a gay
white American man who was diagnosed with HIV in 1995 and who was
then living and had been treated in Berlin. The medical cure offered in both
cases was similar. Each patient was living with HIV and life-threatening
Hodgkin lymphoma. After undergoing a stem cell transplantation during
cancer treatment, their HIV also went into permanent remission. These
are both specific medical cases, highly unlikely to lead to a medical HIV/
AIDS cure that will ever be appropriate, accessible, or scalable. Stem cell
transplantation is far too costly and risky. Its mortality rate hovers between

10 and 25 percent.[1] Yet when this story of a cure broke, it gained major media traction. Medical institutions were inundated with calls from hopeful people yearning for medical cure.

Later that month, on March 31, Los Angeles–based hip-hop artist and entrepreneur Nipsey Hussle was murdered. As news of this tragedy spread, social media chatter about the killer's motivations surfaced conspiracy theories. Chief among them was Hussle's supposed knowledge of an HIV cure. This claim revolves around his relationship with Alfredo Darrington "Dr. Sebi" Bowman, a Honduran herbalist who claimed before his death in 2016 to have cures for HIV, herpes, and other conditions.[2] Hussle was one of an array of celebrities, from Michael Jackson to Lisa "Left Eye" Lopes, taken with Sebi's promises.[3] In "Blue Laces 2," Hussle raps, "They killed Dr. Sebi, he was teaching health."[4] Hussle announced in 2018 that he was making a documentary about Sebi. As he described it, "Dr. Sebi went to trial in New York because he put in the newspaper that he cured AIDS. He beat the case. Then he went to federal court the next day, and he beat that case. But nobody talks about it."[5] There are many factual errors in this account, but what is certain is that Sebi took profitable advantage of desperation. The real tragedy, Kenyon Farrow noted, is that "one quack" claiming the existence of "wholistic African cures" still garnered more airtime than the self-narratives of people living with HIV who face stigma and who still persist in seeking acknowledgment and response from medical providers, politicians, insurance and pharmaceutical companies,[6] religious organizations, and families. Medical cure is almost the only way HIV/AIDS tops, even for a moment, our news feeds. Such media leads to envisioning in our present a fantastical future without HIV/AIDS.[7] Stories of medical cure are grounded in the assumption that chronic illness and disability are tragedies that demand prevention and eradication.[8] Whether entirely mythical or just determinedly rare, AIDS cures delight and affirm cultural ideologies about health, medicine, and ability. Cure is always imbued with politics.[9]

AIDS activists, advocacy organizations, physicians and medical researchers, and individuals living with HIV/AIDS have devoted vast energy and resources to medical cure. Cure names not just the state of being permanently cured but also an investment in processes for which cure is the goal. For example, while no vaccine for HIV exists, the search for one continues. Being cured of HIV/AIDS, even in the limited medical sense, remains elusive despite contemporary political rhetoric about the end of AIDS that posits that the epidemic's terminus is not only imminent but also inevitable. In this chapter, I grapple with cure in an examination of Visual AIDS's Frank Moore Archive Project and its digital counterpart, Artist+ Registry. Since 1994, this community-based archives has documented, preserved, and activated through curation the work of artists with HIV/AIDS. The word "curator" originated from *curatus*, a person entrusted with the care of souls in a parish.[10] Activist-archivists recognized curation and archiving's potential as practices of caring for their community. At Visual AIDS, the archives is integral to cure.[11] This AIDS archives contributes significantly through its archiving and curation to a broadly defined project of cure that can provide a fix for some of the acute losses and marginalizations experienced by artists with HIV/AIDS. Taking up cure means, according to Eli Clare, sitting "inside a knot of contradictions. Cure saves lives; cure manipulates lives; cure prioritizes some lives over others; cure makes profits; cure justifies violence; cure promises resolution to body–mind loss."[12] Reaching for an HIV/AIDS cure saves lives and improves people with HIV/AIDS's life chances; however, medical cure also advances violence against and marginalization of those same persons in ways I detail in this chapter. Visual AIDS's collecting, arranging, describing, preserving, making accessible, and mobilizing records has always been care work performed in service of advancing social justice. I extend archival scholars Andrew Flinn and Ben Alexander's concept of activist archiving, which names a praxis in which archivists are guided by social justice as archival imperative.[13] As I will show, the Archive Project highlights the material and conceptual affordances of archiving as anti-AIDS activism. Its records and their nimble activation hold imaginative capacities for challenging persistent gendered, racialized, and classed hatred, discrimination, and stigmatization faced by those living with HIV/AIDS. The archives also demonstrates the limitations of activist archiving in meeting pressing needs, redressing harms, and effecting cure. However, when grounded in vital nostalgia—activist longings for a past time that questions, contends with, and repairs structural power inequities—activist archiving engenders important measures toward healing, enacts long-term survival, and promises thriving.

I begin this chapter by situating the Archive Project in relation to the messy ideology of medical cure, a cultural imperative routinely taken for granted as necessary and beneficent.[14] Drawing together HIV/AIDS and disability scholarship, I expose how any remedy that would actually make HIV/AIDS livable, as a bodily and cultural experience that has engendered real beauty and real horror, exceeds the bounds of medical cure. A prodigiously holistic cure is requisite to responding in kind to an epidemic that is and has always been political, cultural, and social as much as biomedical. Cure demands dismantling racism, homophobia, misogyny, transphobia, poverty, xenophobia, and ableism—the myriad structural injustices that minoritize and marginalize HIV-positive people and their communities. I trace in three sections reflective of cure's multiplicity the Archive Project and Artist+ Registry's efforts toward holistic HIV/AIDS cure. Through vital nostalgia, the Project provides an archival cure: remedy for artistic death, critical care for HIV-positive artists, and curing, preservation, and curation that ensure the archives' endurance and accessibility. I reframe AIDS archives and cure as more than aspirational epidemic end points.

Aspiring to Cure

In November 2018, I flew to New York for forty-eight hours to attend "Activating the Archive Project." Within a series marking Visual AIDS's thirtieth anniversary, the event celebrated the archives as one of its "most impactful projects."[15] Held at NYU's Fales Library and Special Collections, the intergenerational panel, facilitated by Visual AIDS staffers Kyle Croft and Tracy Fenix, featured early archives members, staff, and contributing artists. Panelists included Eric Rhein, Sur Rodney (Sur), Nelson Santos, Shirlene Cooper, and David Hirsh. My last-minute trip was prompted by Hirsh's name in the e-mail announcement. I had been eager to interview Hirsh, the Archive Project's surviving cofounder, during fieldwork in 2015 and 2016, but neither then–programs director Alex Fialho nor I could find anything about his whereabouts after the mid-1990s. It was not until 2018, when Rhein, an artist, dialed a number found in an old file and discovered that it still belonged to Hirsh, his friend and archive committee collaborator, that he was reunited with Visual AIDS. I arranged to meet Hirsh before the event. On that perfect fall afternoon, I was early. I waited nervously for Rhein and Hirsh in the shadow of a fierce pussy installation outside of the Leslie-Lohman Museum. Seeking a quiet place to talk, Hirsh and I followed Rhein home. Over tea, surrounded by Rhein's wire artworks, we got acquainted. Even in that first conversation, Hirsh offered tidbits about the archives that he alone possessed. Breaking midafternoon and midconversation, we agreed to continue. Hirsh and I would reconvene by phone many times. We discussed over six months, among other things, Frank Moore's *Archive Project (Zine)*.

On the page "The Eternal Question," Moore, painter and cofounder with Hirsh of the Archive Project, queried: "Has anyone seen my ~~AZT?~~ ~~DAT? DDI? DDC? 3TC?~~ QVC?"[16] (Figure 4, top). This list of pharmaceutical acronyms is a concise chronology of the FDA's approved drugs for treating HIV/AIDS. Beginning with AZT in 1987, each new medication, despite high hopes, proved to have limited efficacy and nasty side effects. Experimental conventional therapies failed before 1995, the year Moore drew up this list. It was not until 1996 that a more effective combination therapy became available. With characteristically acerbic wit, Moore ends with "QVC?," referring to the televised home shopping channel, as the only viable remedy left. On a later page, "DIET DEVOLUTION of an artist with 'HASHEVAIDS' (Yiddish for 'where have all the blue skies gone?')" (Figure 4, bottom), Moore expanded his analysis of medical cures attempted. He divvied up the 1990s by treatment protocol, as follows: 1990, three pills and "no more alcohol;" 1991, seven pills and a directive not to consume "yeast, lactose, sugar, good stuff;" and finally, 1995, a veritable handful of capsules labeled "toxic," "doesn't work," "hair falls out," "poison." Hirsh noted the humor and hard truth in Moore's commentary: "It truly, really, it was such an agonizing process."[17] Each failure compounded the reality that until 1987, "there was nothing" at all.[18] Under the subtitle "NEW AIDS THERAPY," Moore charted medical cure's physiology. He rendered the body in a style reminiscent of ACT UP die-ins that featured chalk outlines of demonstrators' bodies on streets, an accusatory invocation that mobilized crime scene investigation aesthetics. In one hand is a palette and in the other a paintbrush. Body parts are segmented, classified. "ACT UP yawn!" scrolls down one arm. Other parts are reduced to medical objects: the legs read "GlaxoSmithKline" and "AZT." The head spins in attempt to wrap itself around "(the latest thing)." The phallus too is marked: "anti hard sauce." The *Zine*'s medical cure analysis still resonated with Hirsh, who recounted to me how for his HIV-positive partner, "there was nothing that could really offer much relief."[19] In the face of unremittingly grave conditions, "we had to invent our own hope."[20]

A disability lens is needed to examine HIV/AIDS's relations to hope and to its assumed counterpart: cure. Whether noun or verb, in the late capitalist United States, when we talk about cure, it inevitably refers to the restoration of health, the eradication of illness, and the removal of disability through medical treatment. In other words, what we mean is *medical* cure. Medical cure ideology first requires "damage," or harm understood as within the confines of individual bodies and minds.[21] Second, medical

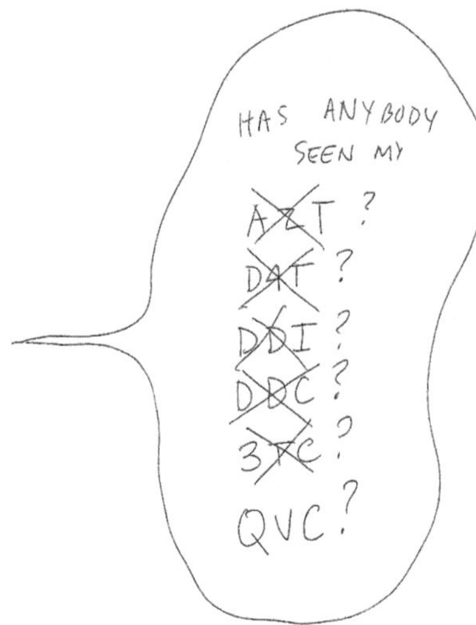

Figure 4. Painter and Archive Project cofounder Frank Moore made a darkly witty commentary in his *Archive Project (Zine)* on HIV/AIDS treatment through 1995. "The Eternal Question" and "DIET DEVOLUTION of an artist with 'HASHEVAIDS,'" *The Archive Project (Zine)*, created for Visual AIDS in 1995. Courtesy of Visual AIDS.

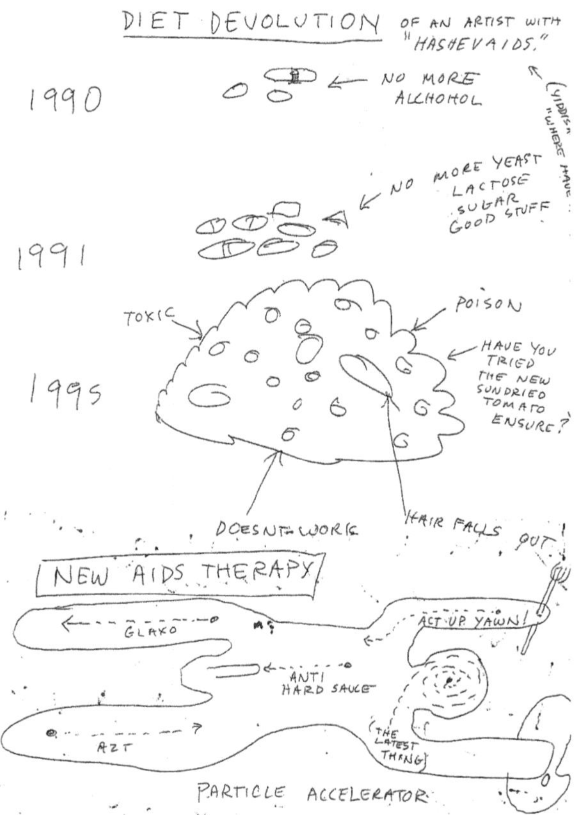

cure asserts that there was an "original state of being," and moreover, Clare notes, that it was superior to what currently exists.[22] Medical cure, finally, aims to restore "what is damaged to that former state."[23] Centered on eradication, medical cure operates in tandem with violence.[24] The means by which cure is practiced is tied to its roots in the Latin *cura,* "care,"[25] and *curare,* "to care for" someone or something.[26] Curing also denotes a treatment process; it is a preservation method undertaken with meats to ensure their long-term viability for safe consumption through smoking, salting, or drying.[27] Figuratively, cure names the "means 'to remedy, rectify or remove (an evil of any kind),'" a definition that illustrates the moral judgments inherent in its logics.[28] Scholarly and activist critiques focus largely on medical cure as part of challenging the medical model of disability that sees it as an individual pathology to be corrected through professional interventions.[29] Disability studies praxis troubles the compulsory assumption that cure is necessary and denounces its prioritization over social and environmental changes that facilitate more livable lives for people with disabilities or illnesses. Clare summarizes, "It is ableism that needs the cure, not our bodies."[30] Cure ideology is rooted in the medical-industrial complex;[31] its investment in curing individual bodies supports neoliberal individual responsibilization and interlocking public–private institutional responses; it propels the inextricability of economic and scientific interests. Even while our cultural fixation remains on medical solution, Eunjung Kim argues that "cure discourses and imagery operate in political, moral, economic, and emotional realms that go beyond individual medical treatments and personal desires for remedy."[32] A focus on medical cure routinely prevents societal contention with violent systems of power and our complicity within them.[33]

Since the earliest instances of HIV/AIDS-related illness, first recognized in 1981, medical cure has been sought. Despite divergences in what an HIV/AIDS cure entails and how to accomplish that, cure and the processes that work toward it are central to the efforts and aspirations of shifting configurations of anti-AIDS constituencies: people living with HIV/AIDS, AIDS activists, biomedical researchers and physicians, public health officials, and government and nongovernmental organizations. Histories of AIDS activism often begin with the 1987 advent of ACT UP and end with the 1996 market arrival of protease inhibitor therapy. However, treatment activism began earlier and continues still. The AIDS crisis is characterized by institutional neglect. It was marked in the 1980s and early 1990s, for example, by racial displacement from property and home, literally and figuratively, in that gay white men were often abandoned by their families of origin and, by extension, denied some privileges associated with whiteness. Community responses, palliative care and support services, education, and attempts at various treatments for what was almost categorically a fatal illness began immediately.[34] Gay community networks and services built in the 1970s enabled early responses.[35] In New York City, Gay Men's Health Crisis formed in 1982 and established a network of services, one initially by and for gay men. Without attaining cure, these early day-to-day stopgap efforts, often on an individual level to remedy suffering, are inextricably associated with failure and death.[36]

Medical cure signals the outright and enduring elimination of impairment; it also encompasses the normalizing treatments and the curative processes that work to assimilate the disabled mind/body into normative society.[37] It is embedded in structures of "diagnosis, treatment, management, rehabilitation and prevention."[38] From the crisis's start, activists sought out treatments that could halt or slow illness and death. ACT UP's famed slogan and campaign, "Drugs into Bodies," a direct-action push for faster clinical trials to result in greater and better pharmaceutical options, is the most widely acclaimed of treatment activists' efforts. Within a cultural imperative that demands resolution, fighting for more and better drugs is presented as the only rational response.

There was a real need for drugs to be developed and made available.[39] Given the lack of viable alternatives, Martin Duberman notes, some "'injected, ingested and imbibed' any new substance that came down the pike," well before it was proven effective or safe.[40] Many suffered not just from AIDS but also from ever-changing drug treatments and overtreatment. Before sharing with me why Moore's dark cure humor still spoke to him, Hirsh took a deep breath, then relayed, almost without pause, that when Abbott Burns, his partner of seven years, "learned his diagnosis, he more or less stopped making art in preparation for what was obviously coming."[41] Burns, he recalled, made one attempt in the late 1980s to locate a medical cure: "There was a doctor on the Upper East Side who was publicizing that he had invented a pill which could cure the disease, or slow [its] progress."[42] He returned "with a vial of little white pills. And he took them for four or five days and felt that they were fake."[43] This experience was not unusual; "there were, of course, many people during this period who were publicizing that they were capable of making inroads into the fault line. That was the only attempt he made to find that inroad. After that, he more or less just put up with the symptoms and diseases."[44]

"Drugs into Bodies" is almost invariably read as a radical success that transformed HIV/AIDS materially as an experience and event.[45] Hegemonic treatment activism narratives teach that cure is accomplishable through the three-pronged approach undertaken by some in groups like ACT UP that Lisa Diedrich summarizes: "(1) work to become scientists, (2) work to speed up drug approval processes, and (3) work with drug companies to make more drugs."[46] Activists' radical reshaping of medical practice by politics[47] contributed substantially to the development of antiretroviral therapies that prolong lives and improve their quality. These pharmaceuticals, part of a curative process, are now assumed to be as good as it gets—to approximate medical cure. In public health, cure names the reduction of HIV transmission rates to what is deemed acceptably low, rather than any solution that would encompass those already living with HIV/AIDS.[48] The potential and partial are routinely rounded up to medical cure.[49]

We are still living with pharmaceuticals developed in the late 1980s through the early 1990s, and with what Diedrich calls the "repercussions" of drug-driven treatment activism.[50] By the early 1990s, rifts developed between activists over cure. Some had a single-minded devotion to engendering pharmaceutical cures, while others construed treatment and cure more broadly. They argued that making drugs accessible and effective would require addressing the structural inequalities that limited minoritized people's health care access[51] and interrogating how race, class, gender, and sexuality intersected with illness and disability.[52] The singular focus on pharmaceuticals by many AIDS activists reflected a capitalist logic that asserted that the more drugs there are to choose from, the better the health care.[53] Drugs into bodies reified the dominant neoliberal ideology of our present, in which pharmaceuticals are positioned, as Diedrich notes, as the only "solution to any and all problems—medical, psychological, and social."[54] Scarce resources are thus directed toward, Clare identifies, "research, cure, and the future,"[55] rather than to meeting present needs—health care, housing, employment, education. Dominant crisis accounts contend that with more effective pharmaceuticals, AIDS has been conquered, thus neglecting a nuanced approach to cure.[56]

During our next conversation, Hirsh skipped detailing the mundane tasks of caretaking to which he devoted many months. Instead, he described Burns's last day. Hirsh and a friend had carried him out of the apartment and into a cab to go to the hospital. Hirsh remembered that "the doctor told me that he was in the end stage." They took Burns home;

"we carried him back up the steps to our apartment and put him to bed." It was "Good Friday. Abbott was thirty-three and he was Jewish, and within a couple hours" of their return, he died. Hirsh continued: "I was at his side, holding him. I recognized the point at which his breathing ceased and there was an abrupt jolt in his body, which I assumed was his heart exploding. And so I made the necessary calls." Hirsh shared this as we sat on the phone, thousands of miles apart. All I could give then was my attention, an offering that still feels inadequate. He circled back, without pausing for my response, to the page of Moore's *Zine* that we had been discussing. "The point to all this is the sense of trying to create hope where there was no hope," he concluded. In the 1980s, there was little choice in his mind; what "we had to do was a make up ways of hoping and caring and political activities. Which would carry on those who were still functioning into the future." Turning to Moore's drug timeline, he said: "And then we reached the '90s, and they started coming up with the different medications, which indeed were toxic and caused all sorts of side effects. And that's where Frank entered the story with his humorous recitations." Ever the coherent narrator, Hirsh wrapped it up: "And since our last talk, the one that resounded with me the most was waiting for the pills, the capsules that really would make a difference."[57]

Even as a disability lens helps bring into focus the complexity of its potential cure, HIV/AIDS has a complicated relationship to disability. "AIDS is a form of disability," many scholars and activists assert; however, claiming disability for people living with HIV/AIDS has been "contentious" and class based.[58] There is no medical cure for HIV/AIDS, just more and better treatment protocols. For persons with the social status, financial means, and security to access and adhere to treatment, HIV positivity becomes a manageable chronic condition without identification with disability. In contrast, for those without such resources, claiming "disability" is routinely requisite to accessing lifesaving social supports.[59] As much as it is a medical solution for disability, cure is a temporal and affective practice that regulates HIV-positive bodies and their social relations.[60] Dominant conceptions of medical cure rely on restoring what Kim terms an "imagined or remembered past" in the near future.[61] This is a return to a time before seroconversion, before disability. For those born with HIV, this time is a restoration of an imagined past in which their parent did not seroconvert or did not transmit the virus in utero. In this temporal regime, what Alison Kafer calls "curative time,"[62] only a past without disability and a future where one is cured matter. The only acceptable disabled person becomes someone who has been cured or who is working toward cure.[63] The assumption that one must function normatively to be eligible for social inclusion goes unquestioned.[64] People with HIV/AIDS are excluded from progress narratives until, Kafer continues, they can be "rehabilitated, normalized and hopefully cured," at which point they become "the proof of progress."[65] Those who are unable or refuse to comply with treatment are marked for social death; without a future, they are denied a present. Even if one day an all-out medical cure for HIV/AIDS is achieved—whether with a vaccine, drug, or other technology yet to be imagined—it would not be wholly eradicated. Kim reminds us that cure always carries "the memory of disability."[66] It does not erase formative experiences. "Moreover," she concludes, medical "cure often does not eliminate the stigma associated with a history of disability and illness."[67] As the case I examine in this chapter will show, a holistic cure for the ills that trouble HIV-positive bodies includes activist archiving.

The Archive Project as Holistic Cure

From the start, Visual AIDS has worked through practices of vital nostalgia—remedy, care, and curing—to engender a holistic HIV/AIDS cure that encompasses but reaches beyond medical cure. In a call with Hirsh, he emphasized for me that "from the beginning," Frank insisted that the organization's development be "organic."[68] Hirsh explained that Moore intended the archives to be flexible, responsive, and community embedded. The Archive Project, then, as he put it, "has been from its inception an examination *for a cure,* both holistic and medical, psychic and grounded in material well-being, and in the support of creating art that strove for answers."[69] In other words, by supporting HIV-positive artists materially and conceptually, Visual AIDS enacted a remedy for artistic loss and death. The challenges they encountered and addressed broadened their scope to ongoing community level care. Activist-archivists also prioritized preserving the records created by their community, documenting both AIDS already past and their AIDS present. They knew a holistic cure required access to the AIDS past. Visual AIDS from the start embraced nostalgia, critically and with intention, in order to enact a just and equitable AIDS present and future.

In a catalog essay for *Arts' Communities, AIDS' Communities,* a 1996 exhibition celebrating the archives' first two years, curator, early Archive Project member, and then–Visual AIDS executive director Nick Debs elaborated on its cure: "We are all too familiar with the grief and suffering caused by AIDS. We can't help but cry," he began.[70] In early 1996, AIDS was even for the most privileged "a death sentence."[71] Debs wrote, acknowledging this reality, "AIDS is a fact: it is a disease caused by a physical agent, it causes death, it has killed many, and will continue to kill more. Cry for those who are in pain but know *crying won't effect a cure.*"[72] These words echo ACT UP's refrain that grief must be transformed into anger to effect social change. Advancing a curative process has, from Visual AIDS's formation, been its mission, and it will continue to be so.[73] It was not yet apparent that 1996 would be the year when combination therapies would prove more effective and become available on the American market. Yet the organization had already emphasized, "*By cure we do not mean a medicine* that will stop the mechanism of HIV within the human body. We mean a cure for the human impulses . . . those which cause the evisceration of social service agencies for those living with AIDS, the censoring of life by the religious right and the theory-obsessed left, and the material impoverishment of the majority of humankind."[74] Debs concluded, "We mean *a cure of cruelty and fear.*"[75] As I will demonstrate, the archival cure they advanced through vital nostalgia not only acknowledged disparities in the distribution of crises but also engendered a process of addressing and redressing harms from stigma to discrimination.

The holistic cure that Visual AIDS demands is essential to responding to an epidemic that is political, cultural, and biomedical. "A part of this cure," Debs asserted, "is the efforts of the Archive Project."[76] The archive committee was founded in early 1994. When partnered with Visual AIDS in fall 1995, it became the Archive Project, and in 2002, it was renamed in Moore's honor.[77] The archives embodies the organization's aims, current executive director Esther McGowan said, as its "heart" and "backbone."[78] Archival labor is understood here as care work and activism for community empowerment and social change.[79] One of the first national initiatives to address and record the AIDS pandemic's impact on the arts, Visual AIDS was established in New York City in 1988 by a group of artists, curators, and arts administrators, many of whom were activists and some of whom were living with HIV/AIDS.[80] Visual AIDS produces and presents artworks, projects, exhibitions, public forums, and publications—art that is public facing, inclusive, and accessible—in order to facilitate and support reflection, dialogue, and action on HIV/AIDS.[81] It provides services to HIV-positive artists, including the archiving and exhibition efforts of the Project and its related digital Registry. Visual AIDS remains committed to "honoring" artists with HIV/AIDS and to "preserving" their artistic contributions.[82] The Archive Project highlights that when done through vital nostalgia, activist archiving has material and conceptual affordances, particularly in its imaginative capacities, to challenge hatred, discrimination, and stigmatization born of structural oppression and fear. It also demonstrates the limits of activist archiving as a curative process. I examine the Archive Project's archival cure in three sections informed by cure's multiplicity: first, as a remedy for death; second, as acts of critical care; and third, as curing that enables long-term survival.

Archives as Remedy

On the *Zine*'s "Mindful/Landfill" page (Figure 5), Moore renders a trash can complete with ubiquitous urban rat. Labeled "life's work," it is captioned, "His name was Robert, cutest boy in the East Village—someone said. Molto Talento (Great Animal Sculpture) Now Landfill." In 1994–95, the Archive Project was concerned that for many artists living with HIV/AIDS, two deaths were imminent: one was the death of the physical body, and the other was the death of artistic practice and career. The toxic combination of poor health and financial issues meant that many slowed or stopped creating work. Moore was diagnosed with HIV in 1985. With few symptoms and a thriving career, in 1994 he described feeling "sort of lucky."[83] However, Moore still noted the arduous health maintenance required: "I now have seventy T cells, instead of a normal count of somewhere between 800 and 1,200 T cells. So there is some background anxiety. I see either of two doctors regularly, I take thirty-three pills a day, more or less, and just keeping track of it all is a time-consuming process."[84] Other artists were spending as much as 40 percent of their time contending with health issues.[85] Moore's 1995 *Zine* wittily illustrates these quotidian realities. Picking up the rotary phone, "Its for you," someone off the page yells: "its your: A) Mother <3, B) Doctor $, C) Pharmacy $, D) Coroner!, E) Collection Agency (Do they collect contemporary art?)." The artist responds, "Tell them I'm: A) Dead, B) Painting, C) Retching, D) Asleep, E) In Love, F) Broke." Hirsh recalled himself and Moore being "extremely conscious" that many artists were "dying without their work having been shown, without any recollection of their work outside of the tiny community around them."[86] Artwork was destroyed by families who found it offensive or objectionable; it was neglected by those who were overwhelmed or unaware of its potential. The Archive Project offered a

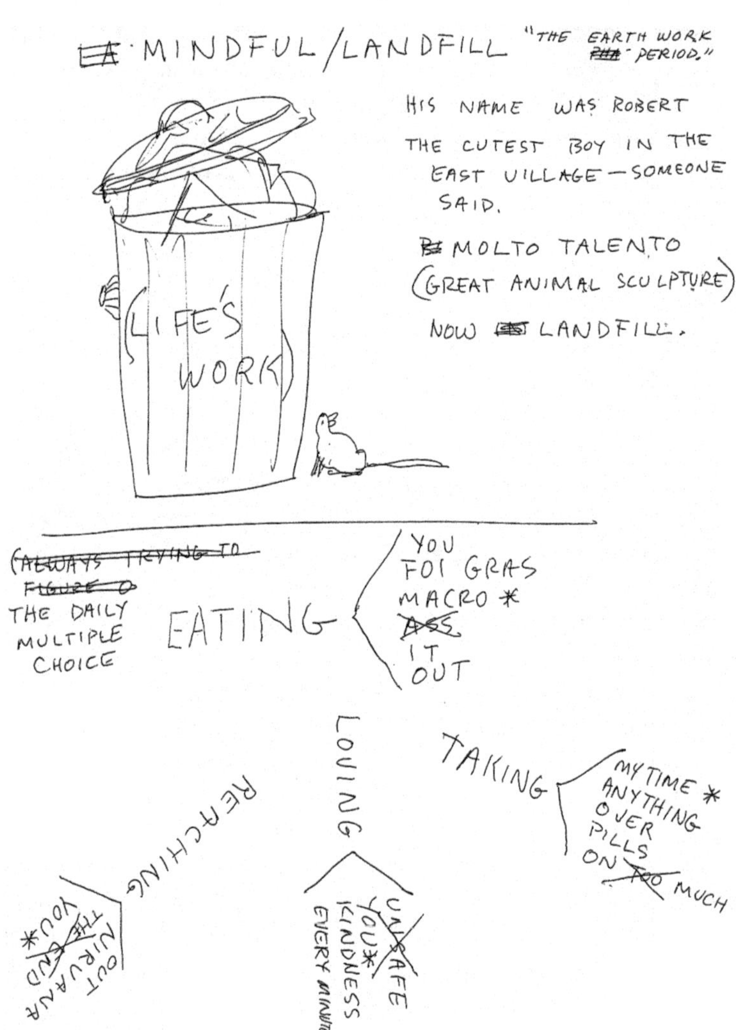

Figure 5. Painter and Archive Project cofounder Frank Moore addressed the artistic death that the Archive Project aimed to remedy in his *Archive Project (Zine)*. "Mindful/Landfill," *The Archive Project (Zine)*, created for Visual AIDS in 1995. Courtesy of Visual AIDS.

measured fix for these "daily calamities."[87] Activist archiving will not eradicate HIV/AIDS, but as a vital nostalgic practice, it offers an "educated
hope"[88] in the face of incurability.

Moore and Hirsh initiated the archive committee in early 1994—an
urgent remedy to ease suffering in a time frequently labeled the crisis's
"deepest darkest point."[89] By 1994, New York City's department of public
health estimated that 13 percent of the city's artists, 8,500 people, were
living with HIV/AIDS.[90] Activists had spent over a decade, Moore wrote,
in "trench warfare."[91] During this decade, Moore described in his sketchbook (now held by the Fales), that "progress (where it has occurred) has
been incremental and riddled with doubt, in which the forces of intoler-
ance and apathy almost always seem to gain the upper hand."[92] Douglas
Crimp described the early 1990s as a period of "setbacks" and "disappointments" in the wake of direct action's early successes in the late 1980s.[93]
There was increasing knowledge of the epidemic's tremendous breadth
and depth, both in populations affected and the extent of the social
change that would be required to improve lives and enable survival.[94]
These conditions, Deborah Gould argues, created an activist landscape
of "despair and desperation."[95] In the same sketchbook entry, Moore similarly emphasized that "burn out" had become "endemic" and that internal conflicts were stalling activism.[96] He highlighted that the hate and
discrimination provoked by AIDS had proven to be powerful political
tools, harnessed by conservative politicians to advance their agendas.
In search of Moore's perspective on the archives, I spent days reading his
correspondence, clippings, and notebooks to little avail before coming
across this note scrawled in red pen. It made explicitly clear that building an archives devoted to collecting, preserving, and making accessible
AIDS information and stories was, for Moore, the most effective means
of redressing the spin and misinformation oppressive political structures
depend on.[97] An AIDS archives could trouble the epidemic's injustices
and inequities. Moore was aware that, even amid loss, creating a repository to hold onto the records of AIDS's present and past was a powerful
move toward a more just present and future. Encountering his words in
the quiet reading room in 2016, and each time I have read them since, I
am struck by the simple power of Moore's concluding line: "Towards an
AIDS ARCHIVE."[98]

Hirsh, then an arts columnist for the *New York Native* and *Bay Area
Reporter*,[99] was enthralled from his first encounter with a painting of
Moore's on a gallerist's desk. He requested an introduction, and the two

became friends.[100] During one of Hirsh's studio visits in January or February 1994, Moore asked, "Would you like to start an archive of slides by artists who have died of or have HIV/AIDS?"[101] At two subsequent meetings, there were, Hirsh recalled, "two primary things going on."[102] First, Moore was determining whether Hirsh was "the person to personify" the archives' "original impulse."[103] Hirsh described for me how at the end of each meeting, as they waited for the elevator, Moore stood "with his head slightly bowed in thought."[104] Hirsh knew that he was considering what they had accomplished. After deliberation, Moore said, "'Okay.' And I knew that meant that we, he and I, were going to proceed."[105] Second, the two discussed in detail the archives' form and function. They decided on "a committee of people who would have various contacts, who would bring fresh viewpoints—a committee of people that would be stronger."[106]

To the archive committee's first meeting at Moore's SoHo loft, he and Hirsh invited artists, curators, and other cultural workers.[107] That early members were drawn from the networks of two professional gay white cismen enmeshed in Manhattan's art scene meant that a majority mirrored these identities. At various moments and for varying durations, David Cabrera, William "Bill" Cohen, José Luis Cortés, Nick Debs, Roberto Juarez, Geoffrey Hendricks, David Nelson, Eric Rhein, Charles Richardson, and Sur Rodney (Sur) were members, along with honorary members John Dugdale, Lyle Ashton Harris, and Martin Wong.[108] Regardless of race, sexuality, or profession, all were men whose lives were, Hirsh said, "transformed dramatically by the AIDS crisis."[109] Some were HIV-positive artists; however, Hirsh argues their selection was not made "on the basis of their status in relation to AIDS in medical terms" but rather "their status in relation to AIDS in their work and in their daily lives."[110] Members knew from personal experiences the urgency of documenting and preserving their community's work and stories before they were forgotten or destroyed. Early on, the committee gathered every other week. Hirsh, who was elected chairperson and led the Project day to day as coordinator, noted that these members "put it together and it worked. So, something happened that was right."[111] Hirsh's organizational capacities are why he believed Moore chose him, rather than "my abilities as an archivist. . . . We projected that in the future, a professional archivist would put things . . . into the proper order."[112] In the meantime, Hirsh told me, "there was the committee to organize, meetings to run, people to meet, information to be gathered, photographers to be located and energized."[113]

The archive committee coalesced in the same period that Visual AIDS was destabilized. By 1994, the "old guard"[114] was, early member Rhein remembered, "burning out," tiring because they were "losing people, care giving," or were "ill themselves."[115] Some needed to step back. Visual AIDS was faced with the decision, Rhein continued, to either "fold" or to "reinvent itself" in order to "to actually provide hands-on, tangible support to artists."[116] In summer 1994, they conducted a national survey of artists and arts organizations. They found that artists with HIV/AIDS were in acute need of professional services, including documentation. Moore, a Visual AIDS board member, proposed joining Visual AIDS and the archive committee, forming the Archive Project in fall 1994.[117] During this transition, Moore created the darkly humorous *Zine,* looking back on the archives' past to envision its future. It offered much-needed release in "a dramatic time," Hirsh recalled, reading it as "one of the first times I had laughed in a couple months. . . . That was a delightful thing that Frank did for us all."[118] The Archive Project was a direct service to artists that would "rescue in some form the works of the many who had died, or were dying," Rhein noted.[119] It became Visual AIDS's driving directive, a position it still holds.

The archives, a remedy for HIV-positive artists' artistic deaths, was attuned to the implications of marginalization in the arts. Generating and collecting photographic documentation of artworks was the primary fix. Hirsh played matchmaker, pairing artists with volunteer photographers. He also set up and attended shoots; then photographs were professionally developed into 35mm slides at the organization's expense.[120] Visual AIDS provided slides to the artist and kept a copy for the archives. In the 1990s, galleries covered the costly documentation process for their artists. The possibilities of loss were most acute for artists without art world recognition, a group more likely to include women, people of color, and outsider artists. The Project used its resources to name and work toward repairing power inequities. Community archives, Michelle Caswell describes, collect in formats reflective of the community's "culture, epistemologies, and values."[121] Slides were all important because they were how work was evaluated and made visible to "venues from galleries to magazines," Hirsh emphasized.[122] Increased visibility greatly improved chances at long-term survival. Juarez argued, "If you don't document things, they just disappear."[123] Interviewed in 1995 about having his work documented, artist Copy Berg reported, "My greatest fear is that I'm going to drop dead and my work will just disappear into some basement or be thrown away."[124] He noted feeling profound relief: "I can't tell you, my anxiety levels just dropped, if I were to die tomorrow, Visual AIDS would finish the job."[125] Within the Project's first year, seventy-five artists' artworks were documented and slides donated, along with other records.[126] The archives thus ensured, as part of an archival cure, that there would be a record of AIDS art past. Their remedy shapes the organization's contemporary abilities to use its records, through vital nostalgia, to redesign the AIDS present and future.

Despite arduous efforts, it proved impossible for the Archive Project's remedy to save many artworks or careers. There were inherent material limitations to what the archives could provide in documentation, preservation, and accessibility in the face of HIV/AIDS's rapid, unrelenting devastation. These limitations shape the AIDS story that can be told. The scope of services that they provided was constrained. Some had hoped to provide permanent exhibition[127] and storage spaces for artworks,[128] but these costly plans never came to fruition. Hirsh had also planned to video interview each artist showing and talking about their work.[129] He had already done hundreds of interviews for his writing but is still haunted by regrets: "The number of video interviews that I did started to decline in my last year or two with the Archive Project because other intense involvements. . . . Looking at the few videotapes that are now available . . . I immediately question why I didn't do more because I really was capturing a moment of historic change."[130] In holding onto this AIDS past, Hirsh, like many survivors of this period, is hard on himself. I was keenly aware that the interview process was emotional and at times difficult for him. The Archive Project became and remains largely a collection of 35mm slides and digital files of artworks, along with press clippings, artist statements, printed invitations, small artworks, and related materials.

On the *Zine*'s title page, Moore's direct address to fellow Project members, a voice chimes in, "DAVID! Look at *MY* Work." This inside joke Hirsh identified as a reference to the immense pressure to work quickly, which meant his attention was needed in "a thousand places at once."[131] He described how, in hopes of documenting as many artists' work as possible, he was "so busy doing this stuff on a daily basis" that "I really took no time to review the material. There may have been emotional reasons for it, but also at the time it was just necessity because of working in a time of compression. . . . There was a rush or urgency. . . . There was always more to do."[132] Not all artists wanted to be or could be reached in time. "He was worried about the disposition of his work," Moore shared about a dying sculptor friend's experience. Then "one day, like a miracle, a dumpster materialized in front of his door. He loaded it all in and went home to his family and died. [The work was] all lost."[133] Juarez similarly remembered, "There were so many people that were losing their lives, and [who] had to worry that their artwork, their life's work, would not continue, would not be cared for. I saw it over and over again. People's families would come and just throw things out. . . . It was real. It was terrifying. . . . It just broke my heart."[134]

The difficult and sometimes unachievable challenges of working against the clock, maintaining momentum, sustaining funding, and just surviving took a toll. On another *Zine* page, "The Archive," Moore depicted the stacks (Figure 6). He classified them: "dead," "he's dead," "deceased," "angel," "dying," or "dead, dead, dead." Archiving the dead's remains, Moore summed up, "sucks." He inquired in an overlay: "When do we get to PARTY?" Examining this drawing during our interview, Hirsh shared, "For an organization as tightly knit and dynamic as we were, we had no parties, no get-togethers, no social events. It was all work."[135] Moore, recognizing the exhausting, heart-wrenching labors of activist archiving, issued to his collaborators a command to "Dance!" If always limited in scope, scale, and thereby impact, the Archive Project's cure nonetheless ensured that there would be a record. Grounded in the political commitments of vital nostalgia—an attunement to power and the importance of the past in dictating AIDS's present and future—the archives created a new and urgently needed home remedy, one generated by, for, and with its community. The Archive Project's remedy eased some of the pervasive hopelessness and fear about the demise of one's artwork and legacy, offering much-needed hope and thereby a measure of cure.

Archives as Care

"AIDS was a fact that had to be faced with a direct stare into the inevitability of death, which was ever present," Hirsh insisted.[136] While the Archive Project provided an initial remedy for its community, the demand for a head-on address of an amalgam of extreme needs marked my interlocutors' responses to the emergency of AIDS. Unable despite their best efforts to ameliorate or resolve embodied experiences of pain, or to stem the parade of deaths, the Archive Project was a form of critical care that they could effectively offer to their community of HIV-positive artists. "AIDS introduced me to a world of constant need, of constant care,"

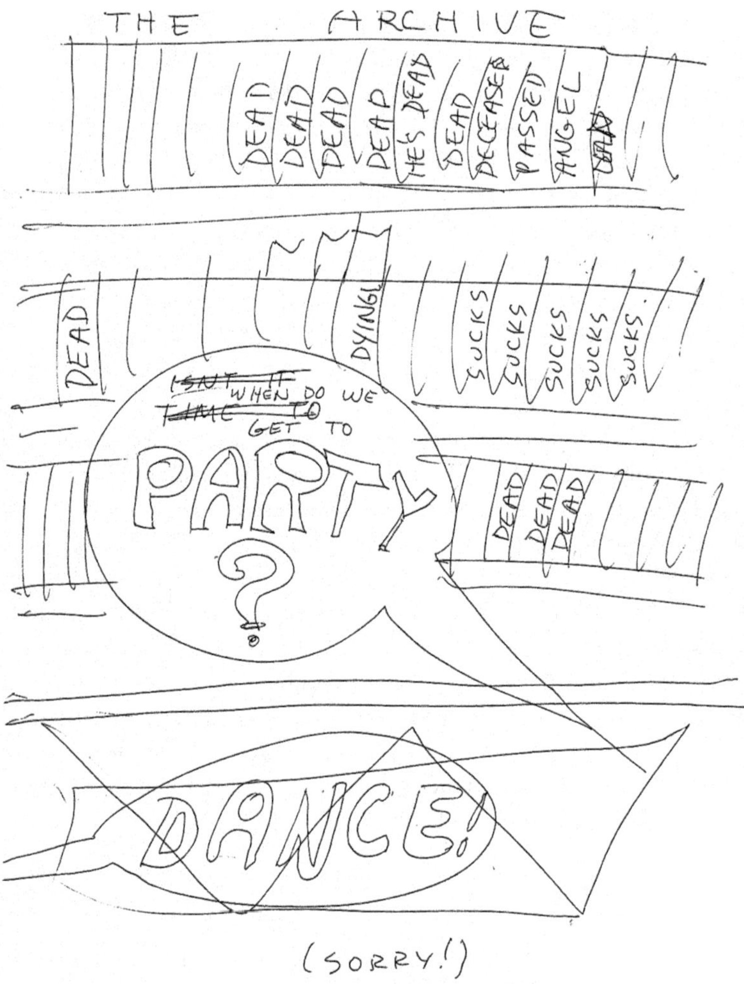

Figure 6. Painter and Archive Project cofounder Frank Moore visually summed up the challenges of archiving records of an endless parade of dead loved ones, acquaintances, and artistic community in his *Archive Project (Zine)*. "The Archive," *The Archive Project (Zine)*, created for Visual AIDS in 1995. Courtesy of Visual AIDS.

Hirsh emphasized.[137] Practices of care and cure are deeply enmeshed. Together, they constitute medicine's aim.[138] For the Archive Project too, cure and care are interlocking practices. Its archival cure includes mitigating damage and countering injury through curative processes of "care, concern, responsibility."[139] Critical caring for artworks, records, and, above all, the people who created them demonstrates how the Archive Project's archival cure is constitutive of vital nostalgia. Moore and Rhein, a fellow artist and early archive committee member, identified the experiences of photographer John Dugdale, an HIV-positive man and honorary member, as inspiration for the archives' centering of care as vital to cure. In the early 1990s, Dugdale's vision had deteriorated from cytomegalovirus.[140] Yet with the privileges of artistic success and whiteness, he could afford assistance; this enabled him to continue making and showing photographs.[141] In summer 1994, Moore, Hirsh, Rhein, and Debs each visited Dugdale's home in Deposit, New York. Rhein's beautiful photographs document Hirsh's interview with Dugdale there about his life and work (Figure 7). Through the archives, the activists extended care's reach through documentation and engendering artistic exposure to other artists living with HIV/AIDS, eventually coming to focus especially on serving HIV-positive women, trans people, people of color, and other artists excluded from more traditional archives.

Given its cultural deficits in glamour, emphasis on interdependence, and inherent failures in the face of imperatives that demand solution for illness and disability, care often does not get its due in accounts of HIV/AIDS activism. In emergent scholarship, Marlon Bailey calls attention to how modes of caretaking within Black cultural workers' communities "were central to forging intimate bonds and enduring relationships and collectivities in the midst of a crisis."[142] Bailey's observation holds true for the Archive Project; it was care that enabled community members' capacities to resist and withstand HIV/AIDS.[143] The Project's activist-archivists, despite never explicitly naming it as such, operated within a feminist ethics of care. They acted and "understood themselves as caregivers," following an ethics of care model in archives that, as Caswell and I have noted, requires archivists to acknowledge how they are "bound to records creators, subjects, users, and communities through a web of mutual affective responsibility."[144] In this section, in order to show how the Archive Project enacted a holistic archival cure through vital nostalgia, I examine how at the archives care work was done, who needed it and who did it, and how it was represented. I also examine where the archives

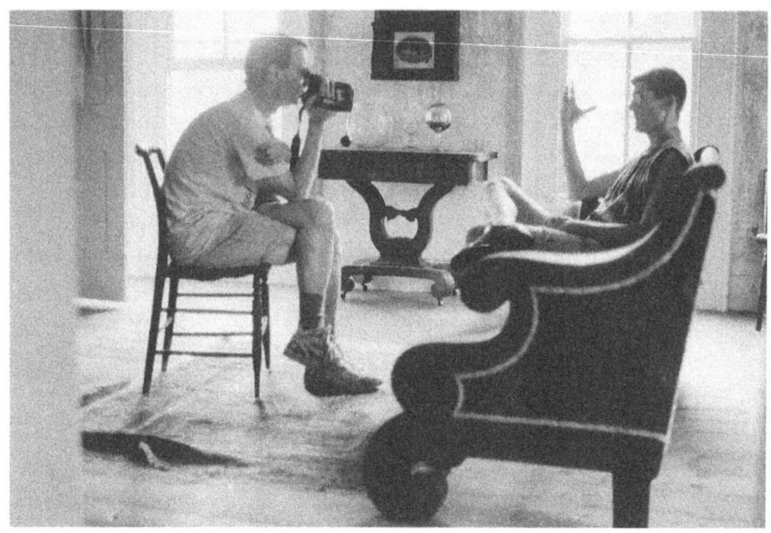

Figure 7. Archive Project cofounder David Hirsh conducting an interview with photographer and honorary Project member John Dugdale at his farm in Deposit, New York, in 1994, as photographed by fellow member Eric Rhein. Toned gelatin silver print, 8 × 10 inches. Courtesy of the artist.

has not provided adequate care, excluding marginalized artists from its archival cure. Activist archiving encompasses strategically mobilizing nostalgia for an AIDS past to enact retroactive justice and contemporary cure.

Tremendous deficiencies in available care and the neglect of caretaking by families and institutions for those with HIV/AIDS who were ill, dying, or dead—conditions that were especially acute for queer, trans, Black, brown, and working-class artists—were experiences my interlocutors repeatedly witnessed. These experiences shaped their motivations to archive and their archival labors. Care encompasses, Caswell and I wrote, "both the often bodily labours of providing what is necessary for the health, sustainment, and protection of someone or something, and the feeling of concern and attachment that provokes such acts."[145] Archiving, then, is a means of caring for bodies—bodies of artistic work as well as physical bodies. "In the balance of things, I tended by necessity towards [the] giving of care," Hirsh reflected.[146] Sur, a curator and early member, was also called to caretaking. He left his gallery job in 1988 because it became intolerable to "pick up the phone and call another artist and find out they can't answer the phone [as] they couldn't get across the room to get a glass of water."[147] He devoted himself to caretaking full time, including assisting artists in organizing their records. Unable to alleviate physical suffering or to forestall death, the Project for early leaders was the manifestation of the ongoing care that they could actually offer loved ones. Their care was an essential component of the archives' holistic AIDS cure, one that worked to counter stigma, discrimination, and fear. The intimate relationships between those doing the archiving and those being archived—their shared situatedness within a community of artists with HIV/AIDS—shaped the content and format of records the archives collected, the language and methods they chose to arrange and describe them, and how the archives was located and accessed within its community of origin.[148]

Many of my interlocutors identified, for themselves or their collaborators, a personal loss as formative to their archiving practice. Early members looked back longingly on the past they shared with a lost beloved in a practice of vital nostalgia; collecting and maintaining AIDS records became a way to advance their activism and to extend beyond the bounds of lifetimes the care they had offered or wished they could have provided to their beloveds. "I came head-on into the crisis with the loss of Brian Buczak, my lover and fellow artist," early member Hendricks shared in conversation with his husband, Sur.[149] Hendricks continued, "He left a legacy, but there was so much more that he wanted to do. With his death there was an initial feeling that somehow, I must carry forth and realize those unrealized dreams."[150] Hendricks was keenly aware that his loss and the responsibility he felt was "just one, a small island in a great sea. There was a whole archipelago of collections."[151] Addressing his husband directly, he observed that Sur was in the "same kind of situation with Andreas Senser. When we came together and got married . . . we realized that this was also a marriage of archives of those we had nursed at their end."[152] As we sat across from one another in his studio on a summer afternoon more than twenty years after the death of Arch Connelly, a close friend and fellow artist, early member Juarez's voice broke and he held back tears as he described how AIDS had "decimated" so many lives.[153] It was overwhelming, he said. "I didn't know what to do."[154] Archiving became part of these men's answers to how to care in incurable time. By preserving and making accessible the AIDS art past, the Archive Project was the "beginning of finding a forum," as Hendricks beautifully put it, "for realizing dreams."[155]

"The goal" of the Archive Project "was to collect the work of as many artists that we could . . . [who] had either died or were still living. Just to see what it would look like. Period. Just to see what we could find. We didn't want it to look a certain way; we didn't know how it would look," Sur reported.[156] The two parameters for placing records in the archives' care were established from the start and remain the same: they collect the records of anyone who self-identifies first as an artist, and second as HIV positive. The latter also implicitly requires an ability and willingness to disclose one's serostatus in a publicly accessible archives. Santos, then the Project's executive director, highlighted the use of HIV serostatus as a collecting parameter as being both "the interesting" and "unusual thing about the Archive Project."[157] Collecting on the basis of serostatus rather than around a theme, artistic medium or movement, or identity category means that the archives holds a wildly disparate range of work, materials, and artists. The collection's breadth is a major strength and counters the normative societal valuation of only those artists who achieve a level of market and institutional recognition; such artists are often white and male. "We see the beauty" in artists' work, "whether that beauty be a representation, an object, or the very act of making," Debs noted.[158] He emphasized that "beauty" should not be confused with standards of artistic merit established by the commercial art world.[159] Many artists, especially minoritized ones, are denied such recognition, and if, Moore wrote, an "artist doesn't believe in himself, and in his work, or if his faith in its value is undermined by having AIDS, being Gay, or by not being able to support her or himself with his or her work as an artist," then "it becomes very difficult to insert this work in our cultural discourse."[160] The Project's unjuried collecting also reflects the temporal register of emergency in which it emerged. "We document what we can get our hands on as quickly as possible. Time is of the essence, for all people, so let the future decide what is 'worthwhile.' We have too much work to do," Debs noted, "to engage in judgment or interpretation."[161] In a period of instability, there was an understanding that notions of quality and value were in flux, providing crucial space to intervene against the art world's perpetuation of structural power inequities. Debs concluded, "We must try to document everything, including the kitchen sink. And we must remember that the kitchen sink is beautiful."[162] In the register of contemporary AIDS time, characterized by chronicity and endurance as much as emergency, the willful "chaos" of the collection,[163] which includes work explicitly about HIV/AIDS as well as pieces and practices that are not in response to HIV/AIDS at all, still feels like a complex and appropriately messy cure— one that contrasts with medical cure's neat sterility.

What began as caretaking confined within an intimate network of lovers, friends, colleagues, and acquaintances evolved quickly into a more expansive communal orientation. "WANTED DEAD or ALIVE," Juarez's 1995 recruitment poster begins, playing on the genre of wanted posters (Figure 8). It is "very provocative, I thought," he shared, "that you don't have to be dead to be in the Archive Project. If you had HIV and were living with AIDS, it was something that could help organize your life and help you with your work."[164] From the start, the Project was open to those who got in touch, at first using Hirsh's home phone and then that of Visual AIDS.[165] Once they began "connecting with artists who none of us had ever known before," Hirsh recalled developing an integration process. He began with a studio visit. Then he would come back with a photographer and be present during documentation. Finally, Hirsh returned to deliver the artist's copy of the slides. He made three visits, and often more. This labor-intensive archival approach illustrates how such visits were not just about collecting but were ultimately a vital form of interpersonal care work, a taking up of responsibility for the life and the work of artist members.[166]

Early leaders' efforts and identities shaped the care the Archive Project provided. Challenges recruiting artists from "minority communities," as Moore wrote—"communities that are, for the most part, cut off from much of the arts activities that go on in Manhattan"—have always been present.[167] Juarez read aloud to me the text he'd written: "ARTISTS and ART BY PEOPLE WITH HIV/AIDS FOR ARCHIVE AND EXHIBITIONS, We need you all: foxgloves, innocences, eyebrights. BE PART OF HISTORY, BE PART OF HERSTORY." There was some institutional awareness that "those artists who have operated at the margins of already marginalized art communities" had needs that were especially acute.[168] The Project aspired to "guarantee their works' survival and exposure" in order to "preserve a tremendous amount of experience and hold it out to the future, saying, 'all of this happened, all of this was real—use the information well.'"[169] The small constituency of cultural workers of color in early leadership worked particularly hard to extend the archives' reach beyond the white, male-dominated Manhattan art scene. Cortés recalled recruiting fellow Puerto Rican artists to have their work documented.[170] Volunteers also developed relationships with organizations embedded in the city's racially and ethnically segregated communities; for example, they worked closely with the Jamaica Center for Arts and Learning in Queens. Personal connections were important in ensuring diverse persons felt welcomed.[171]

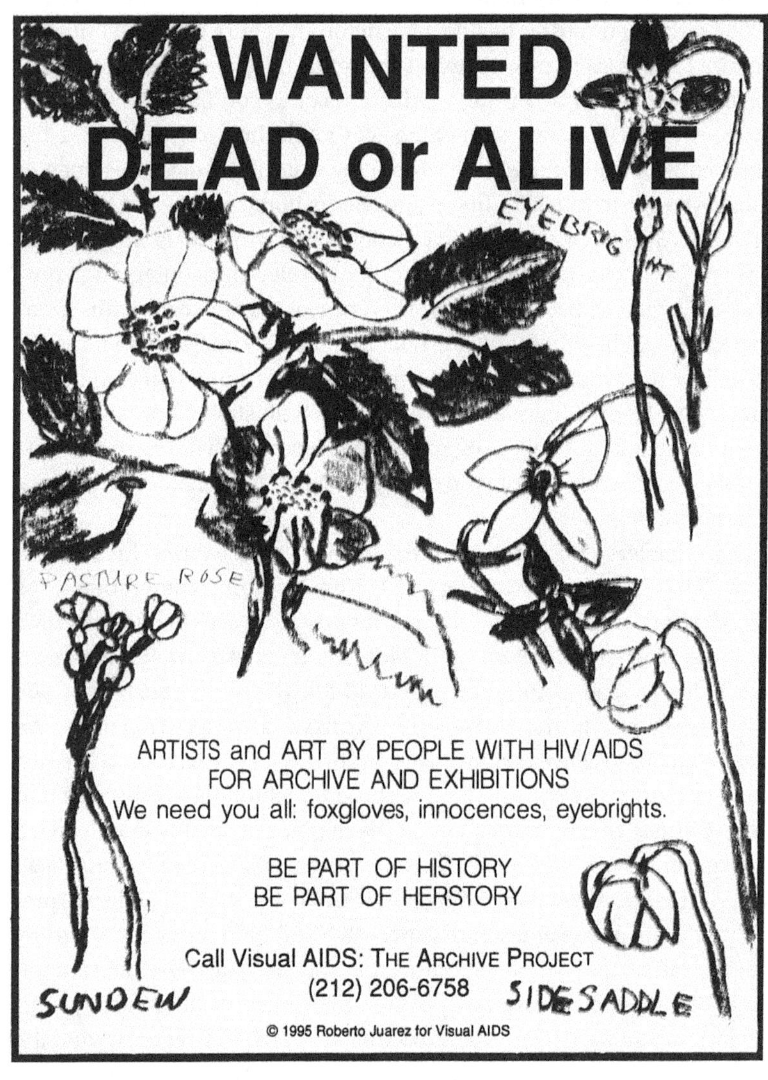

Figure 8. Early Archive Project member Roberto Juarez's *Wanted Dead or Alive* broadside poster was made to recruit fellow artists to join the Archive Project in 1995. Courtesy of Visual AIDS and the artist.

It is by showcasing the plurality of artistic work and artists that the archives "breaks the stigma of who is living with HIV/AIDS," Santos told me.[172] Attesting to the "variety" of people affected and myriad HIV/AIDS experiences and expressions, the collection expands cultural understandings of the pandemic with due attention to particularity, connection, and context.[173] Countering stigma and stereotyping is a significant component of the Archive Project's holistic cure. The archives features many of the most acclaimed of the 1980s' and early 1990s' art AIDS canon: Keith Haring, Félix González-Torres, David Wojnarowicz, Robert Mapplethorpe. Holdings also include artists like Frank Moore, John Dugdale, and Tony Feher, who were well established but lesser known beyond the art world. Yet the Project's unique collection development policy means that unlike other archives collecting on this period's art movements, including Fales's Downtown Collection, it does not subscribe to or reproduce a "canon."[174] It can therefore be activated to disrupt dominant narratives. Rhein identifies it as "vital" that included artists were self-selecting and that it was absent of "hierarchy or criteria."[175] The physical and intellectual arrangement of the analog and digital archives also produces inclusivity. McGowan notes, as an example, that when browsing the online archives, "if someone's last name is Marston, they show up right next to Robert Mapplethorpe and that's an amazing thing. When you look at who is represented in the Registry, you have Keith Haring and then someone who makes a living as a hairstylist in Kentucky who also creates beautiful photographs."[176] In "setting aside fame, acclaim, references or accreditation," the archives captures, she said, "this really amazing breadth of what it means to be an artist. Both what it means to be HIV positive right now in the world, but also what it means to be an artist. . . . It tells a story about who is making art across the U.S. and even the world right now, and how they do it."[177] The archives harnesses through vital nostalgia iconic works and relatively privileged artists to garner greater representation and exposure for marginalized artists and perspectives working toward inclusivity and against dominant AIDS narratives.

Hirsh identified garnering "exposure" as "a type of care, especially when it involves artists with AIDS."[178] Developed by cultural workers invested in the transformative sociopolitical power of visual art and the art world, part of the Archive Project's care has always been serving as a curatorial resource. Garnering artistic exposure through curatorial processes for HIV-positive artists can provide an archival cure for the ailments of shame, stigma, and isolation. Curation is care work, whether it is devoted to objects or people. From the start, early members recognized curation's potential in caring for and working toward a holistic cure for their community. In various configurations, they collaboratively curated shows from the collection, including *The First 10* (1995) and *Arts' Communities, AIDS' Communities* (1996). With the act of curating an "exhibit of viruses or epidemics," Alexander R. Galloway and Eugene Thacker write, "one is forced to 'care' for the most misanthropic agents of infection and disease. One must curate that which eludes the cure."[179] When agential and done with appropriate sensitivity, exposing HIV-positive serostatus in an exhibition or other public program can be "a healing process," Hirsh said.[180] Cortés described to me, "When you have cancer, you don't lie about it or hide it for years. . . . Sometimes it's hard for me to, like, under daily life come out [as HIV positive, but] . . . every time I say it . . . it's like a release."[181] The collective visibility engendered through curatorial care activist-archivists understood as increasing the odds of survival for members and artworks alike. Artistic exposure, Cortés concluded, "for us [is] like a cure."[182]

Access to the archival cure that the Archive Project provides has never been equitable. "Because it's open to anyone, it does provide a more democratic opportunity for someone to join," however, Santos noted, it would be misleading or oblivious "to say it's a complete or fully equal representation."[183] The Archive Project has always had and still has racial, gender, class, and geographic shortcomings in its representation of HIV/ AIDS experiences, activism, and cultural production. These deficits in care's curatorial reach, those who remain uncared for, are produced by and reproduce the ways that Visual AIDS was constituted by "gay white men," part of a tight network that, McGowan emphasized, had the resources to get "some money behind it," and who were privileged enough to "work as artists" professionally.[184] Women of cis and trans experience and artists of color have made powerful contributions to the archives from the Project's start. Some men and women of color were also among the first to have their work documented. However, that early diversity cannot be attributed to intentional, concerted inclusion efforts by early members. The first ten artists, who were featured together in the Project's first major exhibition, were just those who called first. Hirsh remains pleasantly surprised by their diversity; half were underrepresented artists.[185] The collection's foundational biases endure; Santos estimated for me in 2016 that out of the then more than seven hundred artist members, only fifty or so were artists of color. They are also still in majority cismen.

Over the last decade, Visual AIDS has made a concerted effort to do more to document, collect, and promote minoritized artists. They are working through vital nostalgic practices, detailed in the following section, to extend the archives' care to those who have long been neglected by AIDS archives. They do so, McGowan told me, in hopes of resonating with "the nature of how the crisis has changed."[186] Yet the archives' representation is still more reflective of the conceptual realities of "who we imagine is living with HIV" and of "who [has] had the ability," the social and economic security, "to announce that they are living with HIV," former programs manager Ted Kerr emphasized, than of the contemporary epidemic's statistical racialized and classed realities.[187] Kerr detailed strategies he led to redress these stark "silences, and absences in the archive:" identifying, acknowledging, and publicly naming them. By "promoting" their archival absences, the bodies that are not there, the Project highlights them as topics of discussion and possible change; exposing and holding onto past injustices perpetuated by their own archiving practice is thus used as tool to engender different AIDS presents and futures.[188] Citing efforts to collect and engage with more HIV-positive women, McGowan points to the collection development policy's importance.[189] Bringing in these artists often requires first challenging racialized and gendered conceptions of artistic merit and belonging: "You have ten paintings at home, you can have a page on our Registry. It's not about you being a professional artist."[190] They emphasize that "for us, 'you're an artist if you make art.'"[191] Geographic representation for much of the archives' tenure has been largely of artists local to New York City. McGowan is working to expand the archives into what are now crisis epicenters, including the American South.[192] An increased online presence has made the archives more visible and accessible to artists beyond their immediate community; however, further work is needed to provide culturally competent care, to diversify and extend the archives' reach and representation and thereby its cure. Providing curatorial care could lead to forms of material and physical care, mobilizing attention to where care is lacking in the contemporary epidemic.

Archives as Curing

"We knew that there were stories that needed to be preserved and retold—not about 'victims' but about the universes these artists inhabited," Moore wrote two years into building the Archive Project.[193] These records "must be preserved" for their "intrinsic value" and "historic (AIDS) value."[194] Distinct from but encompassed within a holistic cure, the process of curing traces methods used to treat a perishable item so as to prolong its life and ensure its consumption. In an archival sense, preservation and curation are the strategies that materially facilitate now and into the future archival endurance and accessibility. Through curing, the Archive Project makes vital the cultural nostalgia for iconic artists and records of the AIDS art past to engender holistic archival cure. Visual AIDS's communal approach to curing is in contrast to the medical and pharmaceutical establishment's limited focus on curing by treating individual patients. Activist-archivists work instead toward curing harms including stigma, hopelessness, isolation, loss of artistic work, omissions in memory transmission, and community breakdown. Records become tools for artists' individual and collective resilience and empowerment. This approach is strengths based, supporting and celebrating people who are thriving despite, or in some cases because of, their HIV/AIDS experiences. Archival curing meets its community where they are rather than valuing only becoming medically "cured" of HIV/AIDS—a state that still remains unachievable.

In an archival context, curing (although calling it such is a novel intervention) encompasses active preservation processes used to prevent or reduce deterioration and damage in order to minimize the loss of information and extend the life and accessibility of collections deemed archival, and thus of enduring value. Visual AIDS' historical and contemporary materials emphasize a preservation imperative. The Archive Project's About web page notes that it collects "to preserve and honor the work of artists with HIV/AIDS and the artistic contributions of the AIDS movement."[195] Similarly, its digital counterpart, Artist+ Registry, "provides a forum for HIV+ visual artists to display and share their work with viewers worldwide and provides an opportunity for estates of artists lost to AIDS to preserve the work of these artists in a comprehensive online archive."[196]

Preservation of the record for Visual AIDS is a means of transmitting AIDS knowledge and memory to build resilience across generations. Collective memory is central to a holistic archival cure that dismantles stigma, silence, isolation, and marginalization. Archiving AIDS at all, Moore wrote, required "fighting the weariness that sets in when one thinks of preserving a memory of that which one would rather forget."[197] He named a communal fatigue, the "bone weariness of those who deal on a daily basis with AIDS and must then contemplate the effort involved in documenting and preserving not just their own efforts, but the widest possible array of cultural artifacts and information."[198] If endowed with the privilege to do so, it is tempting to forget that AIDS and its attendant pain and suffering "ever happened."[199] Throughout the late 1980s and early 1990s, white activists, to forge a collective consciousness around the horrors of HIV/AIDS, frequently deployed Holocaust iconography.[200] Moore, outlining a vision for the Project's memory practices, connected the archives' preservation aspirations with discovering as a gay man in his late twenties that gay men were systematically targeted by the Nazis. A second challenge was that transmission of memory, traumatic and otherwise, in a community of artists living with HIV/AIDS, many of them queer, traversed social and sexual ecologies where knowledge was not readily passed down through established biological familial channels. Such disruption can prevent it from feeling like such history belongs to you.[201] Early calls to contribute to the Archive Project evoked the mutual responsibility of minoritized persons to record the experiences and events that shape their lives, and of the archives to "preserve these records," ensuring marginalized "stories survive."[202] For people with AIDS, the Project promised long-term survival as a community with a collective history, even before medically facilitated long-term survival for HIV-positive individuals became possible. Preserving records and passing down AIDS memory is vital to curing; it is the only way Moore believed to ensure that genocidal violence "never again" happens.[203] He feared that if denied their history, future generations of gays and lesbians would say, "Never what again?"[204] Activist archiving is a collective memory practice with ambitions at the "preservation of a living voice."[205]

Currently, the Project houses 25,600 35mm slides, artists' statements, exhibition invitations, brochures, catalogs, and other materials in its artists' files.[206] Some activities are undertaken to protect these records by minimizing chemical and physical decay. However, the organization's resources for preserving the longevity of its physical artifacts are limited. Slides are displayed in a custom light box over the neat row of white file cabinets holding the collection (Figure 9). Its records are thus visible where the archives lives in the Visual AIDS office, a small, bustling, artfilled room. The office doubles as a community center; artist members, collaborators, and visitors came in and out during the weeks I spent there, sharing the long worktable. Visual AIDS is on the fifth floor of a Chelsea building with galleries, studios, and nonprofits. The building is not fully

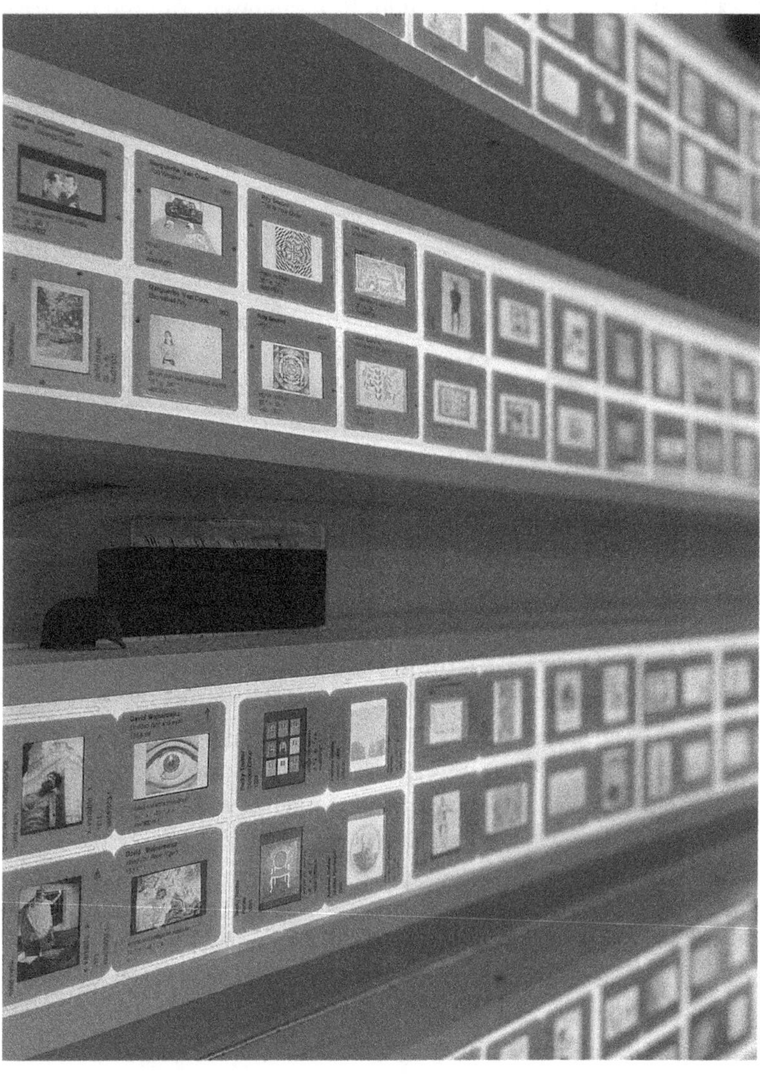

Figure 9. The Lightbox Project featuring slides from the Archive Project's collection as displayed in the Visual AIDS office. The Lightbox Project was curated by Stefanie Nagorka and Sur Rodney (Sur) for Visual AIDS in 2001. Photograph by Tracy Fenix. Courtesy of Visual AIDS.

climate controlled and does not provide the ideal conditions for long-term preservation of primarily photographic records. As early as 1995, there was an awareness that digitization was a promising strategy to make use of limited resources in mitigating loss, and to increase through vital nostalgic efforts accessibility and audience.[207] In 1998, the Estate Project for Artists with AIDS developed Artists with AIDS (https://artistswithaids .org/), the first virtual collection of HIV-positive artists' work. It featured 150 digitized images from the Project.[208] In 1999, Visual AIDS, in partnership with TheBody.com, developed its first website, which included digitized images in rotating, guest-curated web galleries.[209] Curators had to come in and go through binders holding thousands of slides to select twenty or so for their web galleries. Santos, then the associate director, would digitize the selected slides. Between 2002 and 2008, Visual AIDS began accepting digital files from artist members. With the aid of interns, they also began additional digitization, at first just selecting a few slides from as many different artists as possible for in-house scanning.

Digitization forms the groundwork of Visual AIDS's curing, and it is what allows them to curatorially mobilize records through vital nostalgia. In 2008, Visual AIDS developed a strategic plan that called for a digital archives. Making its living archives digital, and thereby adapting to meet its community's needs and realities, was essential in advancing archival cure. It opened the archives to a broader community of artists and garnered greater exposure while paying due attention to the harms its most marginalized members risked. Large-scale digitization was a challenge for a small organization with a budget dependent on fund-raising from public and private institutions and individuals. For most of its existence, Visual AIDS had a staff of two, and although it has grown to the equivalent of three to four full-time positions, it was only for the first time in late 2021 that it included a formally trained archivist.[210] Digitization began in earnest with the Joan Mitchell Foundation's support over a three-year period.[211] Sur noted that digitization provoked questions: "How does it look, how do we promote it, how do we talk about it, who do we include, what do we need, what's missing?"[212] Internally and with artist members over eighteen months, between 2008 and 2010, Visual AIDS developed technical and ethical guidelines reflective of the values of those whose lives are implicated in its records. When the newly christened Artist+ Registry launched in November 2012, it included pages for 272 artist members and 500 images.[213] Though developed from the Archive Project, it got its own name "because 'archive' sounds so final, like a closed box, and we wanted artists living with HIV to feel this is an ongoing, evolving project and resource to them," Santos told me.[214] Technical specifications detailed the number of images from each artist (two minimum, one hundred maximum), file size, image resolution, and format, each informed by constraints from server space to copyright. The organization was meticulous in its commitment to ethically, socially responsible digitization that accounted for the privacy, disclosure, and consent concerns that are especially acute for people living with HIV/AIDS. Within its first year, a hundred new members joined.[215] The Registry as of 2020 features 658 artists (out of the 900 total) and more than 18,000 images, including digital versions of many of the original analog slides and digital documentation of new works described and uploaded directly by artist members through the web portal. Guest-curated web galleries animating work from the Registry continue monthly.

McGowan, Santos, and Kerr completed the Registry's final components at McGowan's apartment in the days following Hurricane Sandy in November 2012, when much of the city and its building were closed. "That weekend was like the Wizard of Oz, [where] like nothing is the same after the storm," Kerr remembered.[216] The storm's wake provided an aptly dramatic moment for the digital archives' launch—a monumental event for the organization and its artists. After going live online, the archives achieved a new level of public exposure that posed in its curing processes great material benefits and risks. Many artists made only a single donation, whether because they lost interest, forgot, were ill, or were not making art anymore.[217] Seeking to ameliorate harm, staff members contacted each artist before the launch. For some, including many artists of color, having their work available online, often for the first time, was thrilling. It was also legitimizing for some contributors, especially those who do not make their living professionally as artists. Having an artist page or being selected for a web gallery, McGowan explained, "validates their belief in themselves as an artist."[218] The launch was not just significant for living artists; it brought artists who had died "back through showing their artwork," Fialho said.[219] Getting in touch with estates often proved impossible. Many artists do not have estates at all, and even if they do, the executor is often not someone with art expertise but instead is someone who is, Fialho noted, "saving their brother's or friend's art as best they can, perhaps in their garage or a storage unit, but isn't thinking about getting the work seen."[220] The team made decisions on an individual basis as to whether to post unreachable artists' work. They erred, as many archives have done, on the side of inclusivity. The "idea is that we preserve this history, and if the history isn't visible," Santos emphasized, "then what's the point of that? So we wanted to put that work up."[221] The reparative solution for artists who had passed was "memorial pages" that explicitly indicated, "This tribute page was created by Visual AIDS."[222] Such pages and any posted work are removed upon request. The development of a digital archives was especially significant in the context of the AIDS epidemic, one that grew up alongside the internet and personal computing. Typically, Fialho found, "if someone died in '89 or '91, they don't really have a web presence."[223] "Mining" critically and intentionally the archives' physical collections and featuring these artists online has powerfully brought many minoritized artists, he emphasized, "back from obscurity, if not complete historical amnesia."[224]

The Registry's digital environment raises distinct preservation, safety, and security needs from its analog counterpart, the Archive Project. The latter has always been publicly accessible, but it occupies the relative privacy of Visual AIDS's office and remains within the community that generated and donated the records. Some artist members declined to join the easily accessible and discoverable Registry, refusing to enter the often-phobic World Wide Web. Aware of how digital platforms routinely amplify racialized and gendered precarity and vulnerability, Visual AIDS does not undermine the rights of community members to stay silent, to refuse to be digitally archived.[225] Previously, in instances where an artist would be publicly identified as HIV positive, such as exhibitions, staff contacted them to obtain consent. Serostatus disclosure is a personal decision; in some contexts, it is a legally mandated one, with material and affective consequences that hold inequitable risks, especially for Black lives.[226] It was most often artists who work with the public who declined. Teachers in particular were concerned that students would Google them before entering the classroom. Some did not want the first thing their students learned about them to be that they are HIV positive.[227] Santos cited one teacher who "comes out to his students early on in the semester every year, both as being a gay man and being HIV positive." Yet he declined to participate because the Registry denied his agency to disclose his serostatus on his own terms.[228] Similarly, some artists with commercial careers did not want to subject themselves to a potential client's biases—biases that might keep them from getting a job.[229] Despite risks of stigma, fear, and discrimination, the majority of artist members gave their consent. Occasionally, Visual AIDS still gets new artist members who wish to donate materials to the archives but do not want to be part of the digital archives. In those cases, artists are registered the "old-fashioned way," creating only a physical file in the office.[230]

The curing that Visual AIDS, as an independent community-based archives, can provide has material possibilities and limitations. Maintaining enduring access to digital information presents serious and evolving technical, social, and ethical challenges. Trevor Owens asserts, "Nothing has been preserved; there are only things we are preserving."[231] Preservation is an ongoing project that demands significant resources. Institutions are often the cultural machinery that makes long-term preservation possible.[232] Visual AIDS is keenly aware of the sustainability challenges posed by the rapid evolution of digital technologies and media obsolescence.[233] It has witnessed some digital archives, such as Artists with AIDS, become diminished and then fully disappear—in this case only to be replaced with a website advertising male enhancements.[234] At Visual AIDS, what will prove sustainable in addressing digital preservation challenges remains an open question, one informed by its community-based status. Many of its preservation challenges—understaffing, underresourcing, and dependence on individual actors[235]—are shared by community archives. These limitations echo those identified by ACT UPers in the mid-1990s as they decided what repository would be able to preserve and make accessible their records (detailed in chapter 2).

Visual AIDS's independence does provide benefits in the curing it provides. The archives "conveys a multifaceted image of the impact AIDS has had, and continues to have, on our culture," Moore wrote in 1996. It "is all the more valuable in that it can be seen straight up, without the filters of government, corporations, academia or mass media."[236] Independence affords a capacity, then–programs director Fialho said, "to stay nimble," to quickly shift priorities, programming, and projects.[237] The archives' ability to sustain itself in the present and for the future has at key moments been carefully evaluated and is likely to be reevaluated again. In the early 2000s, as popular and media attention waned and material resources turned away from HIV/AIDS, Visual AIDS struggled financially. At a town hall meeting, the staff and the community met to determine whether their doors should remain open at all. The question of whether they should deposit the archives at a larger, more formal archival institution arose that night. Santos, then early in his seventeen-year tenure, remembered that it was "the artist members who were most vocal that night about the archives remaining within its community of origin," because "there's no one else doing anything like what Visual AIDS is doing; there's nothing else like the Archive Project."[238] Such responses renewed the board and staff's commitment to independence. The Project does have some meaningful relationships to institutional archives. Fales acquired Visual AIDS's noncurrent organizational records. Within the Downtown Collection, Fales also holds a number of artists' collections whose donations were facilitated by Visual AIDS.[239] They have also worked closely with the New York Public Library on projects, including *Why We Fight*. The archives not only remains within its community but is also "the inspiration for all of our projects," McGowan emphasized.[240] At recent board retreats, they have reaffirmed that the "Archive Project should be the backbone of everything we do and that anything, any event, any book, any exhibition that we do, members of the Archive Project . . . are part of it and are informing it and that their voice, issues that they raise, concerns they have, things they are facing in their lives all are the core of everything we do."[241]

Curing, acts aimed at prolonging the life of objects and the information, memories, and feelings they hold and provoke for contemporary and future access, is a temporal mediation. As the examples I will soon discuss demonstrate, what Fialho termed "looking back to look forward"[242] is a vital nostalgic programming strategy. There is a "human inclination towards preserving because" records had social "currency in the past;" however, such orientation to the past can lead dangerously to what artist and early member Rhein calls out as a "tendency to relegate things to stagnant preservation."[243] When subjected to a historicizing gaze, works can be confined and fixed, closing down alternative interpretations, but a key component of Visual AIDS's curing is the ways that the past is used to draw contemporary attention to and investment from diverse audiences. Building on Moore's emphasis on historical memory transmission, Visual AIDS utilizes its records strategically to situate the epidemic within a genealogy of analogous crisis precedents, invoking the past as a store of resources for constructive contemporary effect.[244] Fialho and Kerr, his predecessor, each emphasized to me that the archives were a forum to address the realities, as Kerr put it, of "how are people on the streets now living with HIV or deeply impacted by it."[245] It is "an engaging, creative challenge," Fialho shared, to mobilize Visual AIDS's long history and reputation "to bring new voices, that maybe haven't been considered in these contexts, in these fields to light."[246]

Generational dynamics inform the archives' critical curatorial use of nostalgia for past AIDS cultural production. Experiences of the longest-term survivors, who acquired HIV before 1996 and spent their early adulthoods believing they would die young and witnessing scores of loved ones die from complications of the health condition with which they too were living, leave an "indelible mark" that affect these artists' mental and physical health, financial stability, and quality of life.[247] Rhein's status as a long-term HIV survivor, "someone who's lost people, and come close to death," shaped his view on the archives' vital nostalgic curation. "There is also a wanting to have what we went through to matter in some real sense that it was that it has some kind of meaning beyond that particular experience," he continued.[248] The archives' curing approach addresses also those with distinctly different generational positions. Santos, McGowan, Fialho, and Kerr highlighted the 2010s' renewal of public interest in 1980s' to 1990s' AIDS cultural production and activism, one largely constrained to canonical artists and arts activism. McGowan described serving younger users who "are nostalgic for activism" and "are actively looking at art from that time to be inspired."[249] She credited political awakenings through the Black Lives Matter and Occupy movements for the resurgence of interest in ACT UP and Gran Fury, and the ways that they strategically deployed "images to get the message across in a way that was really powerful and that worked."[250] Even as Visual AIDS embraces such attention, Fialho described how the organization actively refuses to let its audiences of any generation "get stuck in the historical."[251] It attempts to emphasize through curation the ongoingness and unequal burdens of the current epidemic on Black, Latinx, Indigenous, and trans communities. Visual AIDS promotes a dynamic engagement with contemporary social justice movements through archival activations.

Curatorial resident[252] Ajamu X, a Black British artist and community archivist, offers through the Archiving Activists Portrait Project an example of how Visual AIDS uses a curing process to reach toward holistic cure. Through curation, the archives promotes not just its holdings but also the production of new documentation and use of records to develop cross-generational dialogue aimed at repairing structural injustices.[253] X argued in his proposal, "Rarely is the Black LGBTQ experience explored through the lens of celebration and creativity, individual aspirations and achievement—essentially, the day-to-day lived experience is missing: the layers, the diversity, the individuals are not seen."[254] Through erasure from archival representation, people of color, queers, and HIV-positive persons are denied both history and futurity, relegated to a vulnerable present existence. Holding onto the exclusion of Black lives and joy from AIDS archives, X's March 2016 project used the past as fuel to transform the Archive Project's present and future. X interviewed fourteen young activists of color about their art, inspirations, and "archives activism."[255] He produced a video interview and portrait of each, now held within the archives and published on the Visual AIDS blog.[256] The project centered younger activists: "Some of them were born in '81, '82 when AIDS came into being."[257] In remediating the archives, X documents his subjects of color's activist experiences around HIV/AIDS, ones markedly distinct from his own and from those of many artist members who came of age in the 1970s, 1980s, and early 1990s. To create an intergenerational intervention, he infused the archives with underrepresented histories: "It's about how do we create living archives?"[258] Refusing to imbricate himself into the established hierarchies of power, he used the month-long project to open still exclusionary archival spaces in ways that subvert, undermine, and make possible for others. "Archiving," he asserted, "is about the 'past,' and this 'present' and the 'future' all at once. . . . How do I then archive this now, this moment?" Work that "installs" within the AIDS archives' historical holdings records of contemporary "Black and Brown" HIV/AIDS experiences ensured, X told me, the archives is "moving, alive and fresh." Moreover, such projects made certain that Visual AIDS uses the AIDS past and its power to "speak to a Black and Brown queer futurity."[259] AIDS archives routinely exclude and obscure; however, they are a vital instrument in archival cure that prevents cultural, ontological, or sociopolitical erasure.[260]

For Visual AIDS, digital media has become an important tool for curing through vital nostalgic efforts that look back critically to move toward social justice. "Summoning and connecting with a sense of pastness in the present—for ideological reasons as well as for pleasure," Claire Norton and Mark Donnelly write, is frequently accomplished via "popular media."[261] Mobilizing the archives records of past AIDS cultural production on and across Instagram, Facebook, Twitter, Tumblr, and Vimeo is a means of "reminding folks of the current crisis," Fialho emphasized.[262] In its curing, the archives aims to locate and remember marginalized lives and to evade and contest their ongoing social subordination. Fialho, who directed Visual AIDS's highly active digital presence, described "thinking considerately and consciously about the fact that if I hashtag Keith Haring we are going to get a hundred new followers, but then if I follow that up with photography by Kia LaBeija or Jessica Whitbread, then people are going to know about these artists living with HIV as result of the exposure we get as an organization associated with Keith Haring."[263]

A digital slide show, "Radiant Presence," the 2015 centerpiece of Visual AIDS's annual Day With(out) Art, illustrates how leveraging nostalgia for the AIDS past on new media recenters AIDS's present. Produced collaboratively with ten curators, its lead image, an object of much nostalgia beloved for being "sexy," "flirty," and "fun," is a photograph of a shirtless Haring standing in front a mural depicting a shirtless person that spells out "ARTIST."[264] The face featured is famous, but the person behind the camera, Juan Manuel Rivera, a Puerto Rican artist member and Haring's former lover, is largely unknown. "When we post it on Facebook or we distribute the program information, the promotion evokes Keith." Fialho noted that he knew full well that users "press play because it's a photo of Keith."[265] Yet by utilizing a work from an underrecognized artist of color in the collection, it also broadens attention. Viewers are exposed to fifty other images from the archives in just a few minutes.[266] The video, circulated digitally and projected on buildings from the Guggenheim Museum to the Castro Theater, also featured textual interventions invoking the current epidemic. It offered contemporary statistics and highlighted rampant HIV criminalization.[267]

Preserving and using the records of AIDS past to renew present anti-AIDS activism is a vital nostalgic practice. The archives takes, according to Fialho, a "two-pronged approach" to curing, mobilizing "remembrance but also response."[268] In so doing, they take responsibility for ethically facilitating the passage from present to future.[269] There is a marked recognition within the organization, Rhein shared, "that historical remembrance is a means to informing our future."[270] The archives' ever-evolving commitment to curing bridges the individual and structural; it supports the aspiration to holistic cure and vibrant life for each individual artist; and it assures the long-term survival of the community as a whole by preserving its member's artworks, ideas, and experiences. The archives "brings contemporary vitality to honoring the past. Within this there is vulnerability, resilience and hope for the future." For Rhein, this is where its immense power lies.[271] Visual AIDS's curing draws continual attention, he emphasized, "to what HIV and AIDS have contributed to our humanity. It is both elegiac and a celebration of life. It's very sex positive, its intergenerational, multicultural, queer, expansive."[272]

In the rearranged Fales reading room that November night for "Activating the Archive Project," I sat in the front.[273] In the crowd were current and former staff, artist members, academics, archivists, students, and community members. Greetings and chatter quieted as Visual AIDS staffers Croft and Fenix introduced the Project, event, and panelists. Fenix, a community organizer, had just been hired as the first-ever Artist+ Registry and archive associate. They liaised with artist members, board members, and estates and guided archival, artistic, and professional development services. Fenix posed to the panel and audience the event's central questions: (1) "How can we activate the Visual AIDS Archive Project?" (2) "How have you activated it in the past?" and (3) "Specifically, what does it mean for the archive to be an agent of social change and community building and empowerment?" After each panelist's brief presentation, they circled back to these questions. The audience was also invited to respond, in open conversation toward the panel's end and in writing. We received a handout with the questions, along with instructions to respond through a drawing, poem, prose, or any other way desired. These contributions were collected at the event's end. From the start, the archives was conceptualized as vital in an unfolding HIV/AIDS cure—a means to document and stem loss; offer care; redress stigma, fear, and other cruelties; and engender survival. As the epidemic and lived experiences of HIV/AIDS have evolved, so too has the archives. "Activating the Archive Project" celebrated the archives' past and present, but true to form, it reached also toward the future. We reflected on the political futures of the HIV/AIDS cure that has been promised but has never arrived. The archives' community holds the responsibility for "collectively envisioning the Project's future," Fenix said.[274] A rich understanding of how earlier community archivists—including many of those on the panel and in the room— circulated records and ideas is fundamental to envisioning the archives' next steps. That night, attendees began drawing on history to communally reconceptualize the archives' curative processes for the twenty-first century and to push beyond the ableist confines of medical cure. For me, this work continued long after I exited back into Washington Square. Over the next six months, Hirsh and I continued our conversations, and we unfolded the archives' early propositions at cure.

Medical cure ideology is pervasive, and its legacies shape the contemporary HIV/AIDS pandemic. We are living with the complicated results of drug-driven treatment activism aimed at medical cure by activists, advocates, researchers, physicians, and people living with HIV/AIDS. The antiretrovirals that activists helped bring to market are now sold as an effective, necessary treatment, one routinely rounded up to outright medical cure. Work to eradicate disease appears to drive pharmaceutical development and production, but often saving lives becomes eclipsed by profit making.[275] With great profits, there is little incentive to develop an actual medical cure. Biomedical innovations have gone as far as to render HIV/AIDS sexually noncontagious, yet it is still highly stigmatized, and those infected with the virus remain subject to structural and social discrimination, hatred, and fear. Disability scholarship makes clear that even if a medical cure emerged tomorrow, histories of stigma, violence, and difference cannot and will not be erased.[276] Moreover, individualized medical solutions are often used as a justification for discourse that regularly highlights an approaching resolution, the end of AIDS. Within a culture steeped in medical cure ideology, there is a deep desire to celebrate HIV's defeat. But we are not actually there, and we are unlikely to be anytime soon.

Art as prevention, although laudable, most often reaches an audience with educational and class privileges that may not include those put at greatest risk for HIV. Attention from artists and curators has repeatedly failed to bring about biomedical, cultural, or political cure. Appearing only twenty-five seconds into the "Radiant Presence" digital slide show is artist member Shan Kelley's *With Curators Like These Who Needs a Cure.*[277] The work, a 5 × 7 inch wood block topped with a resin varnish that includes the artist's semen, and an application of his pubic hair, reads, "MY AIDS WON'T FIT IN YOUR MUSEUM." Using semen, a substance that has been deemed dangerous and even deadly under regimes of HIV criminalization that mandate disclosure and punish viral transmission, Kelley speaks to the experience of living with HIV now. HIV/AIDS is an everyday experience too complex, diverse, and contradictory to be adequately contained in a museum, gallery, or archives, or to have its injustices fully redressed by artistic or curatorial acts. The image lingers for a few moments on the computer screen or the exteriors of famed museums on which it was projected. By displaying works such as this, the Project does acknowledge some of its own limits in the face of unrelenting complex incurabilities. Debs noted that while the Project is part of holistic cure, it is "indeed, a very small part."[278] Archives and their curative processes alone cannot end discrimination, stigma, and fear. Yet recognizing constraints does not dismiss the archives' promise as a resource for anti-AIDS activism.[279]

The Archive Project's curative processes, steeped in vital nostalgia, operate on multiple registers: remedy, critical care, curing. It directly remedies the artistic death of those affected by HIV/AIDS by collecting their works. Its acts of care respond to diverse needs in the moment. Its curing works toward enabling livable and vibrant lives for individuals, while also assuring through evolving interventions the long-term survival and thriving of the records's community by preserving and making visible their works, ideas, and experiences. Overall, the holistic cure proffered by activist archiving is a promising means of acknowledging and redressing structural violences. It is a component of HIV/AIDS cure that is actually within our grasp. For more than twenty-five years, Visual AIDS's cadre of activist-archivists' efforts have exposed the complicated curative powers of an activist archiving practice grounded in vital nostalgia.

It is the Archive Project's HIV/AIDS conception and practice of cure as holistic that makes it valuable, if imperfect and limited in execution. Vital nostalgia is constitutive in imagining and enacting the kind of cure that Visual AIDS has always demanded and engendered through the Archive Project and Artist+ Registry. This archival cure values difference. It does not thrive on erasure or normalization; cure does not mandate erasure of the memories, feelings, and experiences of a lingering epidemic past. Cure, which is as much about the past and future as the present, is a demand for structural change and material accountability, care, and response from institutions to support communities and individuals in making more livable lives. What is at stake in its practices is not just the historical past but also historical presents—political authority and agency, the distribution of resources, and equality, equity, and social justice. Archival acts of documenting, collecting, describing, preserving, making accessible, and using records become curative. An archival cure does not offer simplistic or surefire resolution; instead, it provides blueprints toward building different, more just futures. A holistic HIV/AIDS cure requires looking backward as a means to heal and a way to move forward without moving on for affected communities. "Within the pain held by the documents of disease, there is life," Rhein argued. The archives does not aspire to "preserve" its collection "like it's dead, it's history and it's gone. . . . We're preserving it because there is a life and essence there that goes beyond that time and that place, that goes through us and beyond, that wants to inform what we were, what we are, and what we want to become." If there is no present and future value in the archives, Rhein concluded, then we should "just bury it and let it rot."[280]

4 STATUS = UNDETECTABLE

Liminality and Archival Exhibitions in the Age of Survivability

We act as if HIV/AIDS is not in flux, that it's stable. But in fact, if you talk to anyone in the community, that's not the case. We know a lot, but we don't know everything.

—**AVRAM FINKELSTEIN** (2014)

I SPENT A FEW WEEKS of the hot, damp summer of 2015 shivering in the artificial chill of the reading room of the New York Public Library's Manuscripts and Archives Division. My research was then ambiguously about what Sara Ahmed calls affect's "stickiness" in queer archives.[1] Jason Baumann, the Susan and Douglas Dillon associate director for collection development and coordinator of Humanities and LGBT Collections at the NYPL, generously spent an afternoon with me. Our conversation—and his ushering me behind the cubicles dividing the staff-only area to show off the Undetectable Flash Collective's handiwork—changed the course of my research. As Baumann pulled the collective's *What Is Undetectable?* light box out from temporary storage, I skimmed its text: "We've reached a crossroads in HIV treatment. HIV positive and HIV negative are no longer the only possibilities when discussing serostatus. The word undetectable has emerged in this conversation."[2] Undetectability, the subject of the group's site-specific installations and digital media interventions, names the status of a person living with HIV who, enabled by pharmaceutical treatment under medical supervision, has lowered the HIV load in their body to levels that are statistically insignificant and that render it noncontagious. Despite its well-established importance to HIV/AIDS, knowledge of undetectability remains largely confined to AIDS communities, public health actors, and biomedical researchers.

As the virus has become increasingly undetectable in HIV-positive bodies, AIDS has also become increasingly culturally undetectable as a contemporary American epidemic. Cultural undetectability is enabled partly by the activist-driven biotechnical development of effective pharmaceutical therapies. After 1996, these therapies have transformed HIV into a chronic illness for many with the privileges to access and maintain them. AIDS's embodied visibility and attention to HIV/AIDS alike have starkly diminished. When HIV/AIDS surfaces in dominant culture—in films, physical and digital memorials, blog posts, major exhibitions, and scholarly books—it does so almost exclusively in a retrospective register.[3] These cultural productions rely heavily on archival records created by activists and artists during the 1980s and early 1990s. AIDS archival records are increasingly being used by curators within a range of exhibition contexts to develop shows about AIDS and its cultural production during the 1981–96 crisis period. The relentless pastness of these projects' framing threatens to dangerously historicize the American HIV/AIDS epidemic, a prospect that holds deadly threats for those whom Steven W. Thrasher describes as the "viral underclass," minoritized and resource-denied persons and communities who are made continually and needlessly vulnerable to harm not just by the microscopic organisms that make up the virus but by the societal structures that make viral transmission possible.[4] AIDS archives are used to support retrospective narratives, thus acting as an accomplice to the undetectability of the ongoing AIDS crisis in the American cultural imaginary. Through curation that generatively deploys vital nostalgia in its engagement with undetectability, curators and archivists could deploy the AIDS archives in their care work more productively to expose present concerns and needs of those living with HIV/AIDS and to address the open questions about the virus's future.

Curation is an emergent yet crucial space to mobilize undetectability. We need to take undetectability into deliberate account to curate ethically with and about AIDS's archival past because to do so requires critical engagement with HIV/AIDS's present and future. Undetectability's sociotechnical logics offer archivists and curators an entry point for attending to and reigniting urgency around the persistent pandemic. In the archival exhibitions analyzed in this chapter, activist archivists and curators creatively used undetectability with critical intention and care to make the past of HIV/AIDS activism, and its ongoing implications for the epidemic's present and future, newly detectable for the public. The NYPL's exhibition, *Why We Fight: Remembering AIDS Activism*, which included the

Undetectable Flash Collective coproduced with Visual AIDS, made its records of the AIDS past visceral and embodied. *Not Only This, but "New Language Beckons Us,"* held between Fales and Visual AIDS, prominently featured and provocatively activated AIDS records through dialogue with new artworks. Both shows, held in New York City in 2013–14, resulted from generative collaborations between these research sites. Arriving after the events, I drew on exhibition documentation in the archives and on interviews with the interlocutors: archivists and librarians, curators, artists, viewers, and subjects who produced and were intimately involved with these projects. Taking up undetectability offers archivists and curators a crucial means to acknowledge, critique, and redress the gendered, racialized, and classed violences of AIDS's limited dominant representation and to disrupt the erasures inherent in its normative temporal orders. Undetectability informs AIDS archives' capacities for vital nostalgia as a means to meaningfully engage with implicated communities as well as the cultural memory of the AIDS epidemic, and hence to shape the very meaning of HIV/AIDS.

Undetectability in AIDS Time

As the Undetectable Flash Collective proclaimed, undetectability has become more than a descriptor of HIV serostatus. It is a novel identity, experience, and feeling—and, I propose, a curatorial methodology grounded in care work. Undetectability is significant in contemporary HIV/AIDS discourse, (re)producing concerns of temporality, visibility, contagion, bodies, and embodiment central to the twenty-first-century pandemic.[5] Despite the liminality inherent in attaining and sustaining it, undetectability has definitively shifted AIDS's temporal regime, ushering in an age of presumed HIV survivability. HIV/AIDS is thus reconceptualized to include a future—something more than just a past and waning present. In this section, I frame undetectability's emergence and development as a sociotechnical phenomenon with temporal consequences for AIDS, its representation, and its lived experiences. Interrogating conceptualizations of undetectability across medicine, science, public health, the humanities, and artistic and activist engagements lays the groundwork for addressing how to curate AIDS archives with vital nostalgia to bring due attention to and action on the current HIV/AIDS pandemic.

In 1985, the first enzyme-linked immunosorbent assay test kit to screen for antibodies against a specific HIV antigen was approved by the FDA.[6]

This blood test emerged one year after HIV was officially identified as AIDS's etiological agent and five years after the publication of the first cases attributed to the virus in medical reports and the popular press. An HIV-seropositive result means that antibodies to HIV were found in the blood. The test inaugurated a neat binary, HIV positive or HIV negative, that pervades realms of science, medicine, sexuality, politics, culture, and subjectivity.[7] Once people experience seroconversion, given the retrovirus's incurability, their HIV-positive status becomes permanent and fixed. In contrast, as David Caron summarized, "a negative status is far less certain than a positive one."[8] The force of the antibody test is one of many techniques impinging on HIV-positive bodies and subjectivities, including medications, clinical trials, demographics, and insurance.[9]

Undetectability disrupts the binary, established notions of HIV serostatus. Between 1990 and 1996, with AIDS activists' push for faster, more extensive biomedical research and clinical trials, more effective, less toxic combinations of antiretrovirals were developed. It was a full decade after its initial serologic detectability, in 1996, that highly active antiretroviral therapy became available to American consumers. In AIDS parlance, pharmaceutical therapy is "the cocktail"—a combination of medications that offered for the first time an effective treatment for those living with HIV and AIDS.[10] Eventually, antiretrovirals enabled HIV's suppression to undetectable levels. For those with access to such biopharmaceutical intervention, the virus's representation within the human body itself is fundamentally transformed. Already invisible to the naked eye, the HIV virion is made doubly so in the undetectable body through its failure to register its presence in conventional testing.

Undeniably, undetectability has temporal implications. From the start, the epidemic ruptured and reordered standard vectors of human life—place, identity, relation, time.[11] AIDS, as Susan Sontag has noted, is a temporal condition.[12] The virus moves and circulates with a particular rhythm. Untreated, it takes for many a full decade from infection to the development of symptoms.[13] Before the cocktail, a long, relatively healthy life was a near impossibility. AIDS from its initial 1981 medical recognition through the mid-1990s thus had a particular temporal valence. It was as though it had accelerated time,[14] with bodies rapidly aging and deteriorating, a day's death toll eclipsing that of decades. The far-reaching devastation called for, as Marita Sturken emphasized, an "immediate, in the moment, on the street" response.[15] In this period, the presence of visual symptoms marking infected bodies was more common, as it is often only in AIDS's advanced stages that visible identifiers manifest.[16] With improved treatments, AIDS's embodied visibility has largely disappeared, along with its perceived urgency. Undetectability is shorthand for the biomedical interventions that have extended and improved the lives of many persons with HIV, even if doing so is still arduous for many and temporary for some. Currently, undetectability is the pinnacle of biotechnical response. Its development ushered in the advent of a novel AIDS time, one of presumed HIV survivability. Jules Gill-Peterson pronounced this transformation one from "epidemic" to "endemic" AIDS time.[17]

With the rise of undetectability—and alongside it the possibility of stopping contagion—HIV/AIDS is sometimes reconceptualized in scientific, medical, and cultural discourses as less than catastrophic. Undetectability signals a measured sense of safety, security, normality, and containment.[18] In 2008, an early major study in Switzerland found that HIV-positive persons receiving antiretroviral therapy could not transmit the virus through sexual contact if they had virus loads that stabilized at undetectable levels for six months.[19] It built on antiretrovirals' proven effectiveness in preventing gestational parent–fetal transmission.[20] Later that year, a group of people living with HIV/AIDS presented the "Mexico Manifesto," in which they framed the study's conclusions as life affirming. Numerous studies subsequently confirmed that "undetectable equals untransmittable."[21] In the United States, it was not until September 2017 that the CDC publicly concurred.[22] Yet over the preceding decade, health-governing bodies and scientific communities widely articulated cautious support of undetectability's potential. In *Time* magazine, for example, Alice Park described the Swiss statement as "bold and provocative," but Park noted concern about "how this information is going to be used."[23] Health nonprofit NAM in 2008 similarly noted the hope engendered by noncontagiousness, but concluded with the caution that "nothing is risk free."[24] In the age of survivability, select HIV-undetectable subjects are eligible for redemption, becoming "respectable" and "responsible" citizens as their bodies hold the tantalizing promise of halting the virus.[25] Patient advocacy organizations have repeatedly emphasized undetectability's capacities to enhance "quality of life" and social integration.[26] It is their hope, yet unrealized, that undetectability will pose a sufficient challenge to antiquated understandings of HIV. However, despite these biopharmaceutical realities, stigma, discrimination, and violence are still pervasive when HIV/AIDS manages to surface in mainstream discourse.

Undetectability shapes contemporary cultural responses to AIDS, and thereby its meaning. In 1987, Douglas Crimp asserted, "AIDS does not exist separately from the practices that conceptualize it, represent it, and respond to it. We know AIDS only in and through those practices."[27] "AIDS," Paula Treichler wrote, is always "more than an epidemic disease, it is an epidemic of meanings."[28] Official discourses from the state, media, and advocacy groups alike continue to mediate HIV/AIDS in terms of "prevention," "eradication," and "stigma" within which, Octavio R. González shared, "actual people and their creative self-fashionings" can easily "get lost in this structural labyrinth of grand political horizons and inexorable neoliberal forces."[29] Undetectability is, for example, the cornerstone of the treatment-as-prevention model, which dominates contemporary public health. It is central to HIV/AIDS strategies of health-governing institutions, governments, nongovernmental organizations, advocates, major donors, and the pharmaceutical industry. Undetectability is a central pillar of UNAIDS's strategy to end the AIDS epidemic by 2030.[30] Treatment as prevention relies first on dramatically increasing the percentage of persons living with HIV/AIDS who are tested and aware of their serostatus. Second, its success depends on increasing the number of HIV-positive persons receiving antiretroviral therapy and under medical surveillance.

Undetectability can be constitutive of a limited neoliberal individualized HIV/AIDS response. In partnership with its pharmaceutical cousin, preexposure prophylaxis (PrEP), a daily pill ingested to prevent new HIV infections for those deemed by behavior or identity to be at high risk, undetectability is widely positioned as a watershed development in the end of AIDS. It figures discursively into the prevailing understanding that we are in the midst of a slow but inevitable teleological advancement toward the end of AIDS. These crisis solutions reproduce neoliberal responsibilization. Under responsibilization, there is a shift in "responsibility from the state to the subject by responsibilizing them for their own self-help in dealing with increasing uncertainties and potentially traumatic events,"[31] and as Roderic Crooks notes, this is often deployed rhetorically by emphasizing "moral duty and agency."[32] It is on the individual to get tested, practice abstinence or safer sex, or shy away from serodiscordant relations; to seek out, obtain, and adhere to treatment protocols; and, if and when one fails to do so, to be condemned and punished. Blame for new infections is routinely placed on the individual's damning insistence on socially aberrant behavior—sexual promiscuity, intravenous drug use, criminality—despite the fact that "they really should know better."

The U.S. health care system and global sociopolitical realities mean that access to treatment regimens and medical care, and thereby to undetectability, is available only to some. The category of undetectable excludes and further marginalizes members of the "viral underclass" in America, usually poor, Black, Latinx, Indigenous, queer, and/or cis or trans women.[33] HIV vulnerability and AIDS-related suffering and dying are unevenly distributed by race, class, gender, sexuality, indigeneity, carceral, housing, and immigration statuses. It is no accident that those who are most affected are the same persons othered such that Judith Butler asserts they "never counted as lives at all."[34] Systemic violences curtail access to culturally competent education and health care, working against the stability and security requisite to often arduous adherence to lifelong treatment. Undetectability has also been utilized to argue that laws criminalizing HIV transmission, still on the books in more than thirty states, are outdated and that people with "undetectable" virus loads should not be subject to prosecution. This reform approach leaves behind people with detectable virus loads, disproportionately Black and unhoused, who are unable to access expensive medications and thus are still vulnerable to prosecution. Undetectability ultimately depends on a viral underclass.[35] Structural conditions under neoliberalism are conveniently sidelined. Moreover, reliance on the pharmaceutical-industrial complex is a solution characteristic of late capitalism. While reaping tremendous rewards, there is little industry motivation to work toward medical cure. In public health, the end of AIDS has come to mean a significant decrease in HIV transmissions, not a cure for the millions living with the virus. Evoking as it does an impatient wait for their demise, this discourse marks those with HIV or AIDS as the impediment to pandemic's end.[36] A more holistic notion of AIDS cure is rapidly becoming beyond the bounds of the imaginable or enactable.

Curation offers an emergent space to powerfully contest AIDS's cultural and political undetectability in ways that disrupt contemporary endemic AIDS time's normative registers. From treatment protocols' earliest availability, artists have represented medications and explored their complex roles in diverse lived HIV/AIDS experiences.[37] In 2012, Nathan Lee and Rachel Cook curated the first show on this status, entitled *Undetectable,* for Visual AIDS. As Andy Campbell wrote in its catalog, the exhibition was premised on undetectability's specificity "as an embodied identity that warrants consideration as a part of, and apart from, seronegative and seropositive statuses."[38] In the opening essay, Lee described undetectability as "signifying a presence that is absent, predicated on suppression and surveillance, the undetectable occupies an indeterminate space and produces new modes of connectivity, at once increasing the capacity of a body and subjecting it to a relentless regime of control."[39] He highlighted issues of bodily autonomy and political economy inherent in pharmacological solutions. The show raised complex questions about undetectability's affective ramifications, with its "feelings of confidence, defeat, survivorship, guilt, power, love, boredom, dailyness, relief, haunting, imbrication, and trauma," Campbell wrote.[40] In the artwork featured in promotional materials, a 2012 proposal rendering for *Nested Voids: The Conspiracy,* Bradley Pitts combined scientific and architectural approaches to visualize a brightly illuminated vitrine within an expansively gray room. Behind the case stands an anonymized, translucent human figure peering through the glass at the artist's "e-mail correspondence and photos" documenting "the clandestine installation of an imperceptible artwork with in 'Voids,' a retrospective of empty exhibitions."[41] Pitts created an abstract, multilayered archive of the undetectable. The show included artworks explicitly referencing HIV and many that in their citational "obliqueness" gestured to the particularity of undetectable lives.[42] In this chapter, I analyze *Why We Fight: Remembering AIDS Activism* and *Not Only This, but "New Language Beckons Us,"* two exhibitions intentionally curated around undetectability. Both were held with and inspired by AIDS activist archives from the NYPL, Fales, and Visual AIDS in New York City in 2013–14. I examine through these shows how undetectability shapes contemporary cultural practices, policies, and the politics of caring for and connecting with persons living with HIV/AIDS. Its curation simultaneously shapes present feelings, memory practices, and contention with the past of AIDS, thereby holding profound implications for its future that are, as I will show, meaningfully engaged through vital nostalgia.

Curating to Make AIDS Detectable

The curation of the NYPL's 2013–14 exhibition and programming series *Why We Fight: Remembering AIDS Activism* by Baumann with archivist Laura Karas made the historical and contemporary HIV/AIDS crisis newly detectable to the city's public. The exhibition at the Stephen A. Schwartzman Building's Sue and Edgar Wachenheim III Gallery (initially examined in chapter 2) showcased posters, pamphlets, artifacts, and video, drawn primarily from the NYPL's extensive archival collections of AIDS activist organizations and individuals.[43] Vitrines containing a plethora of archival artifacts were arranged topically: "Changing Perceptions of People Living with HIV," "Safer Sex and Needle Exchanges," "Public Mourning," "Healthcare Activism," and, in a final panel, "HIV Today." Ambitious public programming for teens and adults across the five boroughs accompanied the exhibition. Art critics and activists rightfully called out the show's nearly exclusive focus on activism from 1981 to 1996, rather than current anti-AIDS activism. However, despite the limitations the exhibition's normative temporal register imposed, when taken as a whole, *Why We Fight*'s curation demonstrated a generative deployment of vital nostalgia in its engagement with undetectability. In this section, I will demonstrate how *Why We Fight* made HIV/AIDS visible and visceral again. First, I trace curatorial choices that reactivated AIDS activism's affective and embodied nature to disrupt the dominant historicizing representation of AIDS. Second, I demonstrate how the inclusion of the Undetectable Flash Collective, cocurated by the NYPL and Visual AIDS within the show's programming, reflected a deep involvement with the AIDS crisis's present, persistent realities more explicitly than was accomplished in the archival exhibition.

"We're fired up! We won't take no more!" chanted the ACT UP/NY activists on videotape. Their booming voices and bodily actions—feet marching on pavement, hands clapping—formed an ambient cacophony that resonated from the video installation throughout the gallery. The video installation gestured to the show's curatorial methodology, which aimed to counter AIDS's undetectability by producing interactions with the activist past that registered legibly for visitors on bodily and affective levels. *Why We Fight*'s archival mobilizations thus catalyzed possibilities for dissent, now and into the future, through the vital nostalgic activation of historical activist experiences.[44] The gallery's prime location meant that thousands of patrons and tourists wandered past, expanding the encounter with AIDS activism to a general public likely not there for AIDS at all. Visitors were immersed through sound and its affective provocations into the recreated crush of the lively crowd that characterized early 1990s' direct action. The video's sound was not confined within headphones "because activism is noisy," Baumann told me.[45] It ran in an endless loop, operating autonomously, which afforded it a distinctive capacity to affect and hold viewers' attention. Revivifying public interest in HIV/AIDS when it is no longer routinely visually embodied or widely represented requires curatorial engagement that takes undetectability into critical account.

Emphasizing embodiment through AIDS archival records humanized diverse AIDS activism experiences. Vital nostalgia offers a means of engaging AIDS archives in ways that question, confront, and repair the structural power inequities that harm and regulate the lives of people with HIV/AIDS. Activists made, distributed, and wore many of the graphic materials featured. The show reminded visitors repeatedly in its records selection and textual interpretations that human hands held, waved, and passed out these posters and pamphlets, that human bodies donned these T-shirts. Moreover, the exhibition insisted that activists were real, complex people, both gravely ill and resiliently healthful. There was an insistence throughout the exhibition that the relationality between activists' bodies mattered, particularly as many others with privileges, whether heterosexuality, whiteness, middle-classness, or HIV-negative serostatuses, amid an epidemic recoiled from touching those infected.

Archivally oriented exhibitions, Baumann noted, are dominated by "little bits of paper."[46] He continued, "You have the signs. You have the things that people held, but that's not enough" to ensure that the archival records displayed have an emotional impact on viewers that they carry from the gallery into the streets. The show mobilized video's particular potentiality for viscerality. The clips Baumann selected and edited for display on the installation's back wall were culled from digitized records, material shot by activists and held in the NYPL's vast AIDS Activist Videotape Collection.[47] It was not only the format but also the videos' contents that produced my relationship to the past AIDS activism and activists on screen. The footage came from three early 1990s ACT UP/NY–involved demonstrations. The first two events, the 1992 Ashes Action and 1991 Day of Desperation, fit into the now-dominant narrativization of AIDS activism. First, they starred ACT UP/NY, the most famous anti-AIDS activists. Second, they showcased widely recognized aspects of the group's actions at the period of their height in membership and activity: theatricality, intense emotional registers, grand scales, provocative political aesthetics, and media-centricity. In the short Ashes Action segment, for example, we watch activists deposit their deceased beloveds' cremains onto the White House lawn. It was one of the "most dramatic" and "powerful" of ACT UP's political funerals as well as "a pivotal personal moment" for Baumann as a former ACT UP/NY activist who had participated.[48] Although an unsurprising selection, this moving, intimate, and painful footage still brings tears to my eyes, even countless viewings later. The second clip for me works on a different emotional register. In the Day of Desperation footage, a massive action in which thousands of ACT UPers took over Grand Central Station protesting the United States' involvement in the gulf war, we see activists storm the terminal's Beaux arts halls. At the top of the stairs, they unfurl, with an intoxicating, palpable mixture of collective excitement and rage, enormous banners demanding "Money for AIDS not war." The circuits of reference were intensified because Grand Central Station is mere blocks from where visitors stood; many may have walked through the same halls moments before. These two clips play self-consciously on a prevailing ACT UP nostalgia, the present longing for the communal, political, and aesthetic features of that departed activist past experienced both by activists who participated and those of us who wish we had. Yet the final clip disrupts this viewer's simplistic nostalgia for a dominant rendering of AIDS activism. It shows a needle exchange action at City Hall. The action "was really small and it was a little boring," Baumann recounted.[49] The activists on loop are caught in another loop: "they're just walking in circles."[50] Not all of ACT UP's efforts were flashy, grand, or exhilarating. The tedium shown countered the perceived glamour and extraordinariness of direct action, typically shown in documentaries and feature films, as well as elsewhere in the exhibition. Watching the last segment, with its outright denial of voyeuristic pleasure, forced me to pause, questioning my boredom in ways that expose the conflicted politics of AIDS representation now.

For *Why We Fight*, the gallery walls were converted into installations (Figure 10).[51] AIDS in the 1980s and early 1990s was in the public's face, whether evident in the at the time more common visible markings of illness on the body's surface or through the ubiquity of activist interventions in urban spaces. Recreating such embodied visuality was crucial to the exhibition's engendering of bodily and affective engagement for visitors. Reprints of iconic, much nostalgized graphics such as "Silence = Death" and "Kissing Doesn't Kill" were pasted to the walls. Torn and layered, they evoked an earlier moment when posters were inescapable forums for information exchange and public declarations, especially in pedestrian-driven New York City. This form of activist intervention is temporally bounded, targeted into disappearance by Mayor Rudolph Giuliani's mid-1990s' "quality of life" policing[52] and ensuing gentrification. "If I showed the poster in a frame, then it's not really the poster, because the poster would never have been framed; it would just have been slapped onto a street corner, or a lamppost or something. Framing it almost makes them not really what they are," Baumann told me.[53] Reproducing the graphics from digital files and displaying them in less-than-pristine condition was an effort to make these objects and the people who made and circulated them real for visitors.[54] "The only way to turn them back into what they really were," Baumann reiterated, was to restage "what I would have done to the original" in the early 1990s, to "just wheat paste it to a wall, and rip it."[55] Recreation was a means to experiential authenticity. The exhibition's installations used vital nostalgia for certain activist artifacts "to make this moment," Baumann said, "enter people's existence again." The show's curation made HIV/AIDS not only detectable but also made it matter again by activating its archives.[56]

Why We Fight received meaningful critique, including from AIDS activist communities, for its frame of "remembering," reflected even in its title. From the wall texts Baumann wrote to the records featured, the exhibit recentered the period Gill-Peterson calls "epidemic time," 1981–96.[57] The exhibition's temporal framing aligned with the retrospective register and focal period of most contemporary projects about HIV/AIDS in America, from film and television to museum shows and memorials. It is precisely such historicization of AIDS activism that ACT UP/NY contested in its opening night die-in at *Why We Fight*, discussed in chapter 2. The

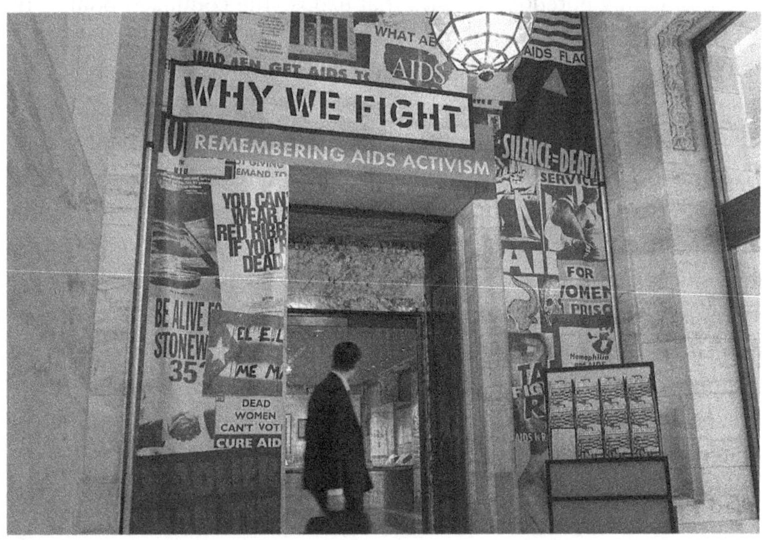

Figure 10. View into to the gallery of the 2013–14 New York Public Library exhibition *Why We Fight: Remembering AIDS Activism*. Logo design and photograph by DresserJohnson. Courtesy of Kevin Dresser and Katie Johnson.

possibility of retrospection at all when it comes to AIDS is dictated by positionality to power that allows those with racial, economic, and cisgender privilege to take for granted many of earlier activists' triumphs and limitations. Emily Colucci's review played with a famous line from activist-artist David Wojnarowicz's exhibited journal on loan from Fales: "If I die of AIDS, don't give me a memorial, give me a demonstration."[58] Of attending *Why We Fight,* Colucci wrote, "I felt that I was watching a long-ago historical event, rather than a demonstration about a crisis that continues to rage on."[59] The show's material coverage of AIDS activism concluded with 1996, the same year as the cocktail's advent. This end point supports the dominant narrative that biomedical innovation signaled the end of AIDS activism, reducing a complex movement to treatment activism and a singular aspiration of getting drugs into bodies.

While AIDS's "endemic time,"[60] which began in 1996 and continues, was not captured by the records displayed, *Why We Fight*'s interpretive descriptions did in measured ways address the contemporary pandemic and its concerns. The label for Gran Fury's "Women Don't Get AIDS: They Just Die from It" poster, for example, highlighted early activists' concerns about women with HIV/AIDS and charted their successful challenge of the CDC's initial AIDS definitions, which excluded symptoms of infections that manifest in female bodies, making it difficult to obtain treatment or state benefits. It concluded, "Early concern for women was prescient, as they now account for half the people living with HIV, and AIDS is the leading cause of death among women of reproductive age worldwide." The final wall text, "HIV Today," also attempted to bring the show's narrative into the present. "The AIDS epidemic is far from over," it noted before enumerating statistics and referencing the World Health Organization and UNAIDS's goals to achieve universal access to HIV prevention, diagnosis, treatment, and care by 2015—goals that were not met. However, the few contemporary-leaning texts did not counter the overarching representation of AIDS activism's pastness. As Colucci wrote, "Wojnarowicz did not want a memorial, and the AIDS crisis and activism shouldn't have one either."[61] Baumann framed the exhibition's temporal constraints as reflective of the AIDS archives' limitations. The show "didn't tell the story of the activism that's happening today" because "I don't have that archive. . . . What's happening today, that's not history yet."[62] Baumann concluded, "In retrospect, I might have wanted to make the show come up more to the present."[63] As an exhibition, *Why We Fight* did not go far enough in engaging archival records in service of redressing the injustices

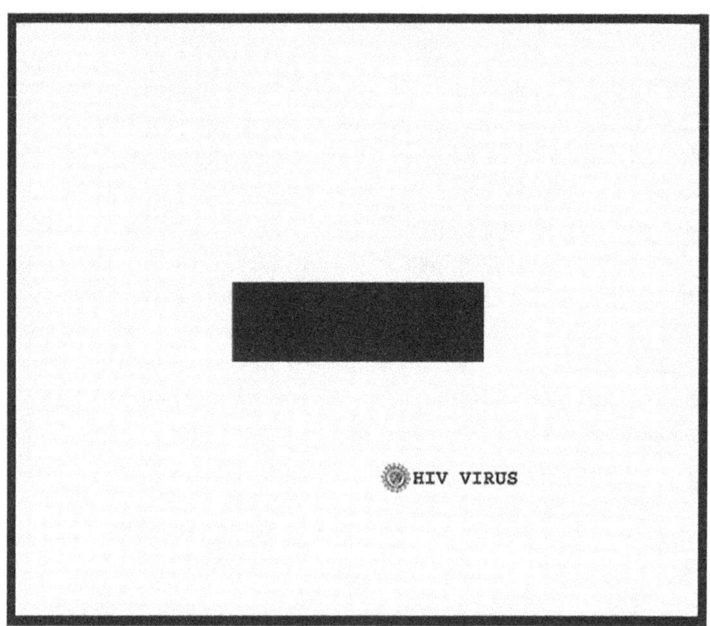

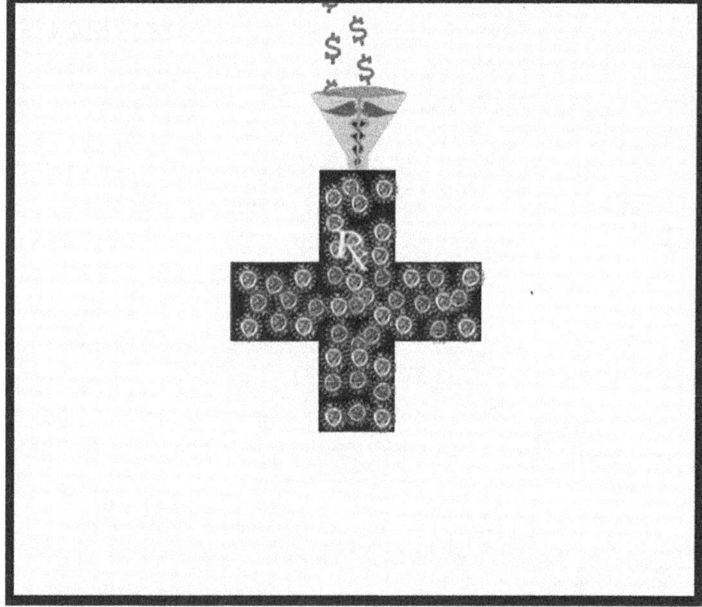

Figure 11. Undetectable Flash Collective member Hucklefaery Ken (Ken Mechler) created this GIF, which circulated on Tumblr during the early stages of the collective's work at the New York Public Library on undetectability. Courtesy of the artist.

that shape the contemporary pandemic. However, the exhibition modeled valuable steps needed to engage diverse publics by making crucially detectable activism's embodied and affective sensations.

Later that year, by developing the Undetectable Flash Collective collaboratively with Visual AIDS, Baumann did extend *Why We Fight* powerfully into the present. Logistical complications meant that the collective's installations opened in four NYPL branches months after the *Why We Fight* exhibition closed in April 2014. The collective became, to use Baumann's term, its "coda."[64] The collective, its process, and its intervention, demonstrated the power of vital nostalgic programming grounded in the AIDS archival past as a means of contesting AIDS's contemporary undetectability in the American imaginary. It utilized site-based installations and social media interventions to begin to renew public attention in hopes of sparking awareness and action within the pandemic's neoliberal present.

I recall my first visit to the Undetectable Flash Collective's Tumblr. A GIF played automatically as I scrolled. I stuck around to watch. On the blacked-out screen, a plus sign bounced. Shifting, one horizontal black bar emerged in the center of the now hospital-green backdrop. An HIV virion, circular with tentacle-like receptors, appeared and moved immediately upward. The retrovirus penetrated the bar, and another appeared. Metamorphosing through infection, the bar became positive, a full-on plus sign (Figure 11). At first, that sign contained only the single virion; however, it rapidly replicated and soon filled the sign, leaving no room to breathe. In the blink of an eye, a funnel marked by a caduceus appeared on top of the sign. Into it, green dollar signs dropped, transfiguring into an "Rx" that in turn multiplied to quickly vanquish the virus. I stayed as the funnel disappeared; on cue, the virion reappeared, and the whole sequence repeated. When only the faded plus sign remained, these words were overlaid:

> Maintaining strict compliance with antiretroviral medication regimens can reduce the risk of opportunistic infections & diseases in HIV Positive People & can significantly reduce the chance of new HIV transmissions (by over 90%). Cost for an individual's HIV antiretroviral medications range from $2,000 to $5,000 a month. Not everyone has equal access to information or treatment further perpetuating socioeconomic divides & HIV stigma. As there is more money in developing expensive, lifelong treatments, profit-driven drug companies have no financial incentive to find a cure.

I had just enough time to read the text before the GIF continued its unremitting cycle. The rhythm was hypnotic, each screen a flash, brief and

sudden. The next screen of text said in AIDS-ribbon red: "BEING 'UN-
DETECTABLE' LENGTHENS LIVES. BUT WHOSE LIVES? & WHO PROF-
ITS? WHERE'S THE CURE?"[65]

Digital media was a training ground and repository for the collective's work. Created by and for the Undetectable Flash Collective, this GIF
and a couple of others were posted, circulated, and remediated on Tumblr. Tumblr in 2014 was a popular digital media platform with a youthful
and queer fan base. Animated GIFs gained initial popularity in the 1990s,
when users were first able to create and host web pages, many choosing
to decorate them with copious animations—a flag blowing in the breeze
or a light flashing.[66] Making and sharing GIFs is a common mode of expression on Tumblr. The GIF's curated movement and transitoriness par-
alleled the collective's formation, their creative process, and the lenticular printing techniques they used. This GIF, still unpolished and unwieldy,
offers a view into the materialization of the collective's agitprop intervention in contemporary AIDS discourse. Its GIFs chart the collective
process of refining a visual message about undetectability's biomedical,
cultural, and political implications and its imbrication in capitalism, in-
equality, criminality and surveillance, medical cure, and the body. The
GIF ended on a summative query: "Undetectable [but at what cost?]."

The Undetectable Flash Collective demonstrated the tremendous contemporary possibilities of earlier activists' graphics and strategies, contained within AIDS archives and displayed in *Why We Fight*, for mobilizing
public recognition of present crisis realities. "We are being told people
don't care about AIDS, but I disagree after a decade of speaking around
the world and having people ask the same question: 'What can we do
now?'" artist and writer Avram Finkelstein, the catalyst for the collective,
shared.[67] He continued, "The answer to the question of how to reengage
a public with the issues surrounding HIV/AIDS in the present doesn't
lie *in looking at* the canon of cultural production from those early days,"
a canon that includes his 1980s' to 1990s' cultural productions with the
Silence = Death and Gran Fury art-action collectives.[68] It is only strategically "*in looking through* these works, to the resistance strategies
that brought them into being in the first place," that AIDS is made visible
for a weary and wary public. He concluded, "That's how we might imagine alternative models for the activation of our social spaces."[69] Finkelstein readily agreed to Baumann's invitation to blog for *Why We Fight*
but offered up a counterproposal to convene one of his flash collectives.
Flash collectives come together for brief durations—a few hours, or in

this unusual case, two months—to engage in a social process of political art and meaning making.[70] Member Nick Kleist noted, "With flash collectivization, there is an instantaneous community that emerges, focused around the intersection of art and activism."[71] Born of much-nostalgized radical political practices and communal affects of earlier direct action AIDS activism, the flash collective model he developed used, Finkelstein noted, "skills drawn on in collective decision making with a surgical and fast-paced format intended to cut directly to the point of the work, content."[72] The collective's addition to *Why We Fight* reflected an emphasis on community-driven programming. Baumann was excited by the project's potential to bring the exhibition "narrative up to date," incorporate "local current voice," and generate "dialogue with the community of people who saw" *Why We Fight*.[73]

The NYPL placed just two stipulations on what became the Undetectable Flash Collective. First, it had to address HIV/AIDS. Second, it had to engage with contemporary AIDS issues. *Why We Fight*, the archival exhibition and its public programming—panels, films, workshops—served as the group's inspiration. Individuals and private funders supported the exhibition and NYPL's LGBT initiative, from which it emerged. Time Warner, for example, was a founding supporter, and the MAC AIDS Fund was *Why We Fight*'s lead corporate sponsor. Private support meant minimal restriction, and Baumann set aside $20,000 for the collective. Finkelstein and Visual AIDS provided curatorial guidance, and together with the NYPL, they issued a call for participation. Flash collective "pedagogy" requires "interdisciplinary" participation, Finkelstein said, that facilitated "diversity in skills and perspectives" in ways that reflected participation in earlier anti-AIDS activism.[74] The fifteen collective members were artists, writers, activists, curators, journalists, policy wonks, and "Radical Faeries."[75] Finkelstein had hoped for greater diversity than was in the applicant pool so as to mirror HIV/AIDS's contemporary racial, class, and gender demographics and vast reach, and to signify that "in any room, there are people who have something to say [about HIV/AIDS] whether they know it or not."[76] All those who applied were invited to join; Baumann said the "participants selected themselves."[77]

The consensus-driven process by which the collective worked was an important curatorial decision. Finkelstein emphasized that it was in this process that characterized direct-action AIDS activism that participants, especially those from younger generations and with less activist experience, gained "tools and the experience of what it is like to be in a community, however curated it might be."[78] At the collective's initial gathering, Finkelstein asked members to consider how art could be an effective space for social intervention,[79] confront difficult ideas, and develop innovative communication strategies. Participation included three meetings at the NYPL and independent tasks. Engagement in the messy realities of the sometimes "painful" process of consensus-driven activism was a central purpose,[80] given that an idealized version of queerly radical communal collectivity is the object of much ACT UP nostalgia. Engaging in a communal process pointed to its value as well as to the realities of its difficulty and the power dynamics that shaped earlier AIDS activists' accomplishments and failures. The process moved participants toward a vital nostalgic engagement with the AIDS past necessary to take present action. "The collective," Kleist described, "is indeed a flash, it is a sudden rush of energy that occurs when all points touch."[81] It "was a little unwieldy, it spun out of control, it got very disagreeable," Finkelstein recalled.[82] Yet working through collectivity's challenges empowered members to find their voice and made them "willing to go on the record, to do it in public space," he said.[83]

The explicit focus on undetectability is significant to the collective's impact and its interrogation of core contemporary HIV/AIDS epidemic concerns: (in)visibility, contagion and transmission, and bodies and their limits. Members developed the theme and produced interventions through mapping exercises aimed at uncovering HIV/AIDS's ontological and epistemological nature. Activities generated possible subjects: the emergent and ongoing status of the HIV/AIDS crisis; pharmaceutical intervention and access; persistent fear, stigma, and discrimination; HIV serostatus disclosure; racialized, classed, and gendered HIV criminalization; and interqueer community serostatus divisions.[84] Undetectability is situated at their very nexus. Member Jano Cortijo called it "a fruitful and challenging experience" by which all "openly contribute[d] and respectfully discuss[ed] each other's ideas to arrive at an agreement about what our message would be."[85] It required the newly christened collective to define undetectability's meaning both medically and politically.[86] "Like HIV/AIDS," member Alina Oswald summarized, "undetectable is not only a medical term, but it involves every aspect of one's life."[87]

The collective's products reflected undetectability's categorical instability as well as the ways it speaks to how the contemporary pandemic is evolving. Oswald reflected, "The face of undetectability will be a fluid one, always changing. It defines a status some people can afford only for finite periods of time. But with advances in technology and medicine, what defines undetectability can change too."[88] Temporariness is significant in conceptualizing the lived experiences of undetectability.[89] Visual AIDS Archive Project early leader Eric Rhein described to me how experiencing undetectability raised troubling questions about his identity and self-conceptualization as an HIV-positive man and artist whose work focused on HIV/AIDS. He asked, "How does that word *undetectable* present me as a more physically desirable being in the world? Do I choose to share [my status now] as much as I did? Do I choose to have that [serostatus] to the front of my identity?"[90] Rhein's final rhetorical question lingered between us: "If my viral load somehow becomes detectable again, does it make me a different person?"[91] He was aware that his undetectable status may be temporary, and he questioned what it might mean in the future. "While an undetectable viral load is a blessing," he concluded, "somehow the term *undetectable* can be equated with *invisible*, that what all I have been through that has informed who I am is erased, and this can feel invalidating."[92] Being HIV positive once meant having to reconceptualize one's life and healthfulness as temporary; living as undetectable shifts and conditionally extends such a lifetime, scaling toward futurity in profound ways. Like undetectability itself, the Undetectable Flash Collective was temporary and produced interventions that were displayed only for brief durations.

At four site-specific installations in 2014, the Undetectable Flash Collective's statement *What Is Undetectable?* was displayed and distributed in ways that also reflect the contingency of undetectability's definition. Their intervention was lenticular prints—36 × 36 inch light boxes, two in English and two in Spanish, and 2,500 outreach postcards in English, Spanish, Chinese, and Russian, the primary languages of NYPL patrons (Figure 12). Since the 1960s, postcards—winking ladies and pinups clothed from one angle and nude from another—have been a popular lenticular product. The collective's outreach postcards were designed to disappear, distributed and dispersed into NYPL patrons' hands. Each light box's postcard read in all caps,

> We're at a crossroads in HIV treatment. HIV positive & HIV negative are no longer the only possibilities when discussing serostatus. The word undetectable has emerged in this conversation. Undetectable originated as a medical term for an "acceptably" low presence of HIV in the bloodstream dependent on strict compliance with "successful" antiretroviral treatments. Maintaining undetectable viral levels significantly reduces HIV transmission, but is

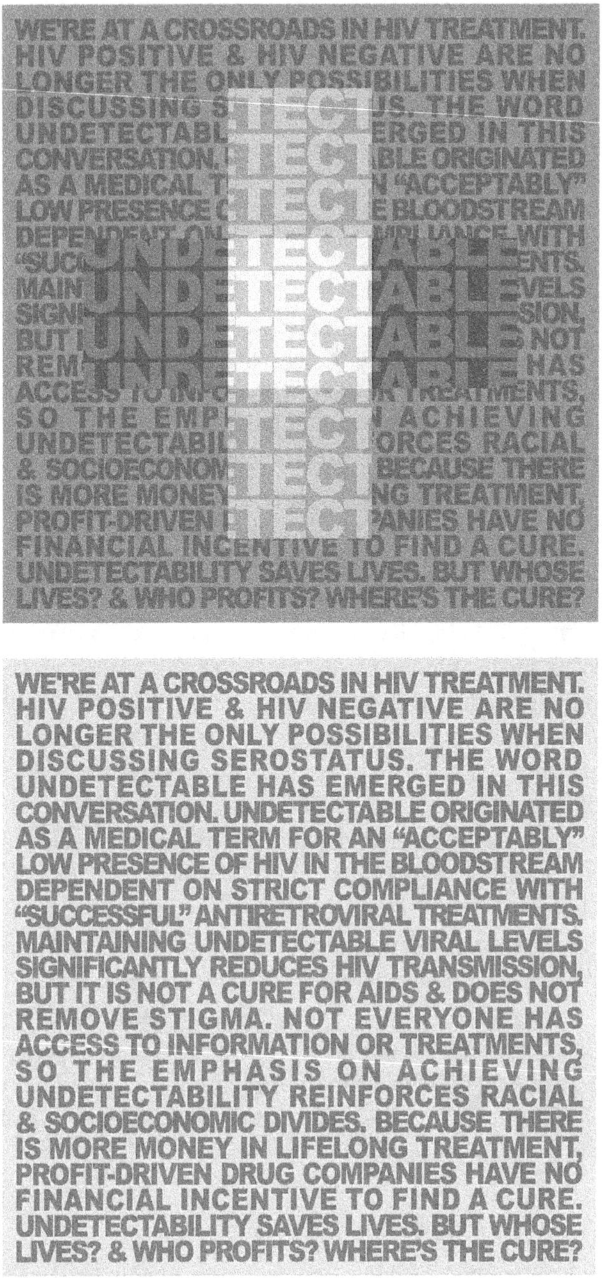

Figure 12. Avram Finkelstein and the Undetectable Flash Collective created this lenticular print of their statement *What Is Undetectable?* for the New York Public Library in 2014. Lenticular light box, 36 × 36 inches. Courtesy of Avram Finkelstein.

not a cure for AIDS & does not remove stigma. Not everyone has access to information or treatments, so the emphasis on achieving undetectability reinforces racial & socioeconomic divides. Because there is more money in lifelong treatment, profit-driven drug companies have no financial incentive to find a cure. Undetectability saves lives. But whose lives? & who profits? Where's the cure?

The words appeared on the familiar bloodred background. Each lenticular print flashed a stylized plus sign, one that evokes religious iconography and the Swiss cross, the West's generic emblem for medicine. The sign's presence and absence reflected that serostatus and its meanings were in flux.[93]

That the Undetectable Flash Collective's digital and analog interventions were public facing meant that they needed to make HIV/AIDS's contemporary relevance broadly legible beyond the tight confines of AIDS communities. They engaged the public at NYPL branches through which thousands circulate every month who are likely neither there for the art nor reflecting on HIV/AIDS. None of the branch libraries chosen had formal galleries; the light boxes and cards were installations that interacted with and interrupted each branch's central space. The collective's activation of public spaces beyond the loaded confines of the Midtown gallery in which the *Why We Fight* exhibition was held crucially broadened its reach and impact. Yet the locations selected for the collective's work also inform the racialized and geographic limitations of their project's reach.

Selecting branches was a point of some contention between the Undetectable Flash Collective and NYPL. Baumann sought geographic distribution and library sites with strong, supportive leadership. Baumann ultimately selected branches in neighborhoods that either had historical AIDS significance or present, peripheral relevance. At Jefferson Market, an English-language light box was displayed along with outreach postcards in four languages, as was the case for each site. It is in Greenwich Village, a neighborhood heavily affected in the crisis's early days and the site of major 1980s' to 1990s' activist demonstrations. Jefferson Market is located only a few blocks from the former Saint Vincent's Hospital, which in 1984 opened the country's second AIDS ward.[94] It is also where The New York City AIDS Memorial subsequently opened in 2016 in a new park across from the complex of luxury condos, complete with rooftop gardens and an underground swimming pool, which replaced Saint Vincent's. As Sarah Schulman has noted, it is no coincidence that the neighborhoods with the highest rates of infection in the 1980s and early 1990s, including the Village, are the same ones that experienced the most marked and rapid gentrification; those who died left openings, and their survivors, lacking rights, were often ousted from rent-controlled dwellings and replaced with straighter, whiter, and wealthier occupants.[95] For the second English-language light box, Baumann selected a very different site. Saint George is Staten Island's largest branch. Displaying the collective's work in a predominately white, politically conservative borough, one with lowest infection rate in the city, was symbolically important to Baumann. The Spanish-language light boxes were displayed in two Latinx-majority communities, Washington Heights and Hunts Point. The latter is in the Bronx, a borough that has some of the city's highest rates of new infections, a significant population of HIV-positive residents, and a striking number of AIDS-related deaths.[96] During the selection process, the collective had visited the proposed sites and conducted demographic research on HIV/AIDS in each neighborhood. The collective unsuccessfully pushed back, noting that none of the four branches were situated directly in the neighborhoods with the highest current rates of new HIV infections, nor within disproportionately affected Black communities. However, reflecting on the project during our 2016 meeting, Finkelstein remembered the locations as ideal: they were "completely mixed class, mixed race, mixed language; it was as close as you could get to a public street in New York."[97]

The Undetectable Flash Collective's creative installations were educational, introducing a broad audience to undetectability, a likely unfamiliar concept. Despite its brevity, their statement complicated the public's newly acquired understanding to bring attention to the inequitable distribution of crises that harm minoritized communities. They also engaged with the inequitable health care access and outcomes that shape the contemporary epidemic's devastation, showcasing for New York City's diverse public that while undetectability promises to prolong and improve the quality of life for HIV-positive persons, it is not an AIDS cure. Undetectability is not a cure biomedically, much less in the holistic ways imagined by Vito Russo in his speech "Why We Fight" or by Visual AIDS's Archive Project.

The collective's work did not end at the NYPL. Visual AIDS extended the Undetectable Flash Collective's existence and discursive reach. Staff were so taken with the collective's productions that they employed them as the basis for a 2015 program at the New Museum's Ideas City festival, themed "The Invisible City."[98] Together, Finkelstein and then–programs director Alex Fialho, himself a collective member, developed a performative "public dialogue." Printed on bright red balloons was the collective's query: "What is undetectable?" At the event, staff and collective members asked the passing crowd that very question. Like the collective's earlier work, this program offered a means "to continue to have that process with people from the general public," Fialho told me.[99] Over three hundred people responded, first writing their words on a balloon's blank side. The answers offered often had little relation to HIV/AIDS, ranging from "I saw five flying saucers when I was 6" to "Inner feelings (and) suppressed emotions." Those that did address HIV explicitly also related to the prompt diversely, from raising further questions, such as "Can undetectable folks transmit HIV?" to relating lived experience under the rubric of "personal goals." The facilitators led one-on-one dialogues about undetectability and its faceted biomedical, cultural, and political meanings. The Undetectable Flash Collective thus became, Fialho stressed, "even more outward facing."[100]

HIV/AIDS is in a crisis of visual representation. Much as the virus is invisible to the naked eye, so too is HIV/AIDS often outwardly undetectable. It is only in the late stages of AIDS that "visually legible symptoms manifest in the body," Patricia Keller and Jonathan Snyder write, whether in the form of "severe weight loss, purplish sarcoma lesions," or "the wasting away of limbs from muscle atrophy."[101] Before the advent of the (more) effective cocktail, in the 1980s until the mid-1990s, the presence of such symptoms that marked infected bodies was much more common, as was media and public attention to the dead, the dying, and their bodies. With improved treatments, AIDS's embodied visibility has decreased even while infection rates in many minoritized communities have not, including in Black, Latinx, Indigenous, and trans communities who are disproportionately subjected to poverty, incarceration, and other institutionalized oppressions. The frequent, willful cultural undetectability of HIV/AIDS has contributed to the contradictory perceptions of the virus as over and as a silent killer, living in the bodies of dangerous others who remain circulating in our networked midst. The Undetectable Flash Collective's interventions act as refusals of the relative invisibility of the American AIDS crisis. *Why We Fight*, especially its affective and embodied resonances and its germination of the Undetectable Flash Collective, rendered HIV/AIDS crucially visible again in New York City and online, albeit only temporarily and on limited communal and geographic scales. The show's curatorial work, grounded in the AIDS archives and vital nostalgia, thus moved us toward greater AIDS visibility requisite to garnering an appropriate response to continuing crisis conditions.

Creating Records to Surface HIV/AIDS

Through curation as a practice of care, activist archivists and curators make previously undetectable AIDS archival records newly detectable. Activist curatorial acts that cull AIDS records from where they are neatly filed in Hollinger boxes in closed archival stacks, seen regularly only by a selective group of archivists and researchers, turn HIV/AIDS, if only briefly, into a contemporary ongoing pandemic visible for the public. In this section, I examine the exhibition *Not Only This, but "New Language Beckons Us,"* held at Fales's Tracey-Barry Gallery in 2013. Curated by Andrew Blackley, this collaboration between Visual AIDS and Fales commissioned new creative works to dialogue with historical AIDS records from the Downtown Collection. The Downtown Collection documents AIDS activism within the arts scene in SoHo and the Lower East Side that flourished from the 1970s to early 1990s. It includes artists, writers, performers, and other creatives' personal papers and organizational records from galleries, theater groups, and art collectives. Then–Visual AIDS programs manager Ted Kerr noted that bringing together Visual AIDS and Fales demonstrated how Blackley understood "that institutions or organizations legitimize your work by cosigning . . . that exhibition which is already powerful and strong was made stronger because it came from these two organizations."[102] By displaying new artworks alongside archival AIDS art-action records, Blackley curated with vital nostalgia in a critical engagement that aimed to make HIV/AIDS newly detectable. As I will show, the records documenting the AIDS past, selected as inspiration and made visible through display, as well as the newly created textual and visual works that animated them reflected a means of engagement with AIDS archives that recognized, contended with, and worked toward rectifying the contemporary epidemic's inequities and injustices. Grasping tightly onto the AIDS past critically and with intention, vital nostalgia is a productive force that engenders possibilities for a more just AIDS present and future.

Offering leather gear, cock rings, portraits commissioned from the Tom of Finland studio, and a wide array of sexual enhancements, the advertisements that Robert Blanchon clipped from the back pages of gay porn magazines constitute the iconography of a much-nostalgized moment of gay sexual, cultural, and aesthetic life. Featured in Blanchon's

1995 photo-based conceptual artwork *Untitled (aroma/1981)* (Figure 13), the ads illustrate the heyday of gay white men's "sexual liberation," bookended by the 1969 Stonewall uprising and 1981 advent of AIDS. This short-lived period, driven by the radicality of following desire and resulting in lots of sex, often casual, anonymous, and in semipublic spaces—bathhouses, bars, discotheques, and resort towns—is much longed for in dominant white gay culture.[103] In *Untitled (aroma/1981)*, the imperative to defend and preserve an already departed moment of gay sex culture faces off against discourse that sought to mollify discrimination against HIV-positive people by "normalizing" gay men's relationships and sexual cultures so as to reassure heterosexuals of their fitness and morality.[104] Blanchon's title referenced "1981," the date of the advent of AIDS, and "aroma" poppers, amyl nitrite inhaled for the euphoric high induced during sex. In the early 1980s, when HIV's cause and means of infection were unknown, some scientists speculated that abuse of unknown chemicals was to blame for "gay cancer's" emergence, pointing to poppers as a likely culprit.[105] By 1995, the poppers accusation was outdated, absurd news, but there was still no cure, or even an effective HIV/AIDS treatment. Blanchon's salient critique of the homophobic, sex-negative blaming of gay men for their illness and death still resonates in a pandemic continually characterized by stigma, racism, homo- and transphobias, neoliberal self-responsibilization, and social death.

Untitled (aroma/1981) was intended by Blanchon to be dynamic, to move from apprehensibility to intangibility. He presented each ad as a fragile sepia photograph left unfixed. The images therefore maintained light sensitivity, fading away with slow deliberation day after day before finally disappearing and becoming undetectable. The artwork made absence sensorially present.[106] The work's previous detectability is renewed only through the archives and creative curatorial effort. Featuring this piece in *Not Only* showcased a careful consideration of AIDS's ongoing need to be made detectable. Since Blanchon's 1999 death at thirty-three from AIDS-related complications, the one hundred negatives he claimed to have made have disappeared; however, fifty-five of the supposedly ephemeral sepia on vellum prints, crafted in the early 2000s by Tania Duvergne, survive.[107] Acquired from Visual AIDS, the posthumous prints are held within Blanchon's papers in the Downtown Collection.

Each transparency was pulled from the archives and painstakingly reprinted by artist and curator John Neff for his 2011 show at Chicago's Golden Gallery and, later again, for a new piece displayed in *Not Only.*

Director Marvin J. Taylor was happy to loan the prints because Neff's exhibition, a process performance, was in keeping with his "desire to take up the cause of artists who had passed away and bring their work back in front of the public."[108] At Golden, Neff displayed on the first wall the borrowed archival records, what Blackley termed the "situationally frozen-in-time version."[109] Within the gallery space, Neff used the records to recreate, one by one, the negative transparencies that constituted Blanchon's original piece. On a second wall, Neff displayed the new unfixed sepia prints, slowly disappearing in the daylight the way Blanchon had intended. As he reprinted and removed the archival prints, Neff left the pins in place on the first wall, providing an elegiac reminder of what had passed and a

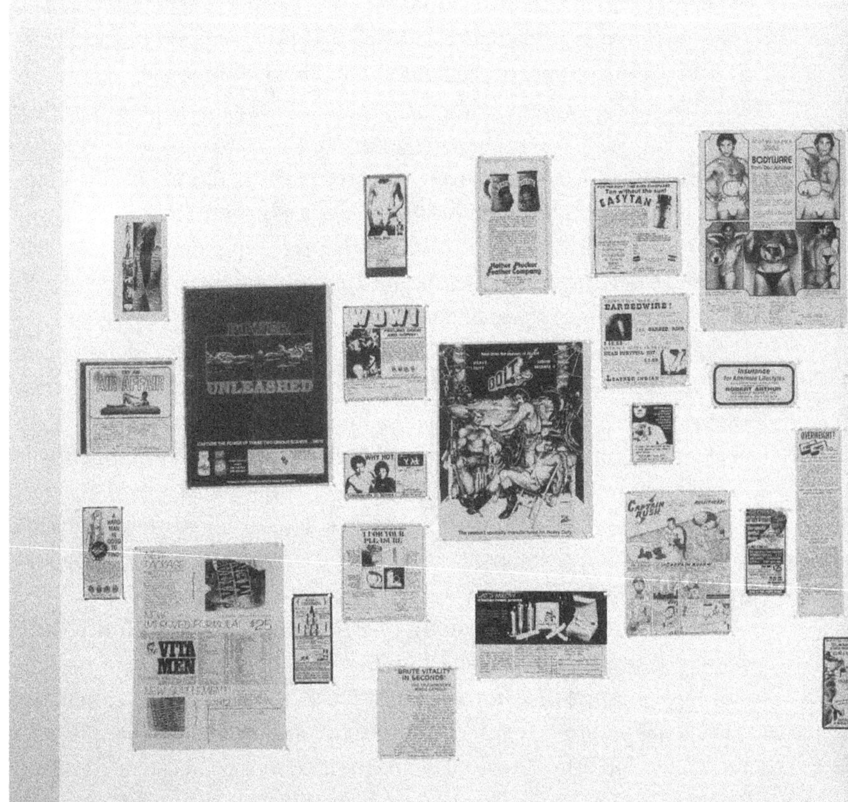

Figure 13. Artist Robert Blanchon's *Untitled (aroma/1981)* is a photo-based conceptual work created in 1995 featuring images of gay life before AIDS. Sepia prints on vellum; dimensions vary. Courtesy of the artist's estate and Visual AIDS.

mapping of new possibilities.[110] The process was "a way to learn about Robert's work, making a new experience of it while keeping alive—a changing and indistinct—memory of the 1995 piece," Neff told me.[111] His effort exemplified vital nostalgia because it did not seek to restore the artwork to an original, past state or to commemorate it. Rather, Neff's activation of the records engaged Blanchon's bold, difficult work on its own terms, with due risk and attentiveness to making process detectable.[112] After his show closed, Neff donated the negatives to Fales. During my first Fales visit in 2015, I photographed his negatives, which reside in two legal-size manila folders in series 8, "Memorials and Posthumous Files," of Blanchon's collection.[113] In 2013, for *Not Only*, Neff returned to

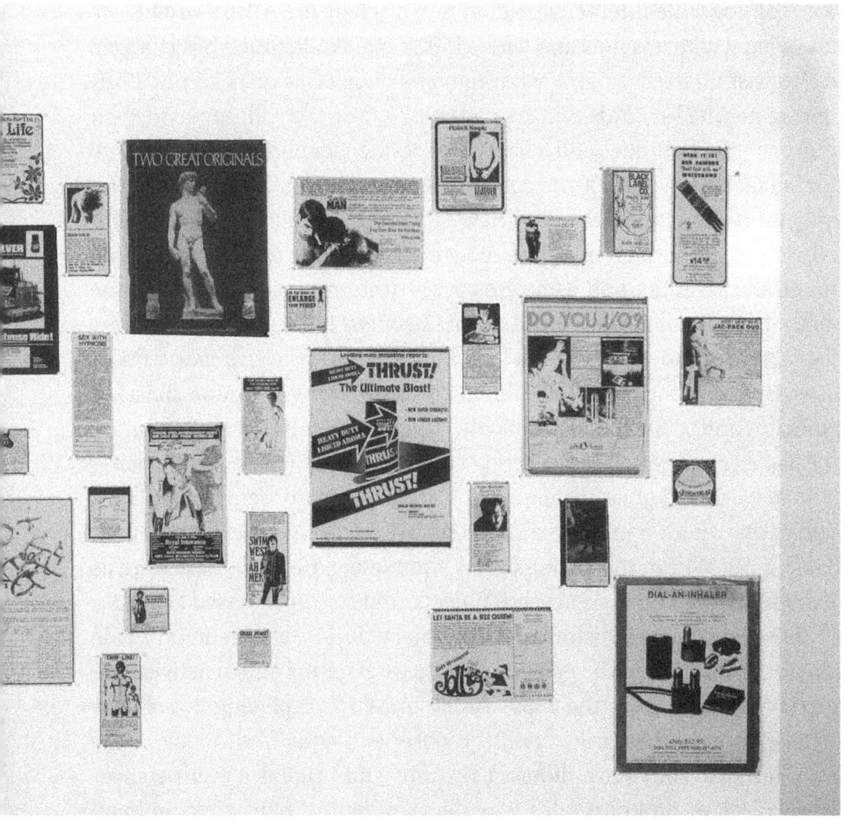

the transparencies, circling back in a written piece to mobilize anew the archival records he had created.

"I'm interested in archives being used to facilitate inquiry or exhibitions in the present moment. I'm less interested in history. I'm interested in what history surfaces in the present day," Blackley explained to me.[114] *Not Only*, in its fastidious composition that coupled Downtown Collection records with commissioned works from contemporary visual artists, filmmakers, writers, and activists, reflected his commitment to curating undetectability, to activating AIDS archives in the present and for the future. It was part of Visual AIDS's *Not Over*, exhibitions and programming marking the organization's twenty-fifth anniversary. The series "contemplated the deep cultural history of the epidemic, along with contemporary realities, in an interactive exploration of where art, AIDS and activism has been, where it is now and where it is going. While much has changed in the past quarter century, what remains is AIDS IS NOT OVER."[115] By pairing archival records and new artworks, *Not Only* illuminated their interpersonal "affinities and adjacencies, influences and recollections," to quote Blackley.[116] In each vitrine, objects created in distinct AIDS times—epidemic time, characterized by HIV/AIDS's confrontational and embodied visibility, and endemic time, where HIV/AIDS is undetectable both in cultural visibility and as a serostatus—were arranged alongside one another in intimate scale. Neff's *Untitled (aroma/1981)* transparencies were displayed, bound in a neat stack and placed next to Neff's new work, a letter he wrote for the event addressed to the show's curator, Blackley, explicitly, and to Blanchon, implicitly.[117] In the exhibition documentation at Fales through which I experienced the show, photocopies of the newly created work and of its accompanying archival record were again placed next to one another in a folder, illuminating, to use Blackley's term, their "kinship."[118] Within the vitrine's glass and metal structure, there were as many as twelve items: six archival objects, and six paper-based artworks.

Showing new and historical AIDS objects in intimate relation made visible continuities in the epidemic's structural harms and in activist creative production from the 1980s to the present. Displaying the objects together meant that "they could be observed, equalized on the same level, but also they have different textures and velocities and perspectives," Blackley emphasized.[119] The development of new works imbued each archival record with a fresh perspective, offering testimony to its enduring relevance. Returning to the transparencies, Neff told me, promised a revivification, a means to make visible the "care and repair, illness and fading at work in the work [Blanchon created] before I entered it."[120] Neff reflected in his letter on layers of "silence" and "ghosts" that occupy the interstices of his recreated prints and Blanchon's vision for *Untitled (aroma/1981)*. Echoing ACT UP's famed slogan, "Silence = Death," Neff articulated how "sometimes, silence equals luxury. Certainly Robert— by all reports a loudmouthed queen—couldn't afford to keep quiet."[121] He continued, analyzing his earlier recreation of the original AIDS art- work: "The challenge is: how to act and talk through the image without presuming to explain, without mystifying, without resorting—in the end— to silence."[122] The show's new works used their voices to demonstrate how AIDS activism and cultural production need to exceed normative elegiac summation. Blackley recalled being "very nervous" as a young curator, trying to do justice to "twenty-five years of an organization," and to more than twenty-five years of AIDS.[123] The curation did not progress in a nor- mative teleology; instead, its circuitous, networked progression moved viewers back and forth in time and space, illustrating the meaningful continuities between the cultural production, activism, and experience of HIV/AIDS—then, now, perhaps always. It needed to be crystal clear that even if it gets less public and artistic attention, Blackley asserted, that "AIDS is as relevant in March 2013 as it [was] in March 1986."[124]

Not Only appealed to Fales as an exhibition that not only used archival materials but also addressed the nature and limits of AIDS archives. The show played self-consciously with and against the AIDS archives' repre- sentational limitations and their profound dangers when it comes to tell- ing the story of AIDS and its arts activism. The Downtown Collection, "no matter how wide and expansive it is or may become, by virtue of being discrete, there are histories it does not, and cannot, include. It is not the history of New York; it's also not *the* history of art; it is not *the* his- tory of activism . . . and yet," Blackley told me, "it is *a* history of New York, of art, of activism."[125] Acclaimed gay white cismale artists are overrepre- sented in AIDS archives, including Fales. Its records could never, Black- ley acknowledged, "tell the full story of Visual AIDS, of HIV/AIDS."[126] He acknowledged the pressing need for "more voices here," voices beyond typical stakeholders—archivist, curator, or records' creator, subject, or donor.[127] By inviting thirty participants, Blackley "asked other people to be in this problem with me."[128] *Not Only* became "a call and response" between the archives and the artists.[129] Each was directed to create in relation to any object of their choosing from the Downtown Collection.[130] Some did their own research; others engaged in research together with

Blackley; for some, Blackley visited the archives and shared digital images. Julie Ault had previously done research and a performance piece involving archival processing at Fales, but Blackley's invitation, "to dive into the archive . . . diving for pearls," still afforded novel opportunity.[131] "There was this freedom to come into the collection, this invitation to be a researcher without the demand of lengthy research or research that would result in any conventional scholarly way," she remembered.[132]

The relations between contemporary artists and archival creators were multiple. *Not Only* showcased how AIDS archives can spark new relationships with persons who lived with HIV/AIDS and make newly resonant diverse experiences of the virus. Some had never met the record's creator. A potent queer "intimacy" developed between Blanchon and Neff, who never met in the flesh, through long-term archival entanglement. Neff described becoming "completely enthralled" with Blanchon after his first online encounter with the artist in Visual AIDS's Artist+ Registry, and remaining so to this day.[133] A letter, a form that "documents and solicits intimate relations," was for him the perfect relational response because it was "simultaneously public and private . . . something Robert would enjoy. An exchange between friends that, publicized, also does a different kind of work."[134] He signed off, "As always, with affection, John."[135] Similarly, John Keene selected painter Martin Wong (1946–99). Keene could still "come to this project and speak to that work," and to AIDS, even as his access to Wong was mediated by archival access, Blackley noted.[136] Others directed their contributions to someone with whom they had a prior relationship outside of the archives, be it fleeting or enduring. Joe Westmoreland wrote a new public letter to Dennis Cooper, jump-starting the form with which they had engaged as pen pals in the 1980s and 1990s. On display alongside his 2012 letter was an open envelope with a 1991 postmark addressed to Cooper in Los Angeles, as well as its enclosed flier for a screening of Westmoreland's film, *Betty Page: Setting the Record Straight*.[137] His new letter moves back and forth between past and present. AIDS is omnipresent, whether in memories of debates about the relation of art and activism in the late 1980s, notes about the crisis's "devastation," his detailing of summer 1995 when he became increasingly ill, his memories of how illness consumed his life, the messy savior of antiretroviral medications, or the power of writing.[138]

The archival records selected by contemporary artists for *Not Only* reflected HIV/AIDS's social, cultural, economic, and technological breadth both in the 1980s to the 1990s and 2010s. The artists' only production confines were the structure of the archives itself and the need, Ault said, to "background," "foreground," or "middle-ground a relation to AIDS."[139] The interpretations of what constituted an HIV/AIDS record varied. For example, Dodie Bellamy had known fellow artist Kathy Acker (1947–97), whose materials she chose. The inclusion of Acker's materials, an artist who "did not live with HIV, and yet—given her life—of course she lived with (within, alongside) it," Blackley emphasized, reflected how AIDS as a category extends beyond the virus's biomedical confines.[140] AIDS, and this show, were "about trauma both social and medical, about art and activism. None stop so distinctly or neatly so as to be able to exclude . . . Dodie Bellamy or Kathy Acker from the conversation."[141] Making AIDS fully detectable now requires loose borders as it lives, he continued, in the "air we breathe, ideologically, institutionally."[142]

Some artists emphasized how sociopolitical issues shaped by HIV/AIDS in the 1980s and 1990s manifested with significant contemporary implications. Ault focused on AIDS and gentrification. She selected from Wong's papers the 1986 press release for *The Last Picture Show*, which was "hand-drawn, handwritten, poetic, and just very exceptional."[143] It was a solo show of Wong's life-size paintings depicting defunct Lower East Side storefronts, each, she wrote, "compassionately rendered casualties of yuppification—from churches to drug establishments to restaurants and a 'poetry store'—sat silent and gated, on the cusp of uninvited redevelopment."[144] Wong described in the release: "It was the best of times. It was the worst of times and the times we had they gone now. They'll never come again. And all those sweet kids used to run the streets with Mikey wonder what they're running now and where . . . and you know if these walls could speak they'd probably be subpoenaed. Even now it's like the moment in these paintings never existed."[145] He documented the gentrification enabled by AIDS's casualties, both the deaths of countless friends and neighbors, and subsequent eviction of their lovers, friends, and compatriots. This document, Ault wrote in her 2013 piece, afforded "glimpses of empirical circumstances, sensations, and reveries that the shuttered facades opened up for him. The evoked embodiments stood for relationships with intimates and friends, and friends of friends, with acquaintances and familiar strangers, many of whom were, by then, lost from Wong's daily life."[146] In other words, it documents undetectability, a disappearance from view. Ault knew Wong and his Lower East Side intimately, and she has an ongoing posthumous relationship with him through his artworks and records. In our interview, Ault described choosing this piece because it contended with gentrification, a topic whose lived, gendered, racialized, and classed poignancy was just as immediately resonant for New Yorkers in the 2010s.[147] The drive to make AIDS detectable again in the contemporary city at the heart of *Not Only* inspired her; it was about "what do you want to talk about, to show people right now, and finding the language to do that in the archive, to engage."[148]

The exhibition's deliberate slow-burning rhythm intervened in the dominant strictures of endemic AIDS time to make HIV/AIDS viscerally detectable in our twenty-first-century AIDS time, where its relevance goes underrecognized. The show's curation powerfully deployed archival logics of undetectability and vital nostalgia to intervene in the velocity of AIDS's temporal registers. The traditional form, vitrines, and dominant format, paper, in the archival exhibition were intentional. Vitrines evoke a profound, enduring sense of preciousness in their preservation and removal of the artifact from direct touch. Paper, however, "is a nexus, a technology that," as Allison Piepmeier writes, "mediates the connection not just of 'people' but of bodies. Paper facilitates affection."[149] *Not Only*'s textual, paper-based form reflected the archives' contents—befitting for a curatorial engagement with the meaning of AIDS archives.[150] Taylor, Fales's director, was enamored of how Blackley "curates art shows that have a lot of writing in them," noting that "he is unapologetic about people having to read." *Not Only* "was the epitome of that," he concluded."[151] Blackley acknowledged that the show's reception was mixed: "A visitor would arrive to the exhibition only to find themselves bending over multiple vitrines, reading some fifty sheets of paper. I understood it might not end up being a 'crowd pleaser.'"[152] There are significant access restrictions to critique in this curation: the many texts were English-language centric, they required high levels of literacy, and people with differing vision and textual processing abilities could easily be excluded from access. Yet for the willing and able audience, the show's persistent power was its requisite slowness. "I was OK with the project being a slower project. You could go into the exhibition and read there, or you could look at it later online or in the archive. . . . No version or mode was necessarily celebratory," Blackley told me.[153] The unhurried pace and quiet reverential space of the gallery privileged contemplation. It created needed space for mourning and melancholy. In an AIDS context, creating contemplative space remediated the rushed pace that dominated the pre-1996 crisis, the period when most of the featured archival records were created. AIDS activism's fast, furious pace permitted little space for sadness, grief, or slow, percolating affects. *Not Only*'s curated temporal intervention made possible deep emotional engagement with HIV/AIDS. In doing so, it recognized and disrupted dominant AIDS time, and thereby the destructive retrospective currents that typically pervade in the contemporary curation of AIDS and its archives.

In curating with AIDS archives, logics of undetectability offer a means to surface that which is also undetectable in the archives, whether records, networked relations, or lives. For example, artist Gregg Bordowitz's 2013 contribution was a text created in response to painter and Visual AIDS's Archive Project cofounder Frank Moore's sketchbook. In documenting the show, Blackley photographed each of the pages displayed from Moore's papers. A copy of that black-and-white photograph was placed next to a photocopy of the contemporary work inspired by it. In this case, Bordowitz's words share an acid-free archival folder with Moore's pages, much as they did previously in a vitrine. The *Not Only* collection Fales acquired is newly networked, providing an entry point to countless other collections, creators, subjects, objects, spaces, and feelings. Such "hidden collections," whether hidden because they are unlisted or listed only under a collective title, or because they are un- or underprocessed records,[154] hold materials that are thus undetectable. Inaccessible records transcend format (print, microform, video, digital file) and raise pressing concerns about representation, security, staffing, institutional memory, and inequities in access.[155] Following, for example, the photocopy of Nancy Brooks Brody's textual 2013 piece with the copy of the six or seven snapshots from Wong's collection that were displayed links a user—someone like me—to the more than seven hundred other snapshots, and far beyond. A user is invited into a constellation of connections that Wong's papers hold with the photocopy of the archival object, the new text, and a piece of paper that tells the location of that archival object, box number, folder number, or series number; this formed, Blackley told me, "paths through the entire collection."[156] This kind of encounter, "start to end," was "about the process of creating primary documentation," Taylor said.[157] Blackley called the entry of *Not Only* into the material constitution of the AIDS archives its "great achievement."[158] In its self-documentation, *Not Only* became "an archival initiative, an intervention in the history of the Fales and the time the Fales documents."[159] Blackley contrasted the brief temporality, the temporariness of detectability in an exhibition that spanned only a few weeks, with the archival acquisition of these materials, "a permanent addition to the Fales Library; it's not going to be their most popular collection ever, but it will always be there for somebody to reference."[160]

Taking Up Vital Nostalgia

My access to the archival exhibitions *Why We Fight* and *Not Only* was through AIDS archives. I arrived in New York, and at this project, years after the shows had taken place in galleries, library branches, and museums. Yet they have an ongoing presence via the AIDS archives—the same archives that curated these shows. Through documentation, the shows that dealt in undetectability are made meaningfully detectable beyond the brief tenure of their display. The presence of archival documentation demonstrates how curatorial care by activist archivists and curators can make AIDS records, and HIV/AIDS, more enduringly detectable for the public. Such a reengineering of AIDS's cultural detectability is required in our endemic AIDS time, as archives are routinely utilized to prop up retrospective narratives that render HIV/AIDS in America as a past tragedy rather than an unfolding emergency.

Typically, AIDS archives are reductively understood as devoted to the enduring preservation of the past. How archives arrange and contextualize the past in ways that produce a society's ability to live in the present and imagine its future go unrecognized by the public. Yet archives shape the ability to construct communal identities and engage in direct action, making them vital to AIDS cultural activism. In this chapter's final section, I illuminate how undetectability as a curatorial strategy grounded in care work moves archives toward serving HIV/AIDS activist communities ethically and fruitfully. *Why We Fight* and *Not Only* showcased through exhibitions and programming the utility of undetectability—a status steeped in the complex interstices between past, present, future—for curation that productively mobilizes vital nostalgia. Through curatorial engagements with undetectability, AIDS archives that hold the epidemic's past can be deployed generatively by curators and archivists to make visible the contemporary concerns and needs of persons living with HIV/AIDS. Such curation not only newly exposes the virus's past and present but also, through its interrogation and reparative address of structural power inequities, opens vital possibilities for remaking HIV/AIDS's future. This curatorial approach calls on archivists to claim a greater activist presence in the interpretation of materials in the exhibitions they curate and facilitate, new works they commission, and cross-institutional collaborations they build. Curating undetectability is a nostalgic practice that emphasizes the longing for past time and space while also attending explicitly to that past's ambivalences, complexities, failures, and violences. Together with undetectability, vital nostalgia disrupts established teleological notions about time's progression. The temporal and affective drag of holding onto the past in a vital nostalgic curation practice with and about AIDS archives is about its generative political potentiality for feeling, imagining, and enacting different, more just presents and futures.

We are now working in a time characterized by HIV's undetectability—not just in individual bodies but also in a culture where HIV/AIDS is often undetectable. This evacuates the crisis of its former urgency, which has serious lived consequences. Curatorial mediations and manipulations of AIDS archives are often complicit in obscuring or obliterating the complexities and inequities of the past, repackaging them for palatable consumption. AIDS has always been a temporal condition. It has damaged and cut short the lives of people affected and infected, in ways made especially visible in the era before cocktail treatment was available. Early activists' HIV/AIDS responses reflected acceleration, the rush requisite to fighting a virus that always seemed a step ahead. AIDS activist archiving is a production of such a temporal context. The biotechnical innovations manifest in undetectability have shifted AIDS time, slowing or stalling the illness's progression for those with persistent access, and along with it the perceived cultural urgency of addressing it. With improved treatments, AIDS's embodied visibility has decreased even while infection rates, suffering, and death in many minoritized communities have not. HIV/AIDS operates always in tandem with poverty, institutional racism and xenophobia, and heterocisnormativity.

How to broaden the public that pays attention to AIDS, that addresses and redresses its violences, is a vital question amid enduring crises. The exhibitions and programming analyzed in this chapter provide a response. Each, with varying persistence and reach, remediated AIDS archives, drawing on records to address the AIDS crisis now. Audience expansion is what the tactics of the Undetectable Flash Collective, for example, have to offer us, along with a view into how institutions and agencies of the state contributed to and mediated these kinds of projects. In this instance, more went right than wrong. It served as a partial antidote to the historical morass that includes the displacement of countless New Yorkers both during the 1981–96 height of the AIDS crisis and well after it, and the gendered, racialized, and classed inequalities and inequities that continue to mark the epidemic. Through affective and visceral experiences created with and through the archives, the exhibitions analyzed made HIV/AIDS substantively detectable, visible again in New York and online. It is here that undetectability really makes sense. Undetectability developed out of the nexus of HIV/AIDS research, public health, treatment, prevention, art, and lived experiences. As a framework, it pays due attention to how "evolutions in the lexicon are important to keeping AIDS visible," González tells us.[161] It can make AIDS culturally detectable, which is why there must be critical attention to undetectability in efforts to make the epidemic more visible, and to renew our fight against its erasure. Curators and archivists hold the power to use their practices to open multiple potentialities for a different AIDS present and future.

Undetectability enables curators to make a temporal disruption with critical intention that is requisite to engendering a contemporary audience's recognition of AIDS as both historical and ongoing crises. Ault described going to Fales for more than information: "For rejuvenation and reinvesting political, social, artistic convergence. . . . It's a certain kind of fortification to go spend time there." The AIDS archives is a "special place, where it's not about, 'OK, I only have a few minutes; I got to race through this material;' I slow down my pace so that I can spend time" with the records, she shared with me. She continued: "I start reading or looking at something and it's like, 'Wow, I didn't know that,' or, 'Look at this,' and I get involved and once that happens, it's like, actually in a certain funny way, the outside world can recede for that time that I'm there, because I get really involved in the contents and in the intangibles that are suddenly tangible in my hands and in my mind through the documents and objects." *Not Only* required from visitors, and trained them in, the same deliberate slowness and critical engagement with AIDS archives that Ault described. Its audience was required to engage with largely textual materials; visitors were forced to slow and stop, bend over to gaze at vitrines, read, and pause and reflect. That slowing down allowed for a nonlinear, noncelebratory narrative of AIDS activism and cultural production. Ault described feeling alienated from current AIDS time and "contemporary promotional culture. . . . The Fales takes me to a different place in my thinking as well as the chance to engage the works and processes of the practitioners and the groups and entities that are no longer active, except in the archive."[162] AIDS archives, curated in a practice of undetectability attuned to vital nostalgia, offer and expand to a broader public such release from the restrictions of living solely in the present; it allows visitors to detect the current presence of the past, and it pushes them to reflect on what that might mean for the AIDS pandemic's present and future.

A crucial part of archives' temporal work is building community and solidarity across space and time. As Brien Brothman notes, archives afford "opportunities to develop understandings of oneself and one's community as proximal to and integrated into past and future generations."[163] The activist curation analyzed in this chapter disrupted teleological, chrononormative expectations of a neat progression from past to present to future. While fair critiques were levied at the *Why We Fight* exhibition for displaying the expected AIDS activist past, thus risking a framing of the epidemic and AIDS activism only as history, the embodied interactions facilitated and the programming that Baumann developed tell another story. The Undetectable Flash Collective worked with an explicit mandate to use *Why We Fight* and the AIDS archives as inspiration. Crucially, however, they were called on to do so in order to better address HIV/AIDS's present. The collective's process and products demonstrated the activist past's material utility for the present. The group drew on image-driven strategies of art-activism, used so effectively during the 1980s and early 1990s, and adapted them for contemporary social, cultural, and political struggles with the virus. *Not Only*, too, moved explicitly between past and present by placing archival materials in dialogue with contemporary creative works. These curatorial strategies made detectable the present realities of the ongoing AIDS epidemic by acknowledging that although the temporality of HIV/AIDS may have shifted, challenging HIV/AIDS's inequities and injustices remains a pressing concern. These archival exhibitions disrupted linear, progressive time; each emphasized, above all, continuity.

Why We Fight and *Not Only* made the past of HIV/AIDS activism newly detectable in 2013 and 2014. They did so in the context of the age of undetectability for HIV not only in science, public health, and medicine but also in cultural discourse. Each exhibition worked with a combination of small-scale installations and public programming to emphasize the partial histories of AIDS activism as well as the links forged with other twenty-first-century social justice movements. Even as their curation sometimes replicated the elisions of the past and reinforced progress narratives, the ways these shows mined the structural, material, and symbolic qualities of the archival records on display meaningfully shapes contemporary understandings of AIDS and of undetectability. Each show activated archival materials to bring the past into critical focus in service of mobilizing for a better HIV/AIDS present and future. These exhibitions narrated the nonlinear relationship between past, present, and future. This is the work of a vital nostalgia, which emphasizes the productive longing for past time and space in order to attend to its ambivalences and complexities. Curatorial gestures called visitors' attention to the contemporary utility of AIDS activism and its projects, now decades old. Each exhibition also emphasized that the archives, and consequently the cultural memory of AIDS, are only partial and contested. These actions serve as a reminder of the continued political necessity for AIDS activism now. The past inserts itself into the present. The past is used by these curators to open multiple potentialities. It is about the process of reflecting on history and the passage of time. Vital nostalgia offers multiple through lines. It explores how to live in multiple times and places simultaneously, presenting ethical and productive challenges. This is a curated nostalgia in which critical thinking and longing are not oppositional or incommensurate approaches.

5

GOING VIRAL

Mobilizing AIDS Archives in Digital Cultures

I wanted to create a bridge that linked thriving and struggling Indigenous communities to taboo issues like HIV/AIDS. In making this poster, I also wanted to challenge other Indigenous artists/activists to speak up and create a space for HIV/AIDS within their communities and ceremonies that simultaneously take into account the impacts of colonization, disease, and government neglect in the hopes of healing. The same goes out to HIV/AIDS and Queer artists/activists: I want all of us to challenge the work we make so it includes the voices of the Indigenous Peoples of this continent.

—**DEMIAN DINÉYAZHI´** (2013)

ANNUALLY ON THEIR TUMBLR "heterogenoushomosexual," Demian DinéYazhi´ marks World AIDS Day. Since 1988, December 1 is recognized as a day of remembrance and action. DinéYazhi´'s December 1, 2015, posts included a link to video footage of ACT UP/NY activist and film historian Vito Russo's 1988 "Why We Fight" speech. The speech demands more than just AIDS action in the present; Russo issues a call to remember AIDS activists' transformative work for social change and justice. The digitized demonstration footage, hosted on YouTube, is ACT UP/NY–affiliated video collective Damned Interfering Video Activist Television's (DIVA TV) creation. The footage is also available on ACT UP/NY's website and is related to the tapes held in the NYPL AIDS Activist Videotape Collection. DinéYazhi´, a nonbinary Diné (Navajo) artist, utilizes microblogging platform Tumblr as the site for art-activist intervention. "Every step I tread in this landscape, Vito Russo is guiding me—along with a long list of brothers and sisters who fought and continue to fight for HIV/AIDS-related issues. Shine on, fabulous lovers!" their caption to the iconic video reads. DinéYazhi´ also applies a slew of hashtags: "#VITO RUSSO #WHY WE FIGHT #ACT UP #HIV/AIDS #HIV/AIDS-RELATED ACTIVISM #AIDS ACTIVIST #HERO #WARRIOR #BABE #BROTHER."[1] The hashtags are a means of collating, processing, and retrieving content; they are intended to incite viral transmission, to proliferate this archival record's rapid spread through Tumblr's currency of liking and reblogging.

At first glance, DinéYazhi´'s caption and hashtags read simply as articulated identification with Russo and ACT UP. Their sentiments seem to conform with a contemporary queer cultural nostalgia for a white-washed AIDS activism for which Russo and ACT UP are appropriated as symbols. Yet when reexamined in the context of the artist's Tumblr, DinéYazhi´'s digital remediation of this archival record's viral potentiality is a more complex political act. DinéYazhi´ transforms AIDS records by putting them into explicit dialogue with the violent histories and ongoing realities of United States genocidal settler colonialism. They demonstrate the power of a vital nostalgia approach: activist longings for a past time and way of critically engaging with AIDS archives that identifies, addresses, and repairs structural power inequities, conducted in and through onlining AIDS archives. DinéYazhi´'s work speaks fluently in digital culture's viral tongues, its AIDS articulations legible from person to person, person to machine, and machine to machine.

AIDS archives hold a powerful, if underacknowledged, significance in contemporary viral media cultures. AIDS records appear frequently on social media, especially on image-driven platforms like Tumblr and Instagram. They are posted and shared, often without contextual metadata, descriptive tags, or acknowledgment of their archival provenances, in ways that shape and are shaped by platforms' sociotechnical affordances as well as social, political, and cultural values. Some scholars, artists, and activists dismiss the liking and sharing of the AIDS canon created during an earlier epidemic era as vapid or trendy. They attribute the digital circulation of AIDS images to anonymous millennials and generation Xers who are merely culling the detritus and troublingly divorcing it from its AIDS context and cultural knowledge. Activist Sarah Schulman, for instance, argues that "grassroots protest is our only hope for survival, not something to be marked and sold, a set of images and memes."[2] Users who curate AIDS-related images online are routinely portrayed by activists deeply invested in HIV/AIDS narratives as embracing past aesthetics rather than seeing the twenty-first-century politics and ongoingness of HIV/AIDS.[3] The viral transmission of AIDS activist records is framed as equalizing the depoliticization of young queer or trans curators and their audiences. Such discourse reproduces an outdated binary between on-the-ground activism and online slacktivism. This oversimplifies the political work and knowledge digital AIDS archival circulations produce.

By digitally manipulating and transmitting oft-nostalgized objects from AIDS archives online, Jess Mac, Kia LaBeija, and DinéYazhi´ reckon with the AIDS past, using it as viral catalyst to actions addressing the epidemic's ongoing gendered and racialized injustices and erasures. These contemporary, marginalized artists transfigure the archival records created during the 1981–96 "epidemic" AIDS time by using digital tools and media platforms. In so doing, they shift temporal contours of our post-1996 "endemic" AIDS time.[4] Whether creatively remediating iconic art-action images or personal video, these artists draw on the aesthetic political languages captured in acclaimed AIDS archives including the NYPL, NYU's Fales Library and Special Collections, and Visual AIDS's Archive Project, an organization each is affiliated with as an artist member or featured collaborator. In epidemic time, HIV/AIDS had a particular valence; a diagnosis before the development of pharmaceutical therapies was practically a death sentence. AIDS activists then were able to draw large crowds and garner critical public attention for the suffering and death at least of select gay white subjects. After the 1996 development of more effective antiretroviral drugs, in our endemic time, the little attention AIDS receives is only retrospective despite its ongoing devastation of marginalized communities. Mac, LaBeija, and DinéYazhi´ strategically perform through their creative vital nostalgia processes what José Esteban Muñoz theorizes as "disidentification."[5] Marginalized people targeted for assault, scapegoated, or otherwise harmed in world-denying ways utilize disidentificatory approaches to reconstruct a dominant cultural text's encoded messages, thereby uncovering that message's exclusionary machinations and reconstituting it to acknowledge, include, or empower minoritarian experiences and identifications.[6] Disidentification uses the dominant culture's objects as raw material to represent a politics or positionality that has been rendered unlivable, disrupting subordination by world making.[7] Mac, LaBeija, and DinéYazhi´, building from Muñoz, take up cultural texts from the dominant power within AIDS culture. The activist-artists situate themselves provocatively through a vital nostalgia grounded in disidentification both within and against the dominant gay, white, middle-class, cismale–centric discourses through which queer and trans people are called to identify with AIDS and its activism now. Mac, LaBeija, and Diné-Yazhí´ refuse the violent temporal registers of dominant AIDS time—ones that marginalize them and their communities into a position out of time.

The digital practices of Mac, LaBeija, and DinéYazhí´ constitute an alternative AIDS archives. These archives are created by and for constituents of those Steven W. Thrasher identifies as the "viral underclass."[8] BIPOC, those denied health and economic opportunities, trans and gender-nonconforming people, incarcerated people, immigrants and refugees, sex workers, and people who use drugs form the viral underclass—people who are harmed not just by microscopic organisms but by the societal structures that render them vulnerable to viral transmission and inadequate care after transmission.[9] In their creative remakings of archival records, the artists generate political discussion that privileges queer, trans, and BIPOC consciousness by unfolding an alternative AIDS time and asserting agency. The possibility of life with HIV/AIDS without violence depends on such vital nostalgic reimaginings of AIDS time and space that recognize and challenge the power relations that govern our records and bodies. Muñoz concludes, "Our charge as spectators and actors is to continue disidentifying with this world until we achieve new ones."[10]

From the 1980s onward, AIDS activists and artists have used computing technologies to construct powerful, life-sustaining political platforms, spaces, and networks.[11] Simultaneously, digital technologies and platforms have produced and reified AIDS phobia and been used to spread misinformation, stigma, and violence.[12] Modeling a vital nostalgia approach, in this chapter I center the visions of Mac, LaBeija, and DinéYazhí´. Enacting a vital nostalgia approach requires giving epistemological weight to records those in oppressed positions create, preserve, and reuse to document and resist their oppression and to imagine and enact liberation.[13] Mac, LaBeija, and DinéYazhí´ powerfully refuse through their digital art-activist practices harm and subordination, including those carried out against HIV-positive people in increasingly pernicious ways in digital cultures. They contend with the AIDS past to reimagine AIDS narratives in ways that engender more vibrant, livable presents and futures for queer, trans, and BIPOC subjects. The ways that the artists remediate with vital nostalgia AIDS archival records through digital tools and in online spaces demonstrates how the alternative AIDS archives they construct afford the means to envision different epidemic endings and engender radical beginnings. Digital practices of transforming and circulating AIDS records that are charged with political and personal meaning expose vital nostalgia's viral workings and urgent promise.

In this chapter, following a discussion of virality, I examine the artists' work. First, I analyze Mac's *Wojnarowicz's SILENCE GIF.* By turning a photograph of the artist's face into a GIF, Mac destabilizes its high-art cachet and establishes cultural associations in their GIF making and sharing. Second, I analyze LaBeija's digital mobilization of her personal AIDS archives in the film *Goodnight, Kia.* Finally, I examine DinéYazhi´'s *NDN Flag,* a digitally rendered poster that appropriates an iconic ACT UP image that in turn appropriated the American flag. Affect accumulates as these records circulate rapidly between networked users.[14] When uploaded and shared in practices of vital nostalgia, AIDS records have the potential to affect those who curate, view, and share them. By manipulating viral digital economies that favor acceleration and real-time interaction, Mac, LaBeija, and DinéYazhi´ remake records of the AIDS past to speak to and transform its present velocity.

Virality in Digital Media Cultures

Digital media creates new affective economies where archival records and cultural productions generated during 1980s and early 1990s AIDS activism in the United States frequently circulate and are powerfully remediated. The legacy of the AIDS crisis's early years plays out significantly in digital worlds that were then in their infancy. However, with a few notable exceptions, there is little critical scholarship on digital media and HIV/AIDS,[15] and even less on digital technologies' productions of AIDS time.[16] I follow AIDS records as activist-artists Mac, LaBeija, and DinéYazhi´ pull them out of their archival boxes and move them into digital platforms, where they transfigure and transmit them. Online AIDS records are frequently transformed into what Hito Stryerl calls "poor images."[17] Such images are "uploaded, downloaded, shared, reformatted and reedited" in ways that users do "for free, squeezed through slow digital connections, compressed, reproduced, ripped, remixed, as well as copied and pasted into other channels of distribution."[18] The transformation of AIDS archival records into poor images makes them newly accessible to a wider public, liberates from them from norms of quality, and subjects them to potent digital uncertainties of viral transmission.[19] In this section, I outline how viral media is shaping digital archival circulations, including how Tumblr provided (at least until 2018) a significant platform for archival work.

Mac, LaBeija, and DinéYazhi´ play on and with the meanings of virus and virality in AIDS and computing cultures. HIV, a retrovirus, is an infective agent transmitted through the exchange of blood or semen that rapidly attacks and multiplies in the cells of a living host, to detrimental effect. In computing, since the 1970s, the word "virus" has been used to describe a piece of code capable of copying itself into other locations, and thereby of propagating itself within a computer's memory or across a network, with detrimental results. Computer viruses are routinely conceptualized as biological viruses.[20] Both are understood as outside "infiltrators" attempting to disrupt a system's healthy operations.[21] With personal computing's rise in the early 1990s, Cait McKinney and Dylan Mulvin chart politicians, computer experts, activists, scholars, journalists, and artists' reliance on viral analogies and explanations honed during the HIV/AIDS crisis to explain "the risks of vulnerability in complex, networked systems." "Virality," they argue, embodied "fears surrounding interdependence, and emergent descriptions of precarity."[22]

HIV has been used to describe how digital media and popular culture works. Douglas Rushkoff argues that by transmitting messages that "attach" themselves to people, viral media are shaping thoughts and perceptions, reproducing themselves.[23] Virality has become a prime organizational logic of networked digital culture. Mac, LaBeija, and DinéYazhi´ comment on, critique, and create viral media, images, and information that are broadly and quickly circulated online. Viral phenomena are characterized by their taking advantage of access to a few nodes in a network, be that network social or technological, to spread to a wide array of connections.[24] Virality in digital cultures is always in close proximity to capitalism; it also emerged from viral marketing, or "the rapid spread of information (esp. about a product or service) amongst customers by word of mouth, e-mail" that developed alongside personal computing.[25] Mac, LaBeija, and DinéYazhi´ self-consciously manipulate AIDS records with digital tools and in digital environments. The viral media content they create is doubly viral because that content is about the nature of, is caused by, and is intimately entangled with HIV/AIDS.

Tumblr was a significant platform for AIDS activist and artistic intervention and archival remediation, including by Mac, LaBeija, and DinéYazhi´. Looking at this platform in 2021 is significant: it appears likely to be outmoded as a primary site of AIDS archival remediation online. In December 2018, after being ousted from Apple's app store platform for hosting sexually explicit images of minors, Tumblr announced an effort to create "a better, more positive Tumblr."[26] It banned "adult" content, including depictions of genitalia, sex acts, or "female-presenting nipples." While producers of sexually explicit content were less than 1 percent of users, its consumers included a quarter of users.[27] The decision pushed away the platform's core constituencies: trans people,[28] sex workers,[29] fans,[30] and artists.[31] Yet for several years, Tumblr, founded in 2007, was an important site of AIDS archival circulation and art-action production. Its youthful user base and the particularities of its design afforded opportunities for the formation of counterpublic spaces for marginalized people. It was a powerful site of media literacy, identity formation, and political awareness.

On Tumblr, images cascade upon images, 37.5 million posts per day, in a seemingly endless saturation.[32] Opening Tumblr, I and millions of users see post after post, traded from one user to another. It is a willfully disorienting space. Users typically offer few explanatory words, there are no standard profiles or friends, and search functionalities offer little straightforward traversing. Immersive temporal experiences on the platform emphasize ephemerality, "liveness," and flow.[33] New images continually appear in personalized feeds, pushing older ones out of sight or dropping them altogether. Each post, comment, or like is readily visible only for a short period. Use practices and social media interfaces reinforce a "nowness" that dictates recalibration of our lived times and attendant social relations.[34] Tumblr offered the unusual social media possibility for users to remain anonymous or pseudonymous. Its "semi-anonymity" made it, Mac said in an interview with Mikhel Proulx, a "cruising ground of aesthetics, porn, politics and selfies."[35] It was wildly popular with queer and trans users. Many of us use digital technologies for expressing identity and articulating connection in ways that temper the acute precarity we feel. Scholars argue that Tumblr's design uniquely engendered the capacities for a multiplicity of identity expressions: nonnormativity, fluidity, ambiguity, and nonlinearity.[36] Tumblr's "context collapsing also implies that one can be multiple; sexuality is not partitioned from one's politics (i.e., the way Facebook controls nipples and butts) and aesthetics." Mac continued, "Gender can be performed in a plethora of ways, as selfies are not a prerequisite to participation."[37] In what Alexander Cho calls its "queer reverb," Tumblr users could readily "resist prescribed narratives" and "change over time without fixed ways of presenting," thus engendering the nonlinear temporalities that permeated the site.[38] Users can also alter the HTML and CSS code to express individuality. Sensing the dangers of social media platforms in advancing white supremacist, heteronormative, transphobic machinic surveillance, many marginalized users selected Tumblr for its alternative, ephemeral, and opaque spaces to locate their feelings, politics, and relations.[39]

Tumblr favors regurgitated media consumption.[40] It is the aspiration of both Mac's and DinéYazhi´'s Tumblr practices to have their graphics go viral, as Mac said in an interview with Claire Paquet, to "show up everywhere."[41] Unlike other image-driven social media platforms that emphasize amateur photography (Instagram) or videography (TikTok), most content on a Tumblr is reblogged from others—or, as Mac described it, it is "reblogging as a quickie—one can touch without forming lifelong bonds, or without one's family and boss seeing."[42] Content appears in a feed, its transmission documented in notes added to a post whenever anyone likes or reblogs it. Tumblr images are often impossible to ascribe to a creator. Proulx argues that deemphasizing authorship reflects a commitment to accessible, mass-market popular media culture.[43] Creatorship on Tumblr is located around the personalized feed as a whole dynamic of constant movement and active selection. In other words, the platform emphasizes curation.

From online social networking's earliest days,[44] people living with HIV/AIDS and their allies have used digital technologies to communicate, organize, build resilience, and access lifesaving resources. Yet even as "virus," "virality," and "going viral" have become buzzwords in computational cultures, attention to HIV/AIDS has nosedived despite the reality that the epidemic rages unabated. The art-activist practices I examine reinsert AIDS into our understandings and mediations of the digital and reconstitute the AIDS archives. Remixing AIDS imagery on Tumblr is about engendering conspicuous online consumption. By using it (as well as by having work circulated on it by other users) as a platform for art-driven activism, Mac, LaBeija, and DinéYazhi´ address AIDS representation within networked media, contending with the central questions of twenty-first-century digital AIDS culture and activism. They are thinking through and manipulating how social media networks are utilized, as well as thinking through what kinds of generative political discourses can be provoked within them.

GIFing AIDS Activism

Wojnarowicz's SILENCE GIF (Figure 14) is one of the earliest posts on
Visual AIDS's Tumblr.[45] The GIF deploys an iconic image of David Wojnarowicz, arguably the most acclaimed artist of the art AIDS canon and
one of the most recognizable faces of an HIV-positive person, claiming
it as another artist's own through digitally facilitated remix. By turning
a photographic still into the popular, accessible GIF format, Mac destabilizes its high-art cachet and its established cultural associations.[46] In
doing so, Mac visually and textually contests the narrative that HIV/AIDS
is white, gay, and consigned to the past. The Wojnarowicz image Mac
takes up, a collaborative self-portrait, is a still from the 1990 documentary *Silence = Death,* about artists' responses to AIDS.[47] Wojnarowicz uses
the footage in his incomplete film, *A Fire in My Belly.*[48] This record is
also featured prominently in Wojnarowicz's papers, held at Fales, and
on his artist page within Artist+ Registry, Visual AIDS's digital archives.
Wojnarowicz, an artist, writer, and AIDS activist, was a gay white man
who died in 1992 of AIDS-related causes in New York City at thirty-seven.

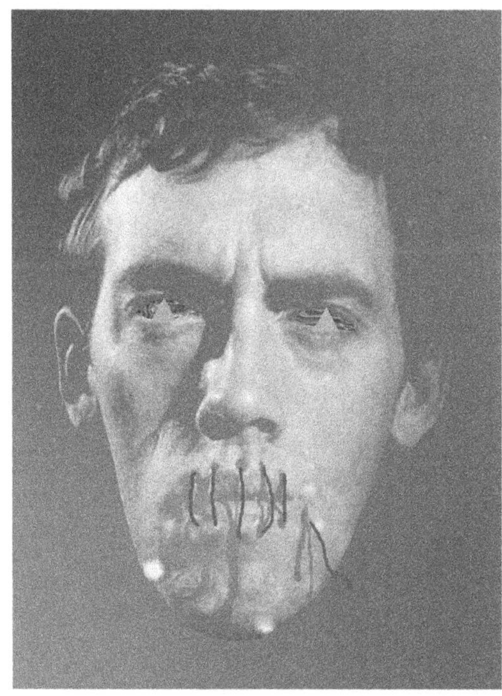

Figure 14. Artist Jess
MacCormack's 2015
*Wojnarowicz's SILENCE
GIF* is a GIF circulated on
the artist's Tumblr.
Courtesy of the artist.

The documentary charts, with eloquence and visceral fury, the myriad silences that have been imposed on Wojnarowicz—silences enacted against queers, and the loud silence of politicians and funders who in refusing to confront AIDS were hastening his demise. As Wojnarowicz speaks, the footage offers an anguishing visual collage. Ants walk over a crucifix; bandaged hands drop bills; and a human mouth is depicted being painstakingly, painfully sewn shut. Drops of blood trickle down the chin from the self-imposed puncture wounds. In the image and GIF, it is clear that this mouth belongs to Wojnarowicz. Five stitches lock his lips, and the needle is rendered still visible in his grasp. The self-inflicted damage announced a more prodigious structural harm. "I think what I really fear about death is the silencing of my voice," Wojnarowicz said in the voice-over. "I feel this incredible pressure to leave something of myself behind."[49]

Jess MacCormack, known by their online persona, Jess Mac, is a Canadian white genderqueer interdisciplinary activist-artist. The short, looping, hypnotic *Wojnarowicz's SILENCE GIF* was made for Mac's Tumblr, a cascade of queer and feminist GIFs created and curated over eight years.[50] Through GIF making and sharing, they critique internet age neoliberalism.[51] Their aim is to saturate Tumblr and Facebook with work ranging from stylized political imagery and slogans to GIFs that transfigure from celebrity selfies to HIV/AIDS art-activism.[52] Critic Proulx noted, "Jess riffs through the visual artefacts of 'Net culture with eyes turned equally to runway fashion, gay porn and tacky blogroll memes.'"[53] Mac utilized Tumblr as a daily ritual. The platform offered an accessible, fast way to integrate art practice into their day-to-day life.[54]

Mac's Tumblr is simultaneously a production of and an intervention against the creep of datafication and digital media virality. "We are all commodities now! We need a following and brand," Mac asserts to Proulx. They describe their digital persona as born of a "curiosity about how one could get reblogged and disseminated throughout the Tumblr 'community,' how to reach vast audiences and go viral."[55] To do so, they take up viral media languages, emulating "memes, symbols, hashtags, representations."[56] There is something powerful and paradoxical about utilizing a corporate digital media platform as the space to critique and contest the dominant economic, social, and political orders that the platform is a product of. The designed affordances and temporal structures of social media platforms are always about data collection and its monetization by the app or third parties. Social networking's business model is built on commercial surveillance. These "profiling machines"[57] collect and process user-generated data in order to effectively target services, advertisements, and content.[58] They willfully obscure the ways that such data uncovers user habits, behaviors, and identities. As it turns out, a refusal to work within the rules of "neoliberal capitalism, and its demands against criticality and inconsistency" makes Mac's actual attainment of "online 'popularity' impossible," in their words, "as it is always a question of power and promotion—the algorithms and those controlling them."[59] The inability to go viral does not dismiss the value found in manipulating virality's meaning and operation to reinsert AIDS into the discursive present.

In the GIF, Wojnarowicz's head floats, a cut from a cut of the film. Wojnarowicz's youthful face is framed by closely cropped dark hair. It appears over an ombré flashing background, hot pink at the top blending into deep purple by the bottom. The action is simple: Wojnarowicz's head moves left to right, seemingly cut and pasted into the frame in a loop without end. Even as Wojnarowicz's is a recognizable face, through its new action, Mac necessarily removes this image from a broader context that would clue the viewer into its original source and message. Mac's reediting mobilized the image to create contemporary resonances for HIV/AIDS by provoking new rhythms of sensation. Making and sharing GIFs is a popular mode of Tumblr expression. Animated GIFs gained initial popularity during popular computing's rise when users began to create and host web pages. Many decorated them with animations—a flag blowing in the breeze, a light flashing.[60] Even as GIF content has evolved with video-hosting sites' emergence, early animation styles like those that Mac deployed remain popular, especially given nostalgia for early web aesthetics. GIFs that evoke earlier technological eras have an alluring kitsch and authenticity attributable to a refusal of smooth sophistication.

Mac makes a few crucial AIDS-specific interventions in their creative remaking of this archival record. The first is to the mouth. In the GIF, the entirety of Wojnarowicz's lower face is marked up in ACT UP's signature hot pink. As the GIF endlessly repeats, viewers are encouraged to focus on the saturation of color into and out of the image that was originally a classy black-and-white gloss. Second, Mac highlights the stitches that knot together Wojnarowicz lips in AIDS signature red. They leave the thread's tail dangling into the void, a lurid trail of pixilated blood. Third, the GIF format's technically limited color palette means that images gain a willfully deteriorated graininess and substandard resolution. The newly rendered imperfections, the degradations in quality, transformed the photograph into a poor image, enhancing the temporal distinctions between the original and the additions made to it. Its digital cultural meaning is made more poignant "through the added emotional value" that Gil Bartholeyns argues is "provided by a temporal distance that is made visible by a dated aesthetic."[61] Fourth, as is characteristic of the format, the GIF runs in an endless cycle. Its loop operates autonomously, affording the creator power to capture and hold attention.

Finally, it is to the eyes that Mac makes the biggest transformation. The metaphorical fire in Wojnarowicz's belly is newly, explicitly visible, his pupils rendered red seconds before filling with pink squiggles. Mac's hand leaves its digital signature. In the cycle's last seconds, pink triangles pop from both eyes, defying the constraints of Wojnarowicz's eye sockets. That hot pink triangle, too, is a symbol provocatively associated with ACT UP and the direct-action AIDS activism of the 1980s and early 1990s. Reclaimed from its history as Nazi insignia that marked gay men's bodies for death, activists turn the inverted triangle.[62] ACT UP featured the pink triangle on a black field as its identifying emblem. It serves as a collective effort to remember a suppressed history of gay men's oppression and annihilation; it also evokes a sense that AIDS too was genocide,[63] one that again targeted queers and marginalized peoples. Drawing on the Silence = Death Project's work, ACT UP's triangle appears over the phrase "Silence = Death," demonstrating in ways that echoed Wojnarowicz's words: silence must be broken, and memory is a matter of survival.

The importance of Mac's critical intervention is complicated and underscored by the digitally driven corporatization of AIDS imagery. On Twitter, the Nike ad features a black sneaker with a hot pink triangle on its heel. The caption reads: "The upside-down triangle used in the 1940s was flipped right-side up in the '80s to promote a bearing of strength and solidarity—a symbol that runs strong through the Nike BETRUE Epic React Flyknit's all-black colorway." In May 2018, Nike issued its annual LGBTQ Pride Month collection. That year's theme, "reclaiming the past, empowering the future," revolved around "colors and symbols that have been reclaimed and historically repurposed by the LGBTQ community." Several designs prominently utilize the pink triangle, including as stylized backdrop in print and digital advertisements. In its press release, Nike describes the pink triangle neutrally as "a shape that has a complex past in LGBTQ culture." They assert in the language of corporate empowerment, "Today, the pink triangle is one of the world's most recognizable symbols of pride, resistance, and solidarity for the LGBTQ community, used to champion action for LGBTQ rights." It is only well into the release that the company acknowledges either AIDS or the Holocaust. Nike is far from the only retailer to appropriate AIDS imagery for profit; a Google search surfaces a pink triangle T-shirt from fast-fashion retailer Hot Topic, and Google's shopping pages showcase a multitude of apparel and accessories featuring the symbol.

Mac's GIF reflects a complex appropriation practice. It walks a precarious, provocative edge, risking being consumable and circulatable without much thought or critical orientation while simultaneously working as a manifestation of vital nostalgia. The GIF is both flashy and cool, its aesthetics aligned with brands like American Apparel, which was then embracing neon colorways. Mac identifies their aim as sheer quantity and obsession with amassing attention. Yet it is also true that the GIF critically remakes a widely recognizable image, one with potent high-art cachet, which is the object of nostalgia for what could have been, for a certain moment and brand of AIDS art-activism. Mac performs in a vital nostalgic practice with needed teeth a disidentification with dominant whitewashed narratives of the AIDS crisis that the original image symbolizes. By turning the image into a GIF, Mac destabilizes its high-art cachet and established a cultural association. Mac's digital practice, as Proulx put it, is "a real commitment to lowbrow viral media culture. . . . There is no allegiance to high-res here."[64] Through their remix, Mac repoliticizes this poor image in ways that speak to the current status of AIDS—a crisis of risk and punishment that, at least in North America, is stacked against trans and queer BIPOC. Mac mobilizes Tumblr and Facebook as cultural platforms and networked distribution mediums for GIFs and digital collages that address in their words the "intersection of institutional violence and the socio-political reality of personal trauma."[65] Working with communities and individuals urgently affected by stigma and oppression, Mac positions art as a tool to engender personal and political agency. Yet it is important to acknowledge the ambivalence in this work and its uptake; The GIF is part of the conditions of possibility for items like Nike's sneakers in its formal strategies. The edge of vital nostalgia can be quite close to conventional nostalgia, rather than opposite or incommensurable to it, and that fine line is part of what makes Mac's work risky and worth analyzing.

Wojnarowicz's SILENCE GIF worked in tandem with their poster for the 2012 AIDS ACTION NOW!'s PosterVirus campaign and their "Silence =

Shutthefuckup" series. The latter makes critical intervention around the criminalization of the HIV-positive body and its implications for relations with the self and the body in digital culture. Mac has focused on HIV/AIDS since 2012, when an HIV-positive man in Ottawa was charged with attempted murder on counts of administering a noxious substance, his semen, without prior disclosure to his sexual partner of his HIV sero-status.[66] Referencing explicitly and drawing on nostalgia for earlier AIDS activism, Mac describes as their inspiration art-action collective General Idea's 1984 "Shut the Fuck Up." The original articulates a seething rage against the art world and mainstream media. Mac draws on that rage and Silence = Death AIDS iconography to form a new pinkish triangle. Their triangle is constituted by imagery of collapsing stars and an eighteenth-century medical Venus. The work is, Mac said in a Visual AIDS interview, a "portrait for each of my friends living with HIV."[67] They draw on the visual and textual rhetoric of an earlier acclaimed AIDS era, but through vital nostalgia, they critique, build critically from, and push beyond the narrow activist objects and subjects of that earlier time. Their digital art-action practice is a reflection on living with HIV/AIDS now when the full humanity of HIV-positive people continues to be, as Mac put it, "in conflict with the law," and where in digital culture "the body becomes a site of control and resistance, identity becomes dissociated, social ties become conflicted, trauma is triggered in everyday, so-called normal activities, access to much needed resources is reduced, uncontrollable feelings of helplessness and rage are acted out."[68] According to Mac, art affords a space to process and articulate these struggles informing how we "tell stories, see ourselves reflected back, shape society and culture, how we resist."[69]

Tumblr offered the ideal site for critiquing the AIDS status quo and the digital platforms and cultures of which they are a constitutive force. Mac hashtagged the GIF "#aids #hiv #decriminalize hiv #fire in my belly #david wojnarowicz." Placed in context in their Tumblr, a veritable catalog of GIFs, each repeating in short but endless looping sequences, the GIF and its curation are powerfully disorienting, political, destabilizing, and world making. Easily sharable, *Wojnarowicz's SILENCE GIF* has accumulated more than four hundred notes on Tumblr and 105,000 views on Giphy, the largest GIF database. Mac's work demonstrates that there is a way through vital nostalgia to do conspicuous but also critical online consumption of AIDS archival records.

Viral Elegy

Only seventeen seconds into *Goodnight, Kia,* Kia LaBeija's (Kia Michelle Benbow) contribution to Visual AIDS's 2017 Day With(out) Art video program, "Alternate Endings, Radical Beginnings," the alarm sounds. Curated by Erin Christovale and Vivian Crockett, the program showcases narratives by Black artists about queer and trans Black experiences amid the ongoing HIV/AIDS epidemic. It is clear that the alarm is not in the room with us, but that it is nearby. Emergency lurks just beyond the frame. Twenty seconds into the soundtrack, the cacophony of unrelenting car alarms is profoundly disquieting. It plays dissonantly over digitally shot footage of grown-up Kia journaling in a window, her solitude resounding in the man-made light of the New York City nighttime. The alarm continues as we shift to the digitized texture of 1990s' home video footage of infant Kia. She is lifted high in her mother's arms, then pulled back earthward for a kiss. Thus begins the video's rapid, nonlinear choreographed shuffle through time and space—a vital nostalgic disruption. In another time, another camera crew snaps a clapperboard, the date 11-3-99, an undisclosed home movie starring nine-year-old LaBeija, who waits, twirling, to deliver her lines. Intercut throughout the five-minute film are archival home video and LaBeija's contemporary crisp high-definition footage. Along with LaBeija, the audience is pulled back and forth in time. The AIDS past is clearly both never fully accessible and never really past.

LaBeija's artistic oeuvre explores and fashions her identities as a Black, Filipina, Native American queer HIV-positive ciswoman and artist. LaBeija invited the film's audience into her moody, intimate, violet-hued dreamworld by mining her privately held, personal AIDS archives. The central subject of *Goodnight, Kia,* and much of LaBeija's repertoire, is her late mother, Kwan Bennett. The film centers grief and memories of Bennett; it investigates the intimate intergenerational connections between them as well as the continual challenges of living with HIV in an era of presumed HIV survivability. The longing and mourning in this elegiac film are militant, political actions driven by vital nostalgia. LaBeija calls her creations "cinematic and theatrical autobiographical works" that "stage, re-imagine, sometimes documenting in real time."[70] In her artist's statement, LaBeija recalls, "At thirteen or fourteen I got my first camera. I remember my mom saying how great it was. 'I want you to tape me so I can tell you everything about my life,' she said. But I never did it."[71] In 2004, the year LaBeija turned fourteen, her mother died of AIDS-related causes. She continues: "By the fall she was gone. That stuck with me for a long time; a regret that kept me up at night for years."[72] Bennett was an activist who worked relentlessly for others living with HIV/AIDS, especially her Filipina and Native American communities.[73] LaBeija frequently draws on these personal histories of activism and on her nostalgia critically: LaBeija felt "incredibly connected to the idea of archiving and capturing. . . . Especially growing up without my mom and knowing there were so many things that we weren't able to capture in photographs, I felt that void and loss."[74] The film continually visually marks absence, what is held out of loss. It includes as many shots without a person as shots featuring someone. Viewers are invited to follow LaBeija in and out of near-empty rooms. She creates an atmosphere in which both intimacy and voids are evident.

Goodnight, Kia reconstitutes through vital nostalgia not just a departed childhood and mother but also the lost environment of LaBeija's first home. In doing so, she centers a distinctly BIPOC vision of what AIDS space was. This film does not feature the widely represented street protests or ACT UP meeting rooms of mainstream AIDS films. We are instead invited into the domestic: the apartment at the Aurora at Tenth Avenue and Fifty-Seventh Street. This site was formative to her being, and LaBeija remains "attached to a space that's no longer mine."[75] It is clear that she still longs for this lost AIDS time and domesticity. LaBeija is invested in "looking back at the spaces where I've existed," but through creative mobilizations of her "own particular history," she works to "reinvent them."[76] Being ousted from the "safe space," the shared world with her mother, she writes, was "so painful that over many years I've blocked most of it out. I only have one or two memories of that time. I can recall sitting in my empty loft looking at friends and family, their faces unsure of what would happen next, slowly and carefully putting things in boxes. Any other thoughts exist only in the spaces in my mind I've chosen to keep locked up."[77] In 2017, her brother gifted the videotapes she features in *Goodnight, Kia:* "All of this footage he had of my old apartment. I was excited and nervous to see it. To hear my mom's voice and to see us in our home again. . . . Once you haven't been around someone in so long, you can begin to lose them a little bit. It's been beautiful reviewing the tapes, tapping into the memories that have seemed long gone." Her vital nostalgia centers on lost humans, times, spaces. Drawing from this alternative AIDS archives is key to the film's disruptive potency.

BIPOC people have long constructed AIDS archives, in forms within and beyond the structures of the normative AIDS archives and paper-based records. The importance of storytelling and embodied practice as archival forms in BIPOC communities remains underexplored. LaBeija, former mother of the iconic ballroom Royal House of LaBeija, in *Goodnight, Kia* indexes movement as a Black queer archival practice. LaBeija is well known for embodying the vogue movements that are her familial legacy. Adopting "LaBeija" as her "character, this persona,"[78] is a means of honoring and activating the rich histories of queer and trans Black and brown ballroom culture, and of the AIDS activism within them.[79] LaBeija notes, "When you hear *LaBeija* you already know what it stands for: resilience and glamour."[80] Will Rawls argues that LaBeija's film is more "dance" than "scripted story."[81] LaBeija describes "voguing in my pictures. To vogue is to tell your story through a series of poses; each pose is an image in itself. I think of my self-portraits as a dance with the camera."[82] Movement—dance—becomes a way for her of "working through the trauma that lives so deeply in the body."[83] In color-saturated contemporary footage, we watch her underwater choreography. Her moves are powerful and fluid in the luminous violet depths. There are almost no words in the film; the elegy of feeling exceeds them. The soundtrack transitions from alarms on city streets to the rich, looping music of her father Warren Benbow's Spiritual Jazz Quartet's performance of "Motherless Child." It is only in the final seconds, after the credit sequence has begun, that LaBeija, age nine, is audible. She faces the camcorder. From off screen, we hear a deep voice proclaim, "OK, and . . . ACTION," to which young LaBeija responds, "Which part?" It is the only audible dialogue; it becomes a punctuating question mark. She asks her audience to think back, to review the gestures, fragments, parts, asking them which seems to embody best the piece's message and subject.[84]

On Tumblr, LaBeija's poster *#Undetectable* circulates.[85] Visual AIDS routinely reposts content created by and about its artist members, including LaBeija. In the reposted digital edition of the poster, her contribution to PosterVirus 2016, LaBeija repeats the slogan "#Undetectable." She cites and mobilizes in form and content virality and undetectability on digital media platforms.[86] LaBeija's oeuvre includes digital self-portraiture and collage as well as film and performance using digital techniques for digital audiences, and she comments on themes of virality, networked relationships, and technical mediations of time and embodiment. In "#Undetectable," LaBeija collages the same digital self-portrait, layering it beneath her words. Her seven identical selves, fixed at seven disparate angles, fill the computer screen. Looking over her shoulder, LaBeija peers at the anticipated audience over her dark sunglasses, eyebrows arched and lips pouted under her neon green coiffure. Each Kia performs a self-fashioned calculated glamour, evoking midcentury femme fatale and punk siren alike. Her self-portrait speaks in the aesthetic language of the selfie that Instagram popularized, playing with a critical self-consciousness on Black women's self-representational practices,[87] and countering depictions of long-term HIV survivors in dominant AIDS culture. Even as LaBeija no longer has an active Tumblr, her work continues to circulate there.

Much of LaBeija's digital self-portraiture and performance challenges representations of long-term HIV survivorship. Long-term survivors are nearly always depicted in popular and AIDS media as gay white cismen who came of age before and during the 1980s, who witnessed the deaths of countless loved ones and acquaintances, and who, thanks to less than critically nostalgized heroic treatment activism and its pharmaceutical fruits, have lived with HIV since the crisis's height. Those we picture "as having survived AIDS," Hugh Ryan notes, are those we can actually conceptualize as "having had AIDS."[88] Dominant representations not only absent women, trans people, BIPOC, and children from the AIDS record but also lead us to believe that they were never there at all.[89] LaBeija was born in 1990 with HIV to an untested mother; both were diagnosed in 1993.[90] "My work gives a voice to issues that I think need to be talked about. I am a representation of a forgotten people—children living with HIV. We have always been left out of the history of AIDS, and now decades later we are still here," she asserts.[91] Of representation in *Goodnight, Kia,* LaBeija writes, "The archival footage in this piece is especially important. Most people see me as an adult living with the virus but how often do they get to see a full life with HIV. I think seeing ourselves as children always contextualizes who we *are*. By allowing viewers to take a peek into intimate moments of my childhood I am reclaiming who I am. I'm still that little girl, just a little bit bigger."[92]

LaBeija works against the dominant order of AIDS signification. Voyeuristic mainstream media spectacles of people with AIDS have long represented positive bodies as alien, ill, and dying, evoking pity, fear, and danger. Phobic images make AIDS visible by showcasing visual identifiers that mark some infected bodies in untreated AIDS's advanced stages. LaBeija offers a counter view from inside, positioning her positive body as vibrant, youthful, and alive—and as belonging to a queer Black milieu. In short, she is portraying, as Laura Stamm writes, a "body that is infected with but not defined by the HIV virus."[93] Mobilizing her archival records for LaBeija is also a means of countering mainstream AIDS representations, which Julia S. Jordan-Zachery documents render Black women simultaneously "invisible and hypervisible."[94] Black women in the aggregate are frequently invoked in AIDS discourse, labeled as the "fastest-growing" or "most at-risk" populations. Individualized selves and Black women's perspectives are omitted. Black women are routinely, as Jordan-Zachery points out, "denied access to care and their plight does not make it to the public agenda—they go unrecognized and unrepresented. While it appears that they are being talked about, in essence they are not being talked about—thus rendering them shadow bodies in the framing of HIV and AIDS."[95] In making herself subject and author, LaBeija, as Lyle Ashton Harris notes, is "not only speaking for" herself but also speaking back to "the history of photography, the history of these kinds of representations, and the power of the image."[96] Fashioning her Black queer femininity as the face of long-term HIV survivorship, LaBeija makes legible embodied experiences of HIV now. Taking up the paradigm of (hyper) invisibility, LaBeija emphasizes her work's service to girls and women: "My attention is on the children that are still around, and women, because it's so taboo for women to talk about it."[97]

I first watched *Goodnight, Kia* in a small theater in Maine during Day With(out) Art programming that my students organized. It was shown that day in hundreds of museums, galleries, campuses, and community spaces across the United States and around the globe. Yet most of its viewers have and will see it only as it circulates in digital media. The film moves in posts, likes, and reblogs on Vimeo, Tumblr, Facebook, and other platforms. Through vital nostalgia for an AIDS activist history that is uniquely hers, LaBeija invents herself as embodying a new AIDS era and futurity: "In ballroom, the idea of being an icon or a legend is key because an icon can never die." Artwork is a "way of creating my own immortality, of consistently being in conversation with people for the rest of time."[98] LaBeija's undetectable body virally transmits only AIDS histories and knowledges as it moves in digital space. She uses digital tools for visibility, to raise awareness, and to contest the social structures that marginalize, endanger, and erase bodies like hers. LaBeija turns to viral media to draw attention to contemporary expressions and experiences of HIV/AIDS, which are reflected and produced by our cultural situatedness in computing and digital cultures. She notes that one of the primary "powers of producing images" is that they "will outlast us. They will be in constant conversation with those who are looking at them and those who need them. For me, that's one of the things I love about art. When I see something and it speaks to me, I feel a sense of belonging, a sense of being understood."[99] Playing in and with nostalgia and virality by deploying a BIPOC queer lens, LaBeija demands through vital nostalgic practice that AIDS be understood as not just of the past but also as an inescapable condition of our immediate present.

Flagging Refusal

In 1989, activists Richard Deagle,[100] Tom Starace, and Joe Wollin created a new graphic to be circulated by ACT UP for Independence Day. The screen print turns the American flag, a long-standing emblem of nationalism, militarism, and imperialism, into a new kind of militant symbol of alarm. Activists posted the rerendered flag on subway cars, walls, and streets. The creators maintain the flag's recognizable blue field and white stars while transforming its stripes. They emblazoned on the red stripes a damning all-caps running text: "Our government continues to ignore the deaths and suffering of people with HIV infection because they are gay, black, Hispanic, or poor. By July 4, 1989 over 55 thousand will be dead. Take direct action. Fight back. Fight AIDS." Appropriating the flag was a timely political strategy given *Texas v. Johnson,* a Supreme Court case earlier that year that had affirmed desecrating the flag as protected speech. That decision prompted right-wing politicians to introduce legislation aimed at "protecting the flag," and in New York City it offered neofascists license to hold violent demonstrations.[101] A print of Deagle, Starace, and Wollin's flag is held within the ACT UP/NY Records at the NYPL.[102] It has been digitized and features prominently in the NYPL's digital collections. The print circulates frequently on Tumblr, including via ACT UP/NY's account.

In another December 1, 2015, Tumblr post, DinéYazhi´ shared their *NDN [Native Indian] AIDS Flag* (Figure 15). They explicitly appropriate Deagle, Starace, and Wollin's agitprop print. They renew it, transforming it into toothsome agitprop of their own. "Influenced by traditional Diné (Navajo) songs, which use repetition as a way to speak of continuity," they regularly utilize repetition, whether of words or images strategically. "There is always retelling, renewal, reimaging, revolution," DinéYazhi´ said of their process.[103] *NDN AIDS Flag* was reposted by Visual AIDS and hundreds of users. DinéYazhi´'s artwork is referential, playing on queer cultural nostalgia for an earlier era of direct-action AIDS activism and its aesthetics. Yet the flag is remade into something distinctly of the now. DinéYazhi´ keeps the archival image's recognizable nationalist American flag imagery, the all-caps proclamation, and attention-grabbing bright colors and patterns. These design elements draw the eye to their provocative decolonial AIDS messaging. Black stripes cross the now-white backdrop; white stars dot the red field. Their updated 2021 running text in all caps reads: "Our government continues to ignore the lives, deaths & suffering of people with HIV infection because we are queer, trans, Indigenous, Black, Latinx, addicts or poor. To date 700,000+ people have died. Take direct action now! Fight stigma! Fight AIDS!" The words are altered to reflect twenty-first-century epidemic conditions, evolved community-based language and identity terms, and new statistics. Moreover, what is novel is that the flag makes in words and images a queer and trans Indigenous critique missing from the earlier intervention—one that was meaningfully absent from the examined purview of 1980s' and 1990s' AIDS activism. Native Americans face significant health disparities, including HIV/AIDS. Between 2005 and 2014, the U.S. Centers for Disease Control and Prevention reported a 63 percent increase in HIV transmission among gay and bisexual Native men alone, as well as an overall HIV rate

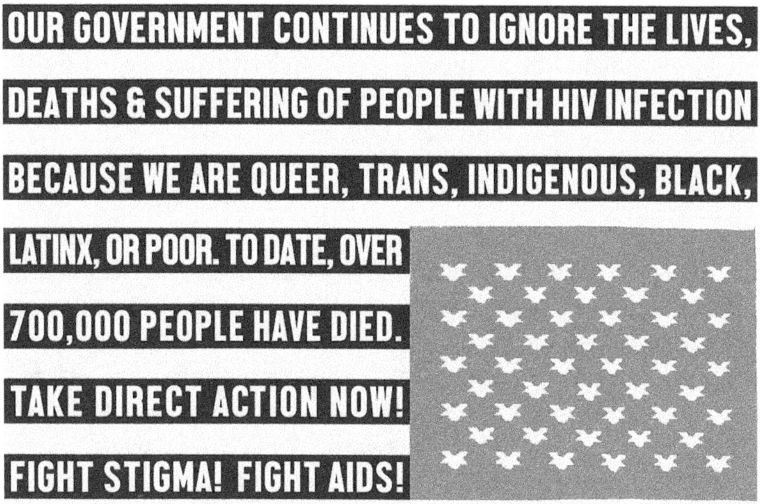

Figure 15. Artist Demian DinéYazhi´'s *NDN AIDS Flag* first circulated in 2015 on Tumblr and in 2021 was updated by the artist to reflect contemporary epidemic realities. Courtesy of the artist and R.I.S.E.: Radical Indigenous Survivance & Empowerment.

increase by 19 percent across tribes.[104] The flag's power is transformed once again in this reclamation of politicized aesthetics, AIDS culture, and the digital self. DinéYazhi´ speaks directly to the continued violence through erasure of nonwhite persons with HIV/AIDS from epidemic narratives. They format that damning critique within the American flag in order to continue to implicate the government in putting these persons at risk and to hold the state accountable for their sickness, suffering, and deaths.

DinéYazhi´ makes strategic reference to a nostalgized white AIDS activist canon while encoding the histories and values of their culture and Indigenous community of artists into their transformation of the dominant AIDS symbol. In this artwork, DinéYazhi´ engages in a long tradition of Native artists remixing the American flag—an emblem used to assert the sovereignty of a settler government on Native lands—as a means to address and redress the violences of settler colonialism and empire.[105] The star's shape mirrors those in the 1991 *Flag Rug*, a Navajo-style wool rug woven by Diné textile artist Bertha Harvey.[106] DinéYazhi´ works within the illustrious tradition of Indigenous artists replacing colonial materials and symbols with visually resonate Indigenous ones.[107] In their captioning of the high-res image shared on Tumblr, DinéYazhi´ notes both the ACT UP agitprop and Harvey's rug "were made around the same time as the HIV/AIDS epidemic and the continued genocide, forced assimilation, and various health epidemics Indigenous Peoples of north america have been faced with since the onslaught of colonization."[108] Manuel arturo abreu writes that the work of DinéYazhi´ "embodies survivance" in its "stewardship of the legacies of Native innovation, as well as nourishing and revitalizing Indigenous culture and forms of knowledge."[109] Similar to the dominant representational status of AIDS in the twenty-first century as only of the past, Indigenous peoples too are often confined to pastness in the popular imaginary. The living presence of Native artists in the art world remains rare, abreu notes, "since it challenges the museum's modus operandi: presenting Native art as artifacts from an idealized past."[110] Through vital nostalgia, DinéYazhi´ inserts the presence of their people and culture in AIDS time, its activism, and its narrativization.

DinéYazhi´'s practice transcends media and form, including curatorial inquiry, social engagement, performance and poetry, image and video production, and digital merchandising. The platform they create gives voice to and provides the means for envisioning a contemporary queer and trans feminist indigeneity. DinéYazhi´ notes, "I started off as a writer, so most of the images that come to mind are text-based. Sometimes I include photography, Native-inspired designs, and appropriated photographs or designs."[111] Rooted always in Diné traditions of storytelling, ceremony, and a recognition of land's sacredness, their work honors and advances these archival practices in digital culture.[112] DinéYazhi´ also interpolates dominant queer culture and its archetypes, troubles "romanticized conceptions of belonging,"[113] and highlights the oppression and alienation experienced by Indigenous and other queer and trans people of color, given centuries of forced assimilation to logics of white supremacy, colonization, capitalism, and heteropatriarchy. DinéYazhi´ plays self-consciously with and on nostalgia, blurring boundaries between past and present. Mediating history and the archives is requisite to facilitating the conditions where imagining a liberatory sovereign future is actually possible. DinéYazhi´ puts AIDS and its activism into explicit dialogue through vital nostalgia with the histories and ongoing presents of genocidal settler colonialism. By drawing attention to the intersectional injustices that AIDS has always been and is still characterized by, they mobilize AIDS archives and Tumblr as a site of contemporary political, economic, and social action.

The reconstituted *NDN AIDS Flag* is part of DinéYazhi´'s project, Radical Indigenous Survivance & Empowerment (R.I.S.E), an activist arts initiative founded in 2014.[114] Through digital work, such as creating downloadable posters, DinéYazhi´ has said, the R.I.S.E. agenda is "survivance" and "empowering our community and dedicating ourselves to our artwork. . . . It's a life-long battle that must be fought in order to ensure the perseverance of land and people, but also to re-establish the relationship of the people to the land. It's not just an Indian thing, it's a human necessity."[115] From 2012 on, DinéYazhi´ has addressed the HIV/AIDS crisis and its disproportionate and underacknowledged implications for both trans and Indigenous lives. They are inspired to fill the meaningful "absence of art production in Indigenous communities that broaches the topic of HIV/AIDS."[116] In a 2016 print, they coined the slogan "POZ SINCE 1492"[117] to reframe AIDS as fundamental to contending with the longue durée of colonialist white supremacist violence. In a United States context, the origin of disease and plague that are products of white colonization are often traced to Christopher Columbus's "New World" arrival in 1492. DinéYazhi´'s poster builds on understandings of the flesh in Indigenous studies as a way conquest is experienced, as both history and as present lived in and through the body, and places it in a specifically trans and queer AIDS context. DinéYazhi´'s effort shifted attention away from now-prevalent AIDS rhetoric of individual responsibility and victim blaming, placing blame squarely on the logics of racialized violence, settler colonialism, and institutional malfeasance. The 2016 print's alternate title, "The First Infection,"[118] points to white imperialism as the root cause of these ongoing genocides and pandemics, these ongoing "infections" that physically and conceptually afflict harm on the bodies and lives of queer and trans BIPOC.

The *NDN AIDS Flag* was posted to coincide with #WorldAIDSDay and #DayWithoutArt. Since 2014, DinéYazhi´ annually creates or updates downloadable posters. These posters focus on HIV/AIDS's devastating effects on Indigenous communities and are an indictment of the stigma imposed from both outside and within Native communities. They post them widely across social media.[119] *NDN AIDS Flag* was accompanied by DinéYazhi´'s instructions: "As with all our posters, feel liberated to, share, print out, wheatpaste, and disseminate at will!" Like its earlier agit-prop counterpart, this poster is intended to intervene in a public space, to move its in-your-face message unpredictably and quickly across urban walls, subway cars, bus stops, and construction zones. It is also distinctly digital, intended to proliferate online through viral media languages of hashtags, likes, and reposts. Users shared the original poster nearly eight hundred times on Tumblr.[120] DinéYazhi´ draws on the powerful but white-dominated strategies of groups like ACT UP and Gran Fury, remixing them to address the rampant and ongoing structural injustices that fuel the HIV/AIDS epidemic. They disrupt the bounds of AIDS time politics through vital nostalgia. Yet when I return to their Tumblr after December 2018, I am repeatedly warned that it may contain sensitive content. I must now click my acknowledgment to accept risk and am required to log in to view the page. The evolutions of the platform's operation promise to change and challenge viral circulation, and with it the meaning of creative political interventions that online AIDS archives.

Platformed Possibilities and Archival Circulations

To tell a queer and trans BIPOC story of HIV/AIDS, then or now, requires looking at sources that have not been considered to be within the normative purview of formal archives. Looking to embodiment, storytelling, and artistic remediations of virality using digital tools, platforms, and approaches offers a novel, urgent perspective that centers the needs and desires of the viral underclass. My examination of the alternative AIDS archives that Mac, LaBeija, and DinéYazhi´ are creating in tandem with fellow activist-artists showcases the power found in activating the records of the AIDS past to generate renewed immediacy for HIV/AIDS. Mobilizing AIDS archives through viral media has political potential to reconstitute AIDS temporalities to emphasize the epidemic's urgent immediacy as well as its structurally informed persistence. A technologically facilitated interruption of the linear chronological relationality of bodies, archival records, and spaces is requisite to remaking sociopolitical realities. By harnessing digital media's affordances of immediacy, persistence, publicness, affective relationality, and self-archiving, as engendered by its features, options, and pacing, these artists are remaking the face of AIDS in America and its temporal orders. Centering queer, trans, and BIPOC consciousness demonstrates how through vital nostalgia archiving can be bound up with outrage, and how outrage in the face of injustice and unbearable loss wields tremendous political potential. Yet the present and future possibilities of such alternative AIDS archives are intimately bound with the constraints and opportunities of the corporate digital media platforms that host them.

Tumblr's adult-content ban has already fundamentally changed the platform—who is using it, how they are using it. My study falls at an in-between moment; as I write in winter 2020, it is clear that Tumblr is no longer the platform du jour for AIDS communities of artists and activists. Mac's most recent GIF on Tumblr is more than a month old; Mac used to update daily. LaBeija has discontinued her social media presence altogether. DinéYazhi´'s Tumblr, while still there, has become increasingly difficult to access, flagged out of ready discovery and accessibility for "sensitive content." Mac and DinéYazhi´ have largely migrated their efforts to other platforms: Instagram, Facebook, Etsy, personal websites. Visual AIDS also no longer bothers to update its Tumblr. Digital communities must grapple with absence, invisibility, and disappearance. There is much more scholarship focusing on the epic rise and long-standing use of certain tech empires: YouTube, Facebook, Twitter. Research has privileged the survival of big platforms over the smaller ones, the survival of the still persistent digital communities over the dearly departed ones. In this conclusion, I address some of the repercussions of what happens when a corner of the AIDS internet fades from favor. I speculate on what Tumblr's less-than-clear successor for the critical digital remediation of the AIDS archives will be.

The lack of a clear alternative for departing Tumblr users suggests that the AIDS and LGBTQ communities formed there will fracture. Tumblr's ban had immediate impacts on the platform's popularity, but to where queer and trans BIPOC users will shift has been less obvious and embodies the often ambivalent relationship of viral tactics' proximity to capitalism. From 2018 to 2019, the number of unique monthly visitors to Tumblr decreased 21 percent. The amount of time that visitors spend on the site and number of pages visited also declined. In the United States in particular, the decline in the average monthly volume of traffic to the Tumblr login page dropped 49 percent.[121] New or smaller sites, like Pillowfort, newTumbl, and BDSMLR, have attempted to fill the void. Some, largely focused on NSFW (not safe for work) content, closely adhere to Tumblr's design, enabling users to quickly post using text, photos, audio, video, or GIFs; some even allow importing from now-defunct Tumblrs. Many queer and trans users appear to have migrated to other large corporate social media platforms: Twitter, Facebook, Instagram. TikTok, the user-generated short-form video-sharing platform, has a growing number of under-twenty-five queer and trans users, though trans users have called out content censorship.[122] There is also evidence of AIDS engagement on the platform, albeit in viral tactics embedded in capitalist contexts. In 2019, TikTok partnered with AIDS charity (RED), which works with the private sector to fund raise and raise awareness. TikTok encouraged users on that year's World AIDS Day to demonstrate their support by using the hashtag #MakeItRed, during which it turned five popular effects "(RED)" for a week.[123] This red-out action, part of a larger red- (and pink-)washing strategy for TikTok, is a far cry from the archival tactics used by artists including Mac, LaBeija, and DinéYazhi´. Yet both methods share an attempt to ubiquitously circulate the same images within a network.

Of mainstream platform alternatives to Tumblr's reign, I see Instagram, the most popular application for social networking through image sharing, as its most likely corporate successor. It has been used alongside Tumblr for art-AIDS action and seems to have become the site for significant viral circulation of AIDS archival records. Along with the usual selfies, pets, kids, and décor and food porn, users are posting and sharing aesthetically inclined yet informative imagery as political action. Instagram, owned by Facebook since 2012, has one billion active monthly users, most under thirty-five. Daily, ninety-five million posts are created, and it has since 2010 shared forty billion photos. Mac (@imgirlurl), DinéYazhi´ (@heterogeneoushomosexual), and Visual AIDS (@visual_aids) maintain active presences on the platform. It is also home to significant archival AIDS content via accounts, including the AIDS Memorial (@theaidsmemorial), the ACT UP Oral History Project (@actuporalhistoryproject), and Gran Varones (@granvarones). Activist groups like ACT UP/NY (@actupny), the Black AIDS Institute (@blackaids), and Positive Women's Network (@postivewomensnetworkusa) also favor it for community engagement. Instagram is an increasingly significant ecosystem for diverse artists to create and users to circulate content through feeds and stories. Through art and design, Instagram functions as a political megaphone. However, although popular, platforms like Instagram do not offer the same possibilities as Tumblr when it comes to "materiality, multiplicity, ambiguity, fluidity"—qualities trans scholars identify as vital to trans world making online.[124]

That Tumblr provided a technology that could meet the needs of queer and trans BIPOC users for art-AIDS action was a fortunate accident. Tumblr, until 2019, was property of Yahoo!, owned by Verizon Media, then sold to Automattic. Its structures always prioritized the company's financial gain, which meant shifting to appeal to the cultural mainstream. An immediate need for digital archival technologies exists for AIDS art-activist communities that are no longer welcome on Tumblr; yet there is also a real need to consider what alternative digital archival technologies might be designed to engender vibrant, livable AIDS futures. Many in AIDS and LGBTQ communities have and will continue to migrate to corporate platforms even as they work to critique and remake the dominant social structures that those platforms reproduce. Yet alternatives exist and might counter some of the power of corporate platforms. Outside of mainstream digital platforms, artists, activists, and people living with HIV/AIDS have always built their own alternative resources and worlds. For example, early bulletin board systems (BBSs) had boards like AIDS Information Bulletin Board Service (AIDS Info BBS), founded in 1986, which circulated information for the community, including mainstream news stories, medical research, community periodicals, and message boards for caregivers. Visual AIDS's Artist+ Registry launched in 2012 to circulate and promote the work of HIV-positive artists; it enables users to curate web galleries. Future technologies—technologies designed by and for AIDS communities, outside of capitalist frameworks, and with policies allowing queer and trans content in the service of intersectional community building—might reimagine social media's contours and make new worlds.

Artists like Mac, LaBeija, and DinéYazhi´ will undoubtedly continue to use digital tools and platforms as an accessible and powerful way to draw on images and material from the past to conjure possibilities for AIDS futures that center the vibrant lives of BIPOC queer and trans people. Marginalized people have and always will build their own AIDS archives. Regardless of platform, it is clear that the digital is fundamentally changing how we access, mediate, understand, and mobilize around HIV/AIDS. Reckoning with the AIDS past is now done within digital cultures. The ways in which the AIDS archive is onlined and remediated through digital practices, platforms, and tools promise to remake AIDS time and the AIDS archives itself. As the archival records of an earlier AIDS time are now moved, remediated, and transformed in the digital, it has become imperative to think HIV/AIDS and viral digital media together.

EPILOGUE

How to Survive Another Plague

In an epidemic that didn't have to happen, and whose continuing to this day to spread virtually unabated is the result of political neglect or outright mendacity, every death is unacceptable.

—DOUGLAS CRIMP (2002)

Most of us are wondering when life will get back to normal but normal is what brought us to such a precarious place. Nothing should ever be the same again and while that is an unnerving prospect, it may also be our saving grace.

—ROXANE GAY, "NOTES ON POWER IN A PANDEMIC" (2020)

"WHAT'S IT LIKE BEING HIV POSITIVE during multiple pandemics?" artist, educator, and HIV-positive transgender woman Glammy asked. Her artist statement continued, "My internalized stigma makes me feel infectious and afraid of getting others sick. Social interactions trigger how I've been demonized and treated like a weapon for being poz. . . . I often hear 'none of us have lived through a pandemic before,' ignoring how HIV is a pandemic we've been living with for almost 40 years." Glammy's words accompany her drawing, *Forest painted with my blood the night before my Covid test.* In the center, out of a many-ringed tree stump grows a sprout. The forest she renders in blood rejuvenates itself. Intertwined, past and present alike continue despite harsh pandemic living conditions. Glammy's piece responded to a May 2020 invitation that Visual AIDS issued to its artist members—people self-identifying as HIV-positive artists. Members were invited to submit artworks that responded to the global Covid-19 pandemic and stay-at-home social distancing measures. Along with their digital submissions, artists shared short narratives addressing how Covid-19 had affected their experiences and art-making practices as people living with HIV/AIDS. Fifty-three responded, and their artworks were featured in Visual AIDS's September web gallery, "Ampler than Loneliness: Documenting Collective Resilience through HIV/AIDS and Covid-19." The works were also added to their respective pages in Artist+ Registry, Visual AIDS's digital archives. As we live through the Covid-19 pandemic, nostalgia helps us make sense of the conjunctures of AIDS, Covid-19, and racism.

I write this in fall 2020 while continuing to shelter in place in Seattle, my home that became the first-recognized epicenter of America's still-unfolding Covid-19 pandemic in March. I watched in horror as we were replaced by New York City, which by April had reached the initial peak of its Covid-19 outbreak, harshly affecting people of color in the city's economically disadvantaged neighborhoods. Glammy demands that we stop to recognize that we are living now simultaneously amid multiple pandemics, that more than one crisis is unfolding, being weaponized, enfolding our bodies. Her words point to how Covid-19 makes the intersecting HIV/AIDS pandemic both detectable and undetectable.

Such visibility and its lack for HIV/AIDS is not new. Julia S. Jordan-Zachery asserts, for example, that Black women are "made invisible and hypervisible" within contemporary AIDS responses. They are painted as those at greatest risk for acquiring HIV, reduced to pandemic statistics and causalities. Yet as Jordan-Zachery argues, Black women are routinely deprived of housing and health care, and queer and trans Black women's existences are often ignored altogether.[1] Similarly, even as parallels proliferate in popular and AIDS media between the Covid-19 and AIDS pandemics, the contemporary needs and realties of people living with HIV/AIDS, especially those with multiply marginalized racial, ethnic, gender, sexual, and cultural identities, are still routinely ignored and neglected. AIDS archives have key temporal interventions to make once again.

HIV/AIDS, as *Viral Cultures* has illustrated, has long had an uneven temporalization in its duration and intensities as a crisis. Its temporal orders are so grossly divided by access to power that it is more accurate, Jih-Fei Cheng, Alexandra Juhasz, and Nishant Shahani write, to describe HIV/AIDS as "long-term and still ongoing global crises."[2] This means that in 2020, we are not just living with multiple pandemics, we are living in multiple AIDS pandemics at once. "Given the advances in research, information and treatment, it seems inconceivable that someone living with the virus today . . . could look as if he had stepped out of the early years of the epidemic. And yet a series of fateful decisions and omissions, dating back to the discovery of the disease, have led to a present that looks like the past—but only for some," Linda Villarosa wrote. Villarosa's 2017 *New York Times* feature, "America's Hidden HIV Crisis," highlighted the conditions that shape the accelerated AIDS-related suffering and death of gay and bisexual Black men in twenty-first-century Louisiana and Mississippi. Although still inadequate, she continued, United States programs like the President's Emergency Plan for AIDS Relief (PEPFAR) have invested over $80 billion in HIV/AIDS pandemic treatment, prevention, and research in sub-Saharan Africa. Villarosa damningly emphasized that "Black America, however, never got a PEPFAR." The people whose stories she shares exist outside of the boundaries of normative AIDS time in the American imaginary—where AIDS exists in America only as past queer tragedy. Villarosa's words powerfully illustrated the 2017 embodied AIDS reality of Jordon, a twenty-four-year-old, HIV-positive Black man in Mississippi: wheelchair leaning on the wall, Ensure on the bedside table, a six-foot-tall man's skeletal frame, pained winces from HIV-related neuropathy, arms scarred from innumerable hospital visits and IVs. His anguish echoes 1980s' archival footage of gay white men gravely ill and dying, such that Jordon looked like he belonged to an earlier epidemic era. Too many Black gay men, too many minoritized people, are still subjected to inhabiting "a present that looks like the past."[3] Since 1996, AIDS in America has been prematurely and repeatedly declared as a crisis that is over thanks to antiretroviral pharmaceutical combination therapies. These declarations evidence a historical, political, and cultural refusal to recognize that AIDS crises can and do have inequitable and catastrophic consequences.

As the scope and scale of what we were and will be facing from Covid-19 in March 2020 became increasingly clear, numerous comparisons began to be drawn between the HIV/AIDS and Covid-19 pandemics. Commonalities from lessons learned to public health proposals to personal essays were made by AIDS activists, journalists, and scholars of epidemiology, political science, and history in AIDS and LGBTQ publications, and mainstream and boutique news outlets. There are similarities worth acknowledging: most importantly, AIDS and Covid-19 remind us that pandemics act on what Jallicia Jolly terms "pre-existing conditions"—that is, along social fault lines, hierarchies, and inequalities.[4] Pandemics thrive on the politics and structures that put socially devalued people at greatest risk for transmission, and in turn they make the same people the most vulnerable for inadequate posttransmission care. Both viruses share the following: a disproportionate impact on Black, Latinx, Indigenous, unhoused, and incarcerated people, immigrants, and those lacking health insurance; the rapid spread of a novel virus through an unsuspecting population as transmitted through activities that had previously been considered safe;[5] inept federal government responses within frameworks of austerity and of individualistic ableism that suggest that individual and national bodies are threatened only by foreign bodies, so people with both viruses are demonized and seen to embody moral failures;[6] the advancement of surveillance infrastructures and technologies despite realities that tracking produces neither safety nor cure; press conferences that initially downplayed the crisis; folkloric "origin" stories;[7] dangerously racialized, blanketed, and changing assessments of how the disease could be contracted; and irresponsible and phobic nicknames[8] that transfer blame to already othered communities, positioning them as disease vectors and aspiring to assure the straight, white, middle-class public of their security. There are some similarities between the biological viruses' operations too. Without treatment, HIV compromises immune systems, and Covid-19 particularly affects people with compromised immune systems. The asymptomatic incubation period for both facilitates transmission.[9] Additionally, there are repeat actors in these American epidemics: Anthony Fauci, Deborah Birx, and activists who have issued vocal responses: ACT UP/NY, Treatment Action Group (TAG), and individuals like Gregg Gonsalves, who said of living with HIV amid Covid-19, "I feel less physical risk than I do the weight of the history of the AIDS epidemic. Another epidemic being mishandled; it's PTSD of a certain sort where you're like, we're really doing this again?"[10] AIDS was once a mysterious deadly new disease that attacked minoritized communities; now, like AIDS, Covid-19 has led to confusion, speculation, and misinformation.[11] There are affective resonances between AIDS and Covid-19 experiences, including fear, loneliness, and social isolation for those infected and most at risk, as well as the foreboding and dread that permeate everyday life.[12] Many of the same anxious questions from the early days of AIDS are being asked about Covid-19: "How many will become infected? How many will die? When will it end?"[13] Both pandemics have caused not just biomedical earthquakes but also social, cultural, and political ones. In upheaval's wake, in the aftershocks, nothing is the same.

Yet the comparisons now often repeated between AIDS and Covid-19 routinely obscure and flatten more than they uncover and expose about

HIV/AIDS. There are meaningful differences between these pandemics. Even at the viral level, HIV and Covid-19 are different viruses with distinct transmission modes. HIV is relatively inefficient, transmitted only through certain bodily fluids, and even when exposed, transmission occurs with relative infrequency.[14] Covid-19, as we are still learning, is more transmission efficient, and it does so in ways HIV does not—via surface traces, respiratory droplets, or casual contact. AIDS activists and people living with HIV/AIDS have chafed at and articulated the problematics of comparing even the early HIV/AIDS years with those of Covid-19. We saw in 2020 a rapid, if grossly inept, Covid-19 response. While resonant concerns have arisen as the pandemic has progressed about its disproportionate impact on people deemed expendable (the elderly, people with disabilities, BIPOC), AIDS, unlike Covid-19, was never painted as an equal-opportunity malady. Long-term HIV survivor Mark King demands a stoppage of comparisons; doing so disremembers that to even begin a conversation during the early HIV/AIDS pandemic required transcending taboos—talking about anal sex, drug use, condoms, and "who God was punishing," which amounted to scaling "mountains of social bias in order to educate people on the basic facts."[15] With Covid-19 there have been sympathetic responses, with a rush to develop and make accessible testing and vaccines that did not happen in the 1980s. Ted Kerr points out that although bungled, inaccurate, perpetuating misinformation, and committed to downplaying the pandemic, Trump actually engaged the nation about Covid-19, unlike Reagan with AIDS, and states and localities implemented some protections. Most importantly, when comparisons are made between HIV/AIDS and Covid-19, many conveniently sideline the reality that the former is still a plague. We thus ignore how institutionalized narrow conceptions of risk groups (homosexuals, Haitians, people with hemophilia, and heroin users) allowed HIV stigma, discrimination, and criminalization to fester and become a social pandemic that still holds the same power, even as lifesaving medications can render HIV undetectable and thus untransmittable. Significantly, talking about AIDS activism as only of the past does a gross if predictable disservice to contemporary AIDS activists, especially BIPOC activists and artists, prison abolitionists, and those fighting for the rights of immigrants and unhoused people. Kerr concludes, "There is as much to compare in the current response to HIV as it relates to the coronavirus as there is to our past response."[16]

Meaningful differences between the HIV/AIDS and Covid-19 crises extend to archiving. Many AIDS activists, as this book has shown, were actively engaged from 1980s onward in documentation and archiving as a means to effect change in their own time and for posterity. Any positive differences we can see between early AIDS and Covid-19 responses—whether personal or structural—should be credited to the momentous efforts of AIDS activists in facilitating collective sharing of information and records, scientific knowledge, and data at a breakneck pace, and their pushes to accelerate clinical trials, refusals to accept neglect whether from government, community, or family, documentation and collection of records, and transformations into experts.[17] Following this precedent, community projects have arisen to document Covid-19 experiences by and for their communities. Big institutions were slower to respond to AIDS. Most of the AIDS archival collections analyzed in *Viral Cultures* became part of academic or public institutions in the late 1990s and 2000s (if they ever did), a decade or more after activists began archiving. In contrast, Covid-19 documentation projects have arisen from major institutions—Duke, Harvard, the Los Angeles Public Library, and the Massachusetts Historical Society, to name but a few—within weeks of the pandemic's arrival in America.

I feel it; I long for and talk about a desire to return to my "normal" life, to the "before times," to aspects of social life and mobility I took for granted in February 2020. It is no surprise that even those of us who have privilege self-isolate for months, as many others continue to risk their lives because they cannot afford to shelter from the virus, are longing for a prior life—a previous life where on average more than a thousand Americans were not dying from Covid-19 every single day, where those of us not on the margins were not facing financial stresses or an imminent eviction crisis, where the news was not filled with white protesters who refuse to mask while demanding that businesses reopen and their personal freedom not be curtailed, and where the division between those who believe in science and those who don't did not seem to grow ever starker. Yet we ought to be critical of this nostalgia for "normal" life. My nostalgia and others like it require close attention to the proliferation of conventional restorative nostalgias amid Covid-19. Here, there are lessons to be learned from the critical mobilizations of vital nostalgia by AIDS activists, artists, and curators. Those of us with the immense privilege to long for the before need to recognize and remember how we arrived at this conjuncture. Angela Hanks of the Groundwork Collaborative asserts, "We can't go back to normal. Normal is what got us here and we can't afford to simply go back to the ways things were."[18]

The biggest stories of 2020 were Covid-19 and the amplification of the Black Lives Matter movement in the wake of George Floyd's murder by police. Both are stories about the urgency of racial justice, about how BIPOC live and die in America. Nationwide, as a result of the socioeconomic structures we have created and the narratives we cling to, Black, Latinx, and Indigenous Americans are contracting and dying of Covid-19 at higher rates. "Normal" created this situation where our country has become ever more pandemic prone but ever less ready to face it, given the conditions of outsized corporate power that has eroded public power and services, given the massive racialized and gendered wealth inequities, and given a criminal justice system that disproportionately incarcerates Black and brown people. It is not just short-term problems like the Trump administration's leadership failures; the virus has exposed myriad vulnerabilities baked into our economic, health care, and social systems. It is once again painfully clear that issues of health and race cannot be differentiated. As Black feminist writer Roxane Gay argues, "Eventually, doctors will find a coronavirus vaccine, but black people will continue to wait, despite the futility of hope, for a cure for racism. We will live with the knowledge that a hashtag is not a vaccine for white supremacy. We live with the knowledge that, still, no one is coming to save us." She concludes, "The rest of the world yearns to get back to normal. For black people, normal is the very thing from which we yearn to be free."[19] It is imperative that we think critically with and about nostalgia now, that we approach it with nuance that differentiates its forms, and that we call for the generation of productive vital nostalgias, like those detailed throughout *Viral Cultures*, as we face questions of how to survive pandemics.

AIDS archives have begun to play an important, if still emergent, role in the remediation of narratives linking AIDS and Covid-19. These acts illustrate the latest manifestation of the political potentiality of archival records activation through vital nostalgia to bring attention to HIV/AIDS now in ways *Viral Cultures* charted. The *What Does a Covid-19 Doula Do? Zine*, supported by the ONE Archives Foundation, is devoted in half to contextually captioned archival objects from the exhibition, *Metanoia: Transformation through AIDS Archives and Activism*. The *Zine's* other half responds to the title prompt. Juhasz introduces it by attesting, as an AIDS activist, scholar, and media maker since the 1980s, that AIDS and Covid-19 share little beyond the basics of being viruses that are "highly communicable, potentially deadly, frightening, initially little-understood, and prone to the dangerous distortions of mis-, under-, and over- reporting." Yet in the space opened by their limited commonalities, she and other contributors—activists, scholars, artists, curators, archivists—find generative ground for art, activism, community building, care, and, I would add, activist archiving. Juhasz asserts that by reexamining the records created during the early AIDS pandemic by Black and women of color activists, we can draw on successful tactics, grieve losses, and find ways to continue to fight, imagine, and build different presents and futures amid multiple crises. Such promising possibilities are born of an archivally substantiated resilience that is engendered by AIDS records not only because such records were created, but because they were collected, preserved, archived.[20]

Across the country, AIDS archives—including the ONE National Gay & Lesbian Archives in Los Angeles, the GLBT Historical Society (GLBTHS) in San Francisco, and Visual AIDS in New York City—are mobilizing their records, resources, and networks to intervene in the prevailing cultural discourse that draws parallels between AIDS and Covid-19. In the wake of Trump's election, the GLBTHS launched "Fighting Back," a platform for intergenerational dialogue between activists, community members, and scholars that explores how strategies and records from the queer past might formulate contemporary resistance. In April 2020, it pivoted quickly to become a weekly online series on "lessons from AIDS for Covid-19." Events highlighted how both pandemics upended daily life, culture, and economies with mounting death tolls and inept governmental responses. The series, with topics from "Direct Action and Government Response" to "Confronting the Stigma of Disease" to "Being Transgender in an Epidemic," was a means to transform our anxiety, despair, or anger into action, and to find in the archives "models for building community and solidarity in the midst of this pandemic."[21] Their website notes, "And as with HIV/AIDS, we not only struggle to survive Covid-19, we learn to thrive within the pandemic, and imagine the world we want to create after Covid-19." This sentiment marks where the AIDS archives can intervene: mobilizing the AIDS past to address the intertwined pasts, presents, and futures of the multiple crises that constrain the lives and life chances of people marginalized at the intersections of HIV stigma, racism, sexism, homophobia, transphobia, poverty, ableism, xenophobia, and other structural injustices.

Visual AIDS has also pivoted to advance conversations on how to care and curate critically amid both HIV/AIDS and Covid-19. Since March 2020, they have provided resource lists and direct support for HIV-positive artists addressing issues from how to get medication to filing for unemployment and finding financial supports to continue making art. Looking at recent guest-curated web galleries showcases how the organization is continuing to use vital nostalgic curation as a model of archival engagement aimed at holistic cure. Through the mobilization of images from its digital archives, curators interrogate pressing issues. For example, critical commenting on how digital memory spaces, including efforts to document Covid-19, already underway in hundreds of archival institutions, universities, and community-based organizations, can learn from the ethics, efforts, and histories of digital AIDS archives like Artist+ Registry to advance an ethos of care that, given the exploitation of vulnerable people by digital platforms, is urgent.[22] Curators have also explored how art offers access to space for grieving through embodied mourning and remembrance rituals for mounting losses;[23] have sought ways that thinking Covid-19 and HIV/AIDS together might afford healing and connection; and have called for attention and action on both pandemics.[24] These archival strategies embody the strategic efforts of HIV/AIDS activists who for decades have brought attention to health disparities, demanded government action and institutional change, and coalesced political power in the archives. We continue to desperately require vital nostalgia as a means of producing and mobilizing community care in the face of gross inequities and shameful neglect. The legacies and present work of activists, archivists, artists, and curators can teach us how to survive even in intensely hostile environments and model ways of living and being in times of pain and possibility.[25] AIDS archives matter more than ever as we learn to live and to thrive with viruses.

Worlds as we know them end every day. Disasters regularly devastate communities, fundamentally altering lives and environments—social, political, technological, affective. Importantly, this devastation is not equally distributed; rather, its effects are often most dire for marginalized peoples.[26] Living among multiple, coproduced crises requires living in the past, present, and future simultaneously. As vulnerable lives are upended, in the wake of such violence and upheaval, of change plodding or sudden, we struggle with, against, and alongside records, information, and data. In drawing comparisons, productive and less so, people are attempting to contend with emergent fears and precarities driven by Covid-19 and with the ongoing pain and trauma born of the HIV/AIDS crises. Kerr writes, "AIDS is not over in terms of new cases, the need for a cure or a response to the ongoing social calamities that come with an

HIV diagnosis. AIDS is also not over in terms of teaching us what there is to know about the human condition. Comparisons are a way of holding multiple and complex thoughts and feelings together at the same time."[27] Conjuring comparisons between these American pandemics is a means to make sense of the profound uncertainty about what is happening to our lives right now by recalling and reigniting our past—using examples of a deadly virus that we already know, and that we might already live with. I suspect such comparisons are here to stay, particularly as Covid-19 ages to take on its own complicated temporal rhythms and registers. It is becoming clear that its time scale, like that of AIDS, will include the endemic, as Covid-19 too becomes a chronic illness and societal condition.

Viral Cultures has offered an account of the players—activists, artists, curators, and archivists—and ideologies—temporal, political, technological, cultural, and biomedical—that have shaped and continue to shape AIDS archives and the historical and contemporary cultural productions that animate AIDS records. It addresses care work, cure, and curation in three AIDS archives in a recognized center of AIDS cultural production, New York City: the New York Public Library, NYU's Fales Library and Special Collections, and Visual AIDS. The formalized AIDS archives in this book are housed within the country's second-largest public library, an elite university, and a community-based arts organization. I have also examined a more prodigious set of AIDS archives: artists' Facebook walls and Tumblrs, major museum exhibitions and gallery installations, personal collections stored lovingly in domestic spaces. Yet this book largely tells the story of archives and records that are widely recognized as such. These archives, while important, should be only but one focus for further action and scholarship. The fault lines that crises from AIDS to Covid-19 exploit make apparent the urgent need for more AIDS archives, alternative HIV/AIDS narratives, and a prodigious definition of what constitutes the AIDS record in research and practice.

Through erasure from archival representation, BIPOC, queers, trans, and HIV-positive people have long been denied both history and futurity, relegated to a vulnerable present existence. It is imperative that we begin to write AIDS archives stories that begin from alternative conceptions of what the AIDS archives even is. We need pathways of engaging AIDS archives that are grounded in the epistemologies of BIPOC communities, whether it is of archives as embodied practices—ballroom, sex, or gesture;[28] storytelling and oral traditions from Indigenous and queer peoples;[29] or trans and queer care praxes.[30] We also need more stories of how formalized AIDS archives and their records are remediated and mobilized by marginalized peoples to locate and remember their lived experiences and to evade and contest social subordination. Despite harsh living conditions, minoritized subjects surpass temporal relegation by willfully utilizing archives to ensure far more than present survival. However, the powerful possibilities of such archives exist in intimate relation to the dangers and violence they reproduce. We do not need a new dominant narrative of the AIDS crisis; we need many narratives. AIDS is many crises that are local, situated, emergent, changing. AIDS activist archiving can become through such vital nostalgia work a response that can redress the denial of culture, knowledge, and care from those who have been long marginalized. Vital nostalgia is a core tactic in efforts to better understand, reinstate, and honor diverse and disparate AIDS knowledges and experiences.

No crisis, uprising, or other devastation is an isolated event. It is essential to examine the structural forces that shape crises and contribute to their immediate and long-lasting effects; we need to delve deeply into what preceded, what comes after, and how we narrate it.[31] This book has examined the transformative aftershocks in the AIDS archives and with it the structural forces that contributed to the devastation of AIDS—state failures, ableism, racism, homophobia, transphobia, genocide, capitalist profiteering, collective trauma. Vital nostalgia in the AIDS archives facilitates generative political possibilities for response, knowledge, and perseverance. Archives are essential forces in how we envision life as and after worlds—individual or collective, material or imagined—cease.[32] When worlds end, we have a significant opportunity to rebuild differently, to create new ones. These new worlds will only be better if we can figure out how to care and mobilize critically. What voices, approaches, and infrastructures are requisite to producing more just and livable futures?[33] There are no easy answers, but the status quo won't do.

It is time to let go of the idea that the life we knew before this Covid-19 pandemic is coming back, to drop our conventional nostalgia for the before. AIDS fundamentally altered the world in ways routinely made visible—and in those that are often hidden. Steven W. Thrasher writes, "This new crisis too will change our way of life. This new crisis will change everything. *Everything.*" Like AIDS before it, it will alter permanently, he continues, "everything about how we work and socialize, everything about how we make love and make politics." Gay notes, "Nothing should ever be the same again and while that is an unnerving prospect, it may also be our saving grace."[34] Activations of AIDS archives have much to offer us during this moment of upheaval to understand what came before, what has happened during, and to work out what will come in the wake of this personal, social, and political upheaval. In conclusion, I ask, what world will come after?[35]

By drawing together past, present, and future, this book does not merely supply etiological, temporal, or spatial corrections to the narratives of the HIV/AIDS crisis to account for its archives. It also invites and incites readers to dream and work our way out of the limits of our artistic, political, technological, and archival imaginations around HIV/AIDS. We need to envision an end to pandemics that, as Douglas Crimp emphasizes, "didn't have to happen,"[36] that do not rely on erasures or violences—or, as Gay writes, a return to a "normal" that "is what brought us to such a precarious place."[37] Doing so, and engaging in the project imagining a future in the aftermath of HIV/AIDS, requires vital nostalgic reimaginings of AIDS time and space. We need vital nostalgia that recognizes, challenges, and redresses governing power relations. How and where we engage with AIDS archives in this present dictates more than HIV/AIDS's past. AIDS archives and their circulations shape possible AIDS presents and futures. Records hold power that is harnessed by activists, artists, curators, and archivists through vital nostalgia to repoliticize AIDS and reinvest AIDS time with palpable urgency. This is the alternative ending we need to HIV/AIDS. More than four decades into the epidemic, it is through the AIDS archives that we can reach toward engendering "radical beginnings"[38] that would center the voices of those most marginalized and affected by HIV/AIDS now.

ACKNOWLEDGMENTS

This is a book about activists, archivists, librarians, artists, curators, and people living with HIV/AIDS. All in their own way have devoted their lives to building social movements, creating and making information and knowledge accessible, and caring for one another. I am honored and deeply grateful to all those who shared their stories and work with me: Julie Ault, Jason Baumann, Andrew Blackley, Mimi Bowling, Ian Bradley-Perrin, Vincent Chevalier, José Luis Cortés, Alexis Danzig, Lisa Darms, Julián de Mayo, Alex Fialho, Avram Finkelstein, Steven G. Fullwood, David Hirsh, Jim Hubbard, Roberto Juarez, Ted Kerr, Debra Levine, Esther McGowan, Mark Milano, John Neff, Eric Rhein, Nelson Santos, Stephen Shapiro, Sur Rodney (Sur), Marvin J. Taylor, James Wentzy, Joe Westmoreland, Maxine Wolfe, and Ajamu X. This book is indebted as well to Tracy Fenix and Kyle Croft at Visual AIDS. I am also grateful for the efforts of the staff and volunteers at the New York Public Library, Fales Library and Special Collections, and the Lesbian Herstory Archives that made this project possible. My gratitude also extends to Frank Moore and many others who passed before this project but whose work continues to shape the collections and archives, as well as the activations of them captured in *Viral Cultures*.

I began work on this project while in the department of information studies at the University of California, Los Angeles. This project would not have been possible without the support of my friend and colleague Michelle Caswell as well as Kate Eichhorn, Anne J. Gilliland, and Jonathan Furner. Michelle and Kate's feedback on transforming this project into a published book has greatly shaped its form and contents.

Viral Cultures would not have been possible without the smarts and keen eyes of many friends and colleagues who read the proposal and/or portions of the book in progress. Many of their words and thoughts are reflected here. Thank you to Michelle Caswell, Ron Day, René Esparza, Laura Foster, Jack Gieseking, Rebecca Herzig, Jan Huebenthal, Jamie A. Lee, Cait McKinney, Mario H. Ramirez, Erica Rand, and Jay Sosa. Jan and René have read nearly every word over the years in our AIDS writing group, and the book is much improved for it. I am also grateful for the generous invitations to workshop chapters of the book from Kristin Veel, Nanna Bonde Thylstrup, and Daniela Agostinho of the Uncertain Archives Group at the University of Copenhagen, and from Jennifer Hamilton and Five College Women's Studies Research Center. The contributions of all workshop attendees greatly improved this text. Thank you as well to Octavio R. González, Alexandra Juhasz, and audiences at the American Studies Association for their feedback.

My fieldwork and early writing were made possible with generous support from the Social Science Research Council's Dissertation Proposal Development Fellowship and University of California, Los Angeles, Graduate Division's Graduate Research Mentorship and Graduate Summer Research Mentorship programs. Writing and publishing were generously supported by my institutional homes, past and present, including the University of Washington Information School, Indiana University School of Informatics, Computing and Engineering, and Bowdoin College through the Consortium for Faculty Diversity Postdoctoral Fellowship.

At the University of Minnesota Press, my three readers (Lisa Diedrich and Alana Kumbier, along with one anonymous reader) supported this project with their intellectual generosity and pushed me to develop and strengthen it in meaningful ways. I have been fortunate to be guided and supported by a brilliant editorial team including Leah Pennywark, Danielle Kasprzak, Jason Weidemann, and Anne Carter. Many people at the University of Minnesota Press made the book come to life, including Ana Bichanich, Karen Hellekson, Jeenee Lee Design, and Mike Stoffel. Anita Welbon created the brilliant index. Laura Portwood-Stacer's close reading and detailed feedback ensured this project's success. Thanks to the artists and curators and/or their estates who generously allowed me to share their works, which have enhanced this text in so many ways: Robert Blanchon, Ian Bradley-Perrin, Vincent Chevalier, Demian DinéYazhi´, DresserJohnson, Roberto Juarez, Jess MacCormack, Alexander McClelland, Eric Rhein, Stephen Shapiro, the Undetectable Flash Collective, and

Jessica Whitbread. I also want to thank the students who helped ready the book for publication: Todd Campbell, Jack Kovaleski, Emma May, Julianne Peeling, and Marie Peeples.

My work and I have benefited tremendously from research collaborations with friends and colleagues from whom I've learned a great deal about feminist scholarship and mentorship. Thinking and working with Cait McKinney have been formative to my understandings of information activism, HIV/AIDS, and digital media. I was lucky to meet Patricia Garcia early in my career; I could not have dreamed up a better person with whom to collaborate and build a feminist information studies community. I am also grateful to our other Border Quants Collaborators—Jacqueline Wernimont, Marisa Duarte, and Jessica Rajko—for pushing my thinking about data, bodies, and critical practice and modeling feminist research processes that make scholarly life worthwhile. With Patricia and support from the University of Michigan's Institute for Research on Women and Gender, I am also fortunate to have been able to create the Feminist Data Workshop: Anita Say Chan, T. L. Cowan, Anna Lauren Hoffmann, Lisa Nakamura, Jasmine Rault, Niloufar Salehi, and Tonia Sutherland. Over the past year, my AfterLab cofounders Anna Lauren Hoffmann, Tonia Sutherland, and Megan Finn have sustained me with their brilliance, humor, and unwavering support.

I am also fortunate to have worked with brilliant, generous people during this book's development at four institutions and places far beyond them, including the Archival Education and Research Institutes, which have given me an academic home. I am especially grateful for Miranda Belarde-Lewis, Kathy Carbone, Ron Day, Annie DeSaussure, Jennifer Douglas, Laura Foster, Jack Gieseking, Andrew Hamilton, the entire Homosaurus editorial board, Erin Johnson, Cricket Keeting, Tara Kohn, Jamie A. Lee, Jin Ha Lee, Sarah Leonard, Purnima Mankekar, Michelle Martin, Carole Palmer, Britt Paris, Miriam Posner, J. Ricky Price, Laura Prieto, K. J. Rawson, David Ribes, Jennifer Scanlon, Rebecka Taves Sheffield, Joe Tennis, Marieke Van Der Steenhoven, Kathy Wisser, and Cleo Wölfle Hazard. I am also grateful to my doctoral students Itza Carbajal, Claire McDonald, and Sarah Nguyễn. My chosen cohort got me through the PhD and still sustains me: Roderic Crooks, Seth Erickson, Patricia Garcia, Robert D. Montoya, Mario H. Ramirez, Sa Whitley, and Stacy E. Wood. I look forward to toasting this book over martinis and french fries at Taix one day.

Friends beyond academia have also provided the love, support, and joy needed, especially Cassady, Karin, Emma, Leah, Daniella, Naomi, Becky,

Steve, Ariel, Sam, Mariah, Lena, Evan, Alex, Rose, and Chessie. My family has offered incalculable love and grounding; thank you to Lynn, Yeva, Pat, Pegi, Steve, Carlye, Cole, and Jerry. Thank you to my daughter, Solenne; the dream of you kept me going in the final months of writing, and your imminent arrival pushed me to finish—and to let go when needed. My husband, Jesse Deshayes, made this book and all good things possible. Jesse has taught me about care and how to enact a commitment to doing work that can make a real, concrete difference in the world. This project would not have been possible without his unwavering support, editorial prowess, and love.

Introduction

1. Red is the AIDS ribbon color. The Visual AIDS Artists' Caucus in 1991 created it to symbolize solidarity. Sarah Schulman, "The Art of Protesting," *T: The New York Times Style Magazine*, April 22, 2018, 41.

2. Day With(out) Art launched in 1989. The December 1, World AIDS Day, event of action and mourning continues. Museums, galleries, libraries, universities, and AIDS service organizations participate. Fierce pussy's 2013 "For the Record" was updated from their 2010 installation, "Get Up Everybody and Sing," for the exhibition *ACT UP NEW YORK: Activism, Art, and the AIDS Crisis, 1987–1993.* "For the Record," Projects, Visual AIDS, https://visualaids.org/projects/for-the-record1.

3. Past fierce pussy members include Pam Brandt, Jean Carlomusto, Donna Evans, Alison Froling, and Suzanne Wright. "About Us," fierce pussy, https://fiercepussy.org/.

4. "Get Up Everybody and Sing," Projects, fierce pussy, https://fiercepussy.org/projects.

5. Edmund White, "The Resurrected," *T: The New York Times Style Magazine*, April 22, 2018, 117.

6. HIV treatment is not a medical cure. It does not result in full immune health. HIV-positive people undergoing treatment are susceptible to complications including cardiovascular disease and cancer. Long-term antiretroviral exposure can also cause toxic effects. Steven G. Deeks, Sharon R. Lewin, and Diane V. Havlir, "The End of AIDS: HIV Infection as a Chronic Disease," *Lancet* 382, no. 9903 (2013): 1525, 1530.

7. Since peaking in 1997, new HIV diagnoses have been reduced by 40 percent. However, reduction has slowed since 2010. Globally, it hovers at two million annually. UNAIDS, "UNAIDS Warns That after Significant Reductions, Declines in New HIV Infections among Adults Have Stalled and Are Rising in

Some Regions," press release, July 12, 2016, https://www.unaids.org/en/resources/presscentre/pressreleaseandstatementarchive/2016/july/20160712_prevention-gap.

8. John Petrus, "Discussing the Undiscussable: Reflecting on the 'End' of AIDS," *GLQ* 25, no. 1 (2019): 69, http://doi.org/10.1215/10642684-7275488.

9. Douglas Crimp, *Melancholia and Moralism: Essays on AIDS and Queer Politics* (Cambridge, Mass.: MIT Press, 2004).

10. Roger Hallas, "Queer AIDS Media and the Question of the Archive," *GLQ* 16, no. 3 (2010): 431.

11. Jules Gill-Peterson, "Haunting the Queer Spaces of AIDS: Remembering ACT UP/New York and an Ethics for an Endemic," *GLQ* 19, no. 3 (2013): 279–300.

12. Andrew Flinn and Ben Alexander, "'Humanizing an Inevitability Political Craft': Introduction to the Special Issue on Archiving Activism and Activist Archiving," *Archival Science* 15, no. 4 (2015): 329–35, https://doi.org/10.1007/s10502-015-9260-6.

13. Normand Fauteux, vocalist, "Zero Patience," track 1 on Glen Schellenberg's *Zero Patience: A Musical about AIDS* (soundtrack for the 1993 film, dir. John Greyson).

14. Randy Shilts, *And the Band Played On: Politics, People, and the AIDS Epidemic* (New York: St. Martin's Press, 1997).

15. Michael Worobey, Thomas D. Watts, Richard A. McKay, Marc A. Suchard, Timothy Granade, Dirk E. Teuwen, et al., "1970s and 'Patient 0' HIV-1 Genomes Illuminate Early HIV/AIDS History in North America," *Nature* 539, no. 7627 (2016): 98–101, https://doi.org/10.1038/nature19827.

16. Susan Leigh Foster, "Choreographies of Protest," *Theatre Journal* 55, no. 3 (2003): 395–412.

17. Theodore Kerr, "AIDS 1969: HIV, History, and Race," *Drain Magazine* 13, no. 2 (2016), http://drainmag.com/aids-1969-hiv-history-and-race.

18. Alisa Solomon, "What Does It Mean to Remember AIDS?," *Nation,* November 30, 2017, https://www.thenation.com/article/archive/what-does-it-mean-to-remember-aids/.

19. Lawrence K. Altman, "Rare Cancer Seen in 41 Homosexuals," *New York Times,* July 3, 1981, https://www.nytimes.com/1981/07/03/us/rare-cancer-seen-in-41-homosexuals.html.

20. The CDC-identified high-risk groups are known as the four Hs: homosexuals, Haitians, heroin addicts, and hemophiliacs. Gregg Gonsalves and Peter Staley, "Panic, Paranoia, and Public Health—The AIDS Epidemic's Lessons for Ebola," *New England Journal of Medicine* 371, no. 25 (2014): 2348, https://doi.org/10.1056/NEJMp1413425.

21. Dan Royles, "Don't We Die Too? The Political Culture of African American AIDS Activism" (PhD diss., Temple University, 2014), x.

22. Royles, "Don't We Die Too?," x.

23. Solomon, "What Does It Mean to Remember AIDS?"

24. Alexandra Juhasz, "Forgetting ACT UP," *Quarterly Journal of Speech* 98, no. 1 (2012): 69–74, https://doi.org/10.1080/00335630.2011.638662.

25. Royles, "Don't We Die Too?," x–xi.

26. Deborah B. Gould, *Moving Politics: Emotion and ACT UP's Fight against AIDS* (Chicago: University of Chicago Press, 2009), 4.

27. Andrew Weiner, "Disposable Media, Expendable Populations—ACT UP New York: Activism, Art, and the AIDS Crisis, 1987–1993," *Journal of Visual Culture* 11, no. 1 (2012): 106–7, https://doi.org/10.1177/1470412911430584.

28. Gould, *Moving Politics*, 4.

29. Lisa Diedrich, *Indirect Action: Schizophrenia, Epilepsy, AIDS, and the Course of Health Activism* (Minneapolis: University of Minnesota Press, 2016); Dan Royles, *To Make the Wounded Whole: The African American Struggle against HIV/AIDS* (Chapel Hill: University of North Carolina Press, 2020).

30. Steven Epstein, *Impure Science: AIDS, Activism, and the Politics of Knowledge* (Berkeley: University of California Press, 1996).

31. Douglas Crimp, "Mourning and Militancy," *October* 51 (1989): 15, https://doi.org/10.2307/778889.

32. Marty Fink, *Forget Burial: HIV Kinship, Disability, and Queer/Trans Narratives of Care* (New Brunswick: Rutgers University Press, 2020), 8.

33. Crimp, "Mourning and Militancy," 15.

34. During *Art AIDS America*'s 2015 Tacoma Art Museum premiere, the Tacoma Action Collective demanded receipts and an end to whitewashing HIV/AIDS cultural narratives. Tacoma Action Collective, "#StopErasingBlackPeople," *On Curating* 42 (2019), https://www.on-curating.org/issue-42-reader/stoperasing blackpeople.html#.XrROaBdKjUo.

35. Jih-Fei Cheng, "AIDS, Black Feminisms, and the Institutionalization of Queer Politics," *GLQ* 25, no. 1 (2019): 169–77, https://doi.org/10.1215/10642684-72 75418.

36. Jan Huebenthal, "Time after Time: Surviving, Remembering, Memorializing, and the Perils of a Post-AIDS Imagination" (unpublished manuscript, January 2019).

37. Marika Cifor, René Esparza, Jan Huebenthal, and David Román, "Resisting Erasure: AIDS and Modalities of Dissent," panel presented at the American Studies Association, Chicago, Illinois, November 12, 2017. As of August 2020, the website is accessible as archived from the Obama administration.

38. Susan Sontag, *Illness as Metaphor and AIDS and Its Metaphors* (New York: Macmillan, 2001).

39. Huebenthal, "Time after Time."

40. Gill-Peterson, "Haunting the Queer Spaces of AIDS."

41. Debra Levine, in discussion with the author, Skype, October 28, 2016.

42. Marita Sturken, "AIDS Activist Legacies and the Gran Fury of the Past/Present," *emisférica* 9, nos. 1–2 (2012), http://hemisphericinstitute.org/hemi/en/e-misferica-91/sturken.

43. Sarah Sharma, "Temporality," in *Keywords for Media Studies,* ed. Laurie Ouellette and Jonathan Gray (New York: New York University Press, 2017), 195.

44. Gill-Peterson, "Haunting the Queer Spaces of AIDS."

45. CDC, "HIV in the United States," reviewed June 10, 2020, https://www.cdc .gov/hiv/statistics/overview/ataglance.html.

46. UNAIDS, "Women, Adolescent Girls, and the HIV Response," press release, March 5, 2020, https://www.unaids.org/en/resources/presscentre/pressre leaseandstatementarchive/2020/march/20200305_weve-got-the-power#:~: text=Almost%2040%20years%20into%20the,years%20acquire%20HIV%20 every%20week.

47. "Women and HIV in the United States," KFF, March 9, 2020, https://www .kff.org/hivaids/fact-sheet/women-and-hivaids-in-the-united-states/.

48. Center for HIV Law and Policy, "Immigration," https://www.hivlawandpolicy .org/issues/immigration.

49. Sandra E. Garcia, "Independent Autopsy of Transgender Asylum Seeker Who Died in ICE Custody Shows Signs of Abuse," *New York Times,* November 27, 2018, https://www.nytimes.com/.

50. CDC, "HIV by Group," last reviewed October 25, 2019, https://www.cdc.gov/ hiv/group/index.html.

51. Linda Villarosa, "America's Hidden HIV Epidemic," *New York Times Magazine,* June 6, 2017, https://www.nytimes.com/.

52. Center for HIV Law and Policy, "Prisons and Jails," https://www.hivlawand policy.org/issues/prisons-and-jails.

53. Alfred Montoya, "From 'the People' to 'the Human': HIV/AIDS, Neoliberalism, and the Economy of Virtue in Contemporary Vietnam," *positions* 20, no. 2 (2012): 562, https://doi.org/10.1215/10679847-1538515.

54. Marlon M. Bailey, *Butch Queens Up in Pumps: Gender, Performance, and Ballroom Culture in Detroit* (Ann Arbor: University of Michigan Press, 2013), 217.

55. Douglas Crimp, "AIDS Cultural Analysis, Cultural Activism," *October* 43 (1987): 3.

56. David Román, "Remembering AIDS: A Reconsideration of the Film *Longtime Companion,*" *GLQ* 12, no. 2 (2006): 281–301, https://doi.org/10.1215/10642 684-12-2-281.

57. Cheng, "AIDS, Black Feminisms, and the Institutionalization of Queer Politics," 171.

58. Sarah Schulman, *The Gentrification of the Mind: Witness to a Lost Imagination* (Berkeley: University of California Press, 2012), 36.

59. Cifor et al., "Resisting Erasure."

60. See Cathy Cohen, *The Boundaries of Blackness: AIDS and the Breakdown of Black Politics* (Chicago: University of Chicago Press, 1999); Simon Watney, *Policing Desire: Pornography, AIDS, and the Media* (Minneapolis: University of Minnesota Press, 1987).

61. See Ann Cvetkovich, *An Archive of Feelings: Trauma, Sexuality and Lesbian Public Cultures* (Durham, N.C.: Duke University Press, 2003); Cindy Patton, *Inventing AIDS* (New York: Routledge, 1990).

62. Juhasz and Kerr periodize inattention to HIV/AIDS between 1996 and 2008 as the "Second Silence." Alexandra Juhasz and Ted Kerr, "AIDS Normalization," XTRA, 2020, https://www.x-traonline.org/article/aids-normalization.

63. See Darius Bost, *Evidence of Being: The Black Gay Cultural Renaissance and the Politics of Violence* (Chicago: University of Chicago Press, 2018); Adam Geary, *Antiblack Racism and the AIDS Epidemic: State Intimacies* (New York: Palgrave Macmillan, 2014); Jih-Fei Cheng, Alexandra Juhasz, and Nishant Shahani, eds., *AIDS and the Distribution of Crises* (Durham, N.C.: Duke University Press, 2020).

64. See Lisa Darms, "The Archival Object: A Memoir of Disintegration," *Archivaria* 67 (2009): 143–55; Ajamu X, Topher Campbell, and Mary Stevens, "Love and Lubrication in the Archives, or Rukus! A Black Queer Archive for the United Kingdom," *Archivaria* 68 (2009): 271–94; Marika Cifor, "Acting Up, Talking Back: TITA, TIARA, and the Value of Gossip," *InterActions* 12, no. 1 (2016), https://escholarship.org/uc/item/9d2007bj; Rebecka Taves Sheffield, *Documenting Rebellions: A Study of Four Lesbian and Gay Archives in Queer Times* (Sacramento, Calif.: Litwin Books, 2020).

65. George Aumoithe, "Privilege and Silence: ACT UP, the Majority Action Committee, and Insurgent Transcripts of the AIDS Clinical Trial Groups," paper presented at the Memory Lives On conference at the University of California, San Francisco, October 5, 2019.

66. Geoffrey Yeo, "Concepts of Record (1): Evidence, Information, and Persistent Representations," *American Archivist* 70, no. 2 (2007): 315.

67. Sharma, "Temporality."

68. Eric Ketelaar, "The Archive as a Time Machine," in *Proceedings of the DLM-Forum 2002, Barcelona, 6–8 May 2002: @ccess and Preservation of Electronic Information: Best Practices and Solutions* (Luxembourg: Office for Official Publications of the European Communities, 2002), 578.

69. Brien Brothman, "Perfect Present, Perfect Gift: Finding a Place for Archival Consciousness in Social Theory," *Archival Science* 10, no. 2 (2010): 159, https://doi.org/10.1007/s10502-010-9118-x.

70. Brothman, "Perfect Present, Perfect Gift," 162.

71. Ann Laura Stoler, *Along the Archival Grain: Epistemic Anxieties and Colonial Common Sense* (Princeton, N.J.: Princeton University Press, 2009), 45.

72. Michelle L. Caswell, "'The Archive' Is Not an Archives: On Acknowledging the Intellectual Contributions of Archival Studies," *Reconstruction* 16, no. 1 (2016), https://escholarship.org/uc/item/7bn4v1fk.

73. Flinn and Alexander, "Humanizing an Inevitably Political Craft," 331.

74. Jimmy Zavala, Alda Allina Migoni, Michelle Caswell, Noah Geraci, and Marika Cifor, "'A Process Where We're All at the Table': Community Archives Challenging Dominant Modes of Archival Practice," *Archives and Manuscripts* 45, no. 3 (2017): 202–15, https://doi.org/10.1080/01576895.2017.1377088.

75. Andrew Flinn, Mary Stevens, and Elizabeth Shepherd, "Whose Memories, Whose Archives? Independent Community Archives, Autonomy and the Mainstream," *Archival Science* 9, nos. 1–2 (2009): 75, https://doi.org/10.1007/s10502-009-9105-2.

76. Michelle Caswell, Marika Cifor, and Mario H. Ramirez, "'To Suddenly Discover Yourself Existing': Uncovering the Impact of Community Archives," *American Archivist* 79, no. 1 (2016): 61, https://doi.org/10.17723/0360-9081.79.1.56.

77. Michelle Caswell, "Inventing New Archival Imaginaries: Theoretical Foundations for Identity-Based Community Archives," in *Identity Palimpsests: Archiving Ethnicity in the U.S. and Canada,* ed. Dominique Daniel and Amalia Levi (Sacramento, Calif.: Litwin Books, 2014), 35.

78. Vladan Vukliš and Anne J. Gilliland, "Archival Activism: Emerging Forms, Local Applications," in *Archives in the Service of People—People in the Service of Archives,* ed. B. Filej (Maribor, Slovenia: Alma Mater Europea, 2016), 18.

79. Verne Harris, "Claiming Less, Delivering More: A Critique of Positivist Formulations on Archives in South Africa," *Archivaria* 44 (1997): 133–34.

80. Joan M. Schwartz and Terry Cook, "Archives, Records, and Power: The Making of Modern Memory," *Archival Science* 2, nos. 1–2 (2002): 119, https://doi.org/10.1007/BF02435628.

81. Hilary Jenkinson, *A Manual of Archive Administration* (Oxford: Clarendon Press, 1922).

82. Michelle Caswell, Ricardo Punzalan, and T-Kay Sangwand, "Critical Archival Studies: An Introduction," *Journal of Critical Library and Information Studies* 1, no. 2 (2017), https://doi.org/10.24242/jclis.v1i2.50.

83. Jacques Derrida, *Archive Fever* (Chicago: University of Chicago Press, 1996), 4.

84. Michel Foucault, *The Archaeology of Knowledge* (New York: Tavistock, 1972), 129.

85. Verne Harris, "Jacques Derrida Meets Nelson Mandela: Archival Ethics at the Endgame," *Archival Science* 11, no. 1 (2011): 121, https://doi.org/10.1007/s10502-010-9111-4.

86. Terry Cook, "The Archive(s) Is a Foreign Country: Historians, Archivists, and the Changing Archival Landscape," *American Archivist* 74, no. 2 (2011): 606, https://doi.org/10.17723/aarc.74.2.xm04573740262424.

87. Verne Harris, "Genres of the Trace: Memory, Archives and Trouble," *Archives and Manuscripts* 40, no. 3 (2012): 147–57, https://doi.org/10.1080/01576895.2012.735825.

88. Cook, "The Archive(s) Is a Foreign Country," 606.

89. Harris, "Claiming Less, Delivering More," 65.

90. Alycia Sellie, Jesse Goldstein, Molly Fair, and Jennifer Hoyer, "Interference Archive: A Free Space for Social Movement Culture," *Archival Science* 15, no. 4 (2015): 453–72, https://doi.org/10.1007/s10502-015-9245-5.

91. Sellie et al., "Interference Archive," 462–63.

92. Robb Hernández, *Archiving an Epidemic: Art, AIDS, and the Queer Chicanx Avant-Garde* (New York: New York University Press, 2019), 6.

93. Tonia Sutherland, "Archival Amnesty: In Search of Black American Transitional and Restorative Justice," *Journal of Critical Library and Information Studies* 1, no. 2 (2017): 11, https://doi.org/10.24242/jclis.v1i2.42.

94. Marika Cifor, "What Is Remembered Lives: Time and the Disruptive Animacy of Archiving AIDS on Instagram," *Convergence* 27, no. 2 (2021): 371–94.

95. "Gay and Lesbian Collections & AIDS/HIV Collections," New York Public Library, https://www.nypl.org/lgbtqcollections.

96. Visual AIDS, http://www.visualaids.org/.

97. Marvin J. Taylor, "'I'll Be Your Mirror, Reflect What You Are': Postmodern Documentation and the Downtown New York Scene from 1975 to the Present," *RBM* 3, no. 1 (2002): 45.

98. Ryan Conrad, *Things Are Different Now . . .*, Vimeo, December 18, 2012, video, 03:46, https://vimeo.com/55874290.

99. Roger Hallas, *Reframing Bodies: AIDS, Bearing Witness, and the Queer Moving Image* (Durham, N.C.: Duke University Press, 2009), 8.

100. Lucas Hilderbrand, "Retroactivism," *GLQ* 12, no. 2 (2006): 303.

101. Katharina Niemeyer, "Introduction: Media and Nostalgia," in *Media and Nostalgia: Yearning for Past, Present and Future*, ed. Katharina Niemeyer (London: Palgrave Macmillan, 2014), 2.

102. Svetlana Boym, *The Future of Nostalgia* (New York: Basic Books, 2001), xvi.

103. Carolyn K. Anspach, "Medical Dissertation on Nostalgia by Johannes Hofer, 1688," *Bulletin of the Institute of the History of Medicine* 2, no. 6 (1934): 376–91, https://doi.org/10.1177/039219216601405405.

104. Leo Spitzer, "Back through the Future: Nostalgic Memory and Critical Memory in Refuge from Nazism," in *Acts of Memory: Cultural Recall in the Present*, ed. Mieke Bal, Jonathan Crewe, and Leo Spitzer (Hanover, N.H.: University Press of New England, 1999), 89–90.

105. Boym, *Future of Nostalgia*, 3.

106. Michael S. Roth, "Dying of the Past: Medical Studies of Nostalgia in Nineteenth-Century France," *History and Memory* 3, no. 1 (1991): 11–12.

107. Spitzer, "Back through the Future."

108. Boym, *Future of Nostalgia*, 7.

109. Boym, *Future of Nostalgia*, xiv, 4.

110. David Lowenthal, "Past Time, Present Place: Landscape and Memory," *Geographical Review* 65, no. 1 (1975): 2, https://doi.org/10.2307/213831.

111. Susan Stewart, *On Longing: Narratives of the Miniature, the Gigantic, the Souvenir* (Baltimore, Md.: John Hopkins University Press, 1984).

112. Spitzer, "Back through the Future," 90.

113. Boym, *Future of Nostalgia*, xvi.

114. Boym, *Future of Nostalgia*, 7, 13.

115. Hilderbrand, "Retroactivism," 307.

116. Christopher Lasch, "The Politics of Nostalgia: Losing History in the Mists of Ideology," *Harper's Magazine* 269 (1984): 65.

117. Raymond Williams, *The City and the Country* (Oxford: Oxford University Press, 1974).

118. Kate Eichhorn, "Feminism's There: On Post-ness and Nostalgia," *Feminist Theory* 16, no. 3 (December 2015): 251–64, https://doi.org/10.1177/1464700 115604127.

119. Hilderbrand, "Retroactivism," 307.

120. Fredric Jameson, *Postmodernism, or The Cultural Logic of Late Capitalism* (Durham, N.C.: Duke University Press, 1991), 18.

121. Maurice Halbwachs, *On Collective Memory*, trans. and ed. Lewis A. Coser (Chicago: University of Chicago Press, 1992), 103–13.

122. Suzanne Vromen, "Maurice Halbwachs and the Concept of Nostalgia," *Knowledge and Society: Studies in the Sociology of Culture Past and Present: A Research Annual* 6 (1986): 77.

123. Eichhorn, "Feminism's There," 253.

124. Nadia Atia and Jeremy Davies, "Nostalgia and the Shapes of History," *Memory Studies* 3, no. 3 (July 2010): 184.

125. Fred Davis, *Yearning for Yesterday: A Sociology of Nostalgia* (New York: Free Press, 1979), 77; Janelle L. Wilson, *Nostalgia: Sanctuary of Meaning* (Lewisburg: Bucknell University Press, 2005).

126. Boym, *Future of Nostalgia*, xvi.

127. Alexandra Juhasz, "Video Remains: Nostalgia, Technology, and Queer Archive Activism," *GLQ* 12, no. 2 (2006): 321–22.

128. Boym, *Future of Nostalgia*, xvii.

129. Ray Cashman, "Critical Nostalgia and Material Culture in Northern Ireland," *Journal of American Folklore* 119, no. 472 (2006): 137–38.

130. Stuart Tannock, "Nostalgia Critique," *Cultural Studies* 9, no. 3 (1995): 456, https://doi.org/10.1080/09502389500490511.

131. Sue McKemmish, Anne Gilliland-Swetland, and Eric Ketelaar, "'Communities of Memory': Pluralising Archival Research and Education Agendas," *Archives and Manuscripts* 33 (2005): 158.

132. Janet Ceja Alcalá, "A Live Finding Aid of Archival Ethnographies," *Reconstruction* 16, no. 1 (2016).

133. R. Stuart Geiger and David Ribes, "Trace Ethnography: Following Coordination through Documentary Practices," 44th Hawaii International Conference on System Sciences, 2011, p. 3, https://doi.org/10.1109/HICSS.2011.455.

134. McKemmish, Gilliland-Swetland, and Ketelaar, "Communities of Memory," 146.

135. Karen Gracy, "Documenting Communities of Practice: Making the Case for Archival Ethnography," *Archival Science* 4, no. 3 (2004): 337, https://doi.org/10.1007/s10502-005-2599-3.

136. Gracy, "Documenting Communities of Practice," 335–36.

137. Annelise Riles, "Introduction: In Response," in *Documents: Artifacts of Modern Knowledge,* ed. Annelise Riles (Ann Arbor: University of Michigan, 2006), 7.

138. Matthew S. Hull, "Documents and Bureaucracy," *Annual Review of Anthropology* 41 (2012): 253, https://doi.org/10.1146/annurev.anthro.012809.1049 53.

1. "Your Nostalgia Is Killing Me!"

1. Vincent Chevalier and Ian Bradley-Perrin, *Your Nostalgia Is Killing Me!,* November 20, 2013, poster, PosterVirus, http://postervirus.tumblr.com/post/67569099579/your-nostalgia-is-killing-me-vincent-.

2. Theodore (Ted) Kerr, in discussion with the author, New York City, May 23, 2016.

3. Notably, much scholarship comes from 1980s- and 1990s-era ACT UPers. Cvetkovich, *Archive of Feelings;* Gould, *Moving Politics;* Alexandra Juhasz, *AIDS TV: Identity, Community, and Alternative Video* (Durham, N.C.: Duke University Press, 1995); Debra Levine, "Demonstrating ACT UP: The Ethics, Politics, and Performances of Affinity" (PhD diss., New York University, 2012); Benita Roth, *The Life and Death of ACT UP/LA: Anti-AIDS Activism in Los Angeles from the 1980s to the 2000s* (Cambridge: Cambridge University Press, 2017).

4. Douglas Crimp, ed., *AIDS: Cultural Analysis, Cultural Activism* (Cambridge, Mass.: MIT Press, 1988), xiv.

5. Gould, *Moving Politics,* 32. Analyses of ACT UP offer the most in-depth engagement with AIDS activism and emotion.

6. Hilderbrand, "Retroactivism," 303.

7. Alexandra Juhasz and Ted Kerr, "Home Video Returns: Media Ecologies of the Past of HIV/AIDS," *Cineaste* 39, no. 3 (2014), https://www.cineaste.com/summer2014/home-video-returns-media-ecologies-of-the-past-of-hiv-aids/; Kerr, discussion; Theodore (Ted) Kerr, "The AIDS Crisis Revisitation," LAMDA Literary, January 4, 2018, https://www.lambdaliterary.org/features/oped/01/04/the-aids-crisis-revisitation/.

8. Theodore (Ted) Kerr, "AIDS 1969: HIV, History, and Race," *Drain Magazine* 13, no. 2 (2016), http://drainmag.com/aids-1969-hiv-history-and-race/.

9. Juhasz, "Forgetting ACT UP," 72.

10. Avram Finkelstein, in discussion with the author, Brooklyn, New York, May 19, 2016. Subsequently, *Your Nostalgia* appears in Finkelstein, *After Silence: A*

History of AIDS through Its Images (Berkeley: University of California Press, 2018).

11. Finkelstein, discussion.

12. Kerr, "AIDS 1969."

13. Jason Baumann, in discussion with the author, New York City, July 21, 2015.

14. ACT UP, leaflet, "Media Advisory: Hundreds of AIDS Activists Dump Human Ashes on White House in Shocking Political Funeral," October 9, 1992, ACT UP New York Records, Reel 13, Box 18, Folder 10, Manuscripts and Archives Division, New York Public Library.

15. ACT UP, leaflet, "Media Advisory."

16. Baumann, discussion, 2015.

17. Baumann, discussion, 2015.

18. Jason Baumann, in discussion with the author, New York City, August 25, 2016.

19. Baumann, discussion, 2016.

20. Hilderbrand, "Retroactivism," 310.

21. Steven Kerry, January 5, 2018, comment on Kerr, "AIDS Crisis Revisitation," LAMDA Literary, https://www.lambdaliterary.org/features/oped/01/04/the-aids-crisis-revisitation/.

22. Kerr, discussion.

23. Juhasz, "Forgetting ACT UP," 69.

24. Dan Royles, *To Make the Wounded Whole: The African American Struggle against HIV/AIDS* (Chapel Hill: University of North Carolina Press, 2020).

25. M. Alfredo González, "Latinos ACT UP: Transnational AIDS Activism in the 1990s," North American Congress on Latin America, June 29, 2008, https://nacla.org/article/latinos-act-transnational-aids-activism-1990s.

26. Juhasz, "Forgetting ACT UP," 71.

27. David Harvey, "Neoliberalism as Creative Destruction," *Annals of the American Academy of Political and Social Science* 610 (2007): 22.

28. Wendy L. Brown, "Booked #3: What Exactly Is Neoliberalism?," interview by Timothy Shenk, *Dissent Magazine*, April 2, 2015, https://www.dissentmagazine.org/blog/booked-3-what-exactly-is-neoliberalism-wendy-brown-undoing-the-demos.

29. Robert McRuer, "Cripping Queer Politics, or the Dangers of Neoliberalism," *Scholar and Feminist Online* 10, nos. 1–2 (2012), https://sfonline.barnard.edu/a-new-queer-agenda/cripping-queer-politics-or-the-dangers-of-neoliberalism/.

30. René Esparza, "'Qué Bonita Mi Tierra': U.S.–Latinx Third-World AIDS Activism" (unpublished manuscript, 2020).

31. Montoya, "From 'the People' to 'the Human,'" 562.

32. Gilbert Elbaz, "Sociology of AIDS Activism, The Case of ACT UP/New York, 1987–1992 (Volumes I and II)" (PhD diss., City University of New York, 1992).

33. Mark Milano, in discussion with the author, New York City, August 31, 2016.

34. Juhasz, "Forgetting ACT UP," 72.

35. Hilderbrand, "Retroactivism," 310–11.

36. Hilderbrand, "Retroactivism," 309.

37. Hilderbrand, "Retroactivism," 305.

38. Gould, *Moving Politics,* 209.

39. Hilderbrand, "Retroactivism," 313.

40. Milano, discussion.

41. Milano, discussion.

42. Hilderbrand, "Retroactivism," 313.

43. Ian Bradley-Perrin, in discussion with the author, Brooklyn, New York, September 1, 2016.

44. Myrl Beam, *Gay, Inc.: The Nonprofitization of Queer Politics* (Minneapolis: University of Minnesota Press, 2018).

45. Esparza, "Qué Bonita."

46. René Esparza, "'Qué Bonita Mi Tierra': Latinx AIDS Activism and Decolonial Queer Praxis in 1980s New York and Puerto Rico," *Radical History Review* 2021, no. 140 (2021): 127.

47. Hilderbrand, "Retroactivism," 313.

48. Milano, discussion.

49. Juhasz, "Forgetting ACT UP," 72.

50. Foster, "Choreographies of Protest," 404.

51. Tara Burk, "From the Streets to the Gallery: Exhibiting the Visual Ephemera of AIDS Cultural Activism," *Journal of Curatorial Studies* 2, no. 1 (2013): 34.

52. Hilderbrand, "Retroactivism," 310.

53. Product Red, styled as (RED), founded in 2006 by Bono and Bobby Shriver, engages corporations in awareness and fund-raising to end HIV/AIDS in Africa, and in 2020 expanded to include Covid-19.

54. Chevalier and Bradley-Perrin, *Your Nostalgia Is Killing Me!*

55. "About PosterVirus," PosterVirus, http://postervirus.tumblr.com/AboutPoster Virus.

56. "About PosterVirus."

57. "PosterVirus 2013," PosterVirus, http://postervirus.tumblr.com/2013.

58. "PosterVirus 2013."

59. "PosterVirus 2013."

60. "PosterVirus 2013."

61. Gus Caims, "PrEP Wars: Debating Pre-exposure Prophylaxis in the Gay Community," *HIV Treatment Update,* February 14, 2013, https://www.aidsmap .com/news/feb-2013/prep-wars-debating-pre-exposure-prophylaxis-gay -community.

62. Treatment as Prevention relies on antiretroviral medications to attain undetectable virus loads for people with HIV/AIDS that render HIV noncontagious. Jon Cohen, "HIV Treatment as Prevention," *Science* 334, no. 6053 (2011): 1628.

63. Bradley-Perrin, discussion.

64. Bradley-Perrin, discussion.

65. Bradley-Perrin, discussion.

66. Bradley-Perrin, discussion.

67. Finkelstein, *After Silence,* 208.

68. Finkelstein, *After Silence,* 209.

69. Vincent Chevalier, in discussion with the author, Skype, August 2, 2016.

70. Chevalier, discussion.

71. Chevalier, discussion.

72. Chevalier, discussion.

73. Chevalier, discussion.

74. Chevalier, discussion.

75. Chevalier and Bradley-Perrin, *Your Nostalgia Is Killing Me!*

76. Chevalier, discussion.

77. Chevalier, discussion.

78. Chevalier, discussion.

79. Chevalier, discussion.

80. Chevalier, discussion.

81. Chevalier, discussion.

82. Chevalier, discussion.

83. Ian Bradley-Perrin, Facebook, January 10, 2014, 8:18 a.m., comment on ACT UP/NY Alumni page, https://www.facebook.com/groups/ACTUPNYAlumni/permalink/10151868083787747/.

84. Bradley-Perrin, discussion.

85. Kerr, discussion.

86. Bradley-Perrin, Facebook, January 10, 2014, 8:18 a.m.

87. Chevalier, discussion.

88. Chevalier, discussion.

89. General Idea issued the design on billboards, prints, stamps, and wallpaper. Kim Conaty, "*Print/Out:* General Idea," Inside/Out (blog), MoMA/MoMA PS1, April 18, 2012, https://www.moma.org/explore/inside_out/2012/04/18/printout-general-idea/. This piece also inspired the cover art for this book.

90. Chevalier, discussion.

91. Chevalier, discussion.

92. Donald G. MacNeil, "HIV Arrived in the U.S. Long before 'Patient Zero,'" *New York Times,* October 27, 2016, https://www.nytimes.com/.

93. AZT, or azidothymidine, was an early medication for treating HIV/AIDS that was toxic and ineffective when provided alone.

94. J. Scott Applewhite, "AIDS Protest," October 11, 1988, photograph, https://mic.com/articles/138264/the-history-of-hiv-aids-in-the-united-states-that-everyone-should-know#.uPwkcyCT9.

95. Chevalier and Bradley-Perrin, *Your Nostalgia Is Killing Me!*

96. Bradley-Perrin, discussion.

97. Bradley-Perrin, Facebook, January 10, 2014, 8:18 a.m.

98. Chevalier, discussion.

99. Bradley-Perrin, discussion.

100. Bradley-Perrin, discussion.

101. Bradley-Perrin, discussion.

102. Chevalier, discussion.

103. Chevalier noted: "[my first reaction] was, 'Oh, brother' . . . I know that Justin Bieber didn't know anything about it, and his audience would be like, 'ACT UP, like, totally. ACT UP,' but not know what it was." Chevalier and Bradley-Perrin did not learn until the NYPL panel that Bieber's Opening Ceremony T-shirt was a fund raiser. Chevalier also highlighted the setting: "It's a teenager's bedroom, so she had to have a picture of a pop star." Chevalier, discussion.

104. Bradley-Perrin, discussion.

105. Guy Trebay, "In Your Face (The Birth of Queer Nation)," *Village Voice*, August 14, 1990.

106. Bradley-Perrin, discussion.

107. Bradley-Perrin, discussion.

108. Chevalier, discussion.

109. Chevalier, discussion.

110. Before the web's ubiquity, building exteriors were public information exchange forums. Political image activism declined as Mayor Rudolph Giuliani (1994–2001) targeted noncommercial wheat pasting under "quality of life" policing. Burk, "From the Streets to the Gallery," 35.

111. Jim Hubbard, in discussion with the author, New York City, August 31, 2016.

112. Theodore (Ted) Kerr, "NYPL Presents Why We Fight Film Series, Curated by Jim Hubbard," Visual AIDS Blog, Visual AIDS, December 20, 2013, https://visualaids.org/blog/on-organizing-and-your-nostalgia-is-killing-me.

113. Kerr, discussion.

114. Kerr, discussion.

115. Kerr, discussion.

116. Commenter, Facebook, January 10, 2014, 9:31 a.m., comment on ACT UP/NY Alumni page, https://www.facebook.com/groups/ACTUPNYAlumni/permalink/10151868083787747/.

117. Finkelstein, discussion.

118. Finkelstein, discussion.

119. Jason Baumann, in discussion with the author, New York City, August 25, 2016.

120. Baumann, discussion, 2016.

121. Commenter, Facebook, January 12, 2014, 8:08 a.m., comment (since deleted) on ACT UP/NY Alumni page, https://www.facebook.com/groups/ACTUPNY Alumni/permalink/10151868083787747/.

122. Simon Watney, Facebook, January 10, 2014, 5:51 p.m., comment on ACT UP/NY Alumni page, https://www.facebook.com/groups/ACTUPNYAlumni/permalink/10151868083787747/.

123. Kerr, discussion.

124. Ian Bradley-Perrin, Facebook, January 11, 2014, 1:11 p.m., comment on personal page, https://www.facebook.com/photo.php?fbid=10152138863616488&set=a.10150710680671488.454104.589811487&type=3&theater.

125. Kerr, discussion.

126. Kerr, discussion.

127. Finkelstein, discussion.

128. Finkelstein, discussion.

129. Finkelstein, discussion.

130. Finkelstein, discussion.

131. Kerr, discussion.

132. Theodore (Ted) Kerr, "On Organizing, and Your Nostalgia Is Killing Me," Visual AIDS Blog, Visual AIDS, March 1, 2014, https://www.visualaids.org/blog/detail/on-organizing-and-your-nostalgia-is-killing-me.

133. Baumann, discussion, 2016.

134. Baumann, discussion, 2016.

135. Christopher Conry, "Your Nostalgia Is Killing Me," YouTube, March 18, 2014, video, 1:28:07, https://www.youtube.com/watch?v=krD1iEZpBEw.

136. Finkelstein, discussion.

137. Finkelstein, discussion.

138. Bradley-Perrin, discussion.

139. Bradley-Perrin, discussion.

140. David Lowenthal, *The Past Is a Foreign Country* (Cambridge: Cambridge University Press, 1985), 9.

141. Finkelstein, discussion.

142. Finkelstein, discussion.

2. How to ACT UP

1. Vito Russo, "Why We Fight," ACT UP demonstration, May 9, 1988, Albany, New York, speech transcript, http://www.actupny.org/documents/whfight.html.

2. Russo, "Why We Fight."

3. Román, "Remembering AIDS," 282.

4. Russo, "Why We Fight."

5. Flinn and Alexander, "Humanizing an Inevitably Political Craft."

6. Hilderbrand, "Retroactivism."

7. Russo, "Why We Fight."

8. Russo, "Why We Fight."

9. Charles E. Morris III, "ACT UP 25: HIV/AIDS, Archival Queers, and Mnemonic World Making," *Quarterly Journal of Speech* 98, no. 1 (2012): 50, https://doi.org/10.1080/00335630.2011.638658.

10. Douglas Crimp, ed., *AIDS: Cultural Analysis, Cultural Activism* (Cambridge, Mass.: MIT Press, 1988).

11. Burk, "From the Streets to the Gallery;" Foster, "Choreographies of Protest.

12. Scott Wald, interview by Sarah Schulman, ACT UP Oral History Project, June 1, 2012, 42, http://www.actuporalhistory.org/interviews/images/wald.pdf.

13. Jon Greenberg, "ACT UP Explained," ACT UP/New York (1992), http://www.actupny.org/documents/greenbergAU.html.

14. Román, "Remembering AIDS," 282.

15. Solomon, "What Does It Mean to Remember AIDS?"

16. Solomon, "What Does it Mean to Remember AIDS?"

17. Jan Huebenthal, "Injury and Resistance: Centering HIV/AIDS Histories in Times of Queer Equality" (PhD diss., College of William and Mary, 2019).

18. Levine, discussion.

19. Maxine Wolfe, in discussion with the author, telephone, August 18, 2016.

20. Flinn, Stevens, and Shepherd, "Whose Memories, Whose Archives?"

21. Andrew Flinn and Mary Stevens, "'It is nohmistri, wi mekin histori': Telling Our Own Story: Independent and Community Archives in the U.K., Challenging and Subverting the Mainstream," in *Community Archives: The Shaping of Memory,* ed. Jeanette Bastian and Ben Alexander (London: Facet, 2009).

22. Flinn and Alexander, "Humanizing an Inevitably Political Craft," 330.

23. Hallas, "Queer AIDS Media," 431–35.

24. Gill-Peterson, "Haunting the Queer Spaces of AIDS," 279–300.

25. Román, "Remembering AIDS," 285.

26. Levine, discussion.

27. Levine, discussion.

28. Alexis Danzig, in discussion with the author, New York City, September 12, 2016.

29. Danzig, discussion.

30. Danzig, discussion.

31. Danzig, discussion.

32. Catherine Saalfield and Ray Navarro, "Shocking Pink Praxis: Race and Gender on the ACT UP Frontlines," in *Inside/Out: Lesbian Theories, Gay Theories,* ed. Diana Fuss (New York: Routledge, 1991), 363.

33. Juhasz, *AIDS TV,* 3.

34. Juhasz, *AIDS TV,* 3.

35. Ron Goldberg, interview by Sarah Schulman, ACT UP Oral History Project, October 25, 2003, 22, http://www.actuporalhistory.org/interviews/images/goldberg.pdf.

36. Goldberg, oral history interview, 22.

37. Wolfe, discussion.

38. Levine, discussion.

39. Danzig, discussion.

40. Laurie Ouellette, "Will the Revolution Be Televised? Camcorders, Activism, and Alternative Television in the 1990s," in *Transmission: Toward a Post-television Culture*, ed. Peter d'Agostino and David Tafler (Thousand Oaks, Calif.: Sage, 1994), 165–85; Rebekah Willett, "In the Frame: Mapping Camcorder Cultures," in *Video Cultures*, ed. David Buckingham and Rebekah Willett (London: Palgrave Macmillan, 2009), 1–22.

41. Wolfe, discussion.

42. Wolfe, discussion.

43. Goldberg, oral history interview, 22.

44. Juhasz, *AIDS TV*, 1.

45. Goldberg, oral history interview, 22.

46. Danzig, discussion.

47. Hubbard, discussion.

48. Hubbard, discussion.

49. Danzig, discussion.

50. Juhasz, *AIDS TV*, 3.

51. Weiner, "Disposable Media, Expendable Populations," 105.

52. Weiner, "Disposable Media, Expendable Populations," 105–6.

53. Hilderbrand, "Retroactivism," 303.

54. Cifor, "Acting Up, Talking Back"; Cvetkovich, *Archive of Feelings;* Gould, *Moving Politics;* Levine, "Demonstrating ACT UP."

55. Alexandrina Buchanan and Michelle Bastian, "Activating the Archive: Rethinking the Role of Traditional Archives for Local Activist Projects," *Archival Science* 15, no. 4 (2015): 429–51, https://doi.org/10.1007/s10502-015-9247-3.

56. Hubbard, discussion.

57. X, Campbell, and Stevens, "Love and Lubrication," 294.

58. Levine, discussion.

59. Levine, discussion.

60. X, Campbell, and Stevens, "Love and Lubrication," 294.

61. Wolfe, discussion.

62. Wolfe, discussion.

63. Finkelstein, discussion.

64. Bill Dobbs, interview by Sarah Schulman, ACT UP Oral History Project, November 21, 2006, 39, http://www.actuporalhistory.org/interviews/images/dobbs.pdf.

65. Sean Strub, *Body Counts: A Memoir of Activism, Sex, and Survival* (New York: Simon and Schuster, 2014), 202–3.

66. Strub, *Body Counts*, 203.

67. Finkelstein, discussion.

68. Finkelstein, discussion.

69. Finkelstein, discussion.

70. Stephen Shapiro, e-mail message to author, November 10, 2017.

71. Lisa Diedrich, "Doing Queer Love: Feminism, AIDS, and History," *Theoria* 54, no. 112 (April 2007): 28–30, 37.

72. Levine, discussion.

73. Levine, discussion.

74. Levine, discussion.

75. Juhasz, *AIDS TV.*

76. Polly Thistlethwaite, interview by Sarah Schulman, ACT UP Oral History Project, January 6, 2013, 44, http://www.actuporalhistory.org/interviews/images/thistlethwaite.pdf.

77. After a police strip search of activists at a Target City Hall action was deemed illegal, the activists, including many women, were awarded a settlement, some of which was donated to the LHA. Thistlethwaite, oral history interview, 37.

78. In her oral history interview, Thistlethwaite named ACT UP men's contributions to the LHA: "Charlie Barber donated his office equipment, and John Kelly worked with the archives. He was a good carpenter . . . and I actually learned how to plaster from Alexis Danzig and John Kelly" (48–49). Along with Zoe Leonard, they erected the plaster ceiling at the LHA's Brooklyn brownstone (49).

79. Danzig, discussion.

80. Levine, discussion.

81. Cvetkovich, *Archive of Feelings,* 158.

82. Wolfe, discussion.

83. Thistlewaite, oral history interview, 22–23.

84. Wolfe, discussion.

85. Levine, discussion.

86. Stephen Shapiro, in discussion with the author, Skype, December 11, 2015.

87. Shapiro (2015 discussion) recalled the first workspace being on Fourteenth Street and that ACT UP had been forced to move after a fire. The group "could not find anyone to rent to them," so they called on Larry Kramer's brother, who worked in real estate, to secure the location on West 29th Street.

88. Shapiro (2015 discussion) attributed volunteers' abilities, including Rygor's, to commit to AIDS activism full time to their receipt of state disability benefits.

89. Jason Baumann, in discussion with the author, New York City, July 21, 2015.

90. Robert Rygor Papers, 1953–94, Department of Special Collections and Archives, Queens College, http://archives.qc.cuny.edu/finding_aids/RobertRygor. Exact dates of Rygor's tenure as workspace manager are unknown. Diagnosed with HIV in 1990, he devoted his final years to AIDS activism. Rygor died January 16, 1994 (Shapiro, 2017 e-mail).

91. Baumann, discussion, 2015.

92. Shapiro, discussion, 2015.

93. Wolfe, discussion.

94. Shapiro, 2017 e-mail message.

95. Anna Blume, interview by Sarah Schulman, ACT UP Oral History Project, January 25, 2010, 19, http://www.actuporalhistory.org/interviews/images/blume .pdf; Sarah Schulman, *Conflict Is Not Abuse: Overstating Harm, Community Responsibility, and the Duty of Repair* (Vancouver: Arsenal Pulp Press, 2016).

96. Shapiro, discussion, 2015.

97. Stephen Shapiro, 2004 interview by Sarah Schulman and Jim Hubbard, ACT UP Oral History Project, October 23, 2004, 57, http://www.actuporalhistory .org/interviews/interviews_11.html#shapiro.

98. He became involved with the workspace collection while tracking down ACT UP network accounts. Shapiro (2015 discussion) described investigating an issue with funds generated by 1990 compilation album, *Red, Hot + Blue*. Its producer, the Red Hot Organization, donated proceeds to AIDS organizations, including ACT UP and the Treatment Action Group (TAG), constituted by former treatment and data committee members who splintered off in 1992. When ACT UP/NY stopped receiving funds, and amid an array of financial issues, Shapiro began investigating why by using the group's archives. Red Hot, he remembered, claimed that ACT UP failed to thank them and that it had mismanaged funds. Shapiro discovered that the proceeds were going entirely to TAG, who had claimed to be ACT UP's successor. ACT UP received, he recalled, one more payment as a result of research that turned up proper accounting, and a thank-you letter.

99. Shapiro, discussion, 2015.

100. Mimi Bowling, in discussion with the author, telephone, July 9, 2015.

101. Shapiro, discussion, 2015.

102. Shapiro, 2004 interview.

103. Shapiro, 2004 interview.

104. Wolfe, discussion. ACT UP materials were included in the NYPL's 1994 exhibition, *Becoming Visible: The Legacy of Stonewall.* ACT UP's response, as Bowling noted to me in our 2015 discussion, "baffled me to this very day, claiming that we conflated sex with AIDS, which we did not." By 1995, the NYPL had acquired related organization records and personal papers.

105. Wolfe, discussion. Fire is the safety concern that Wolfe and Shapiro emphasized. Likely both were reflecting on an October 1974 arson that had destroyed the interior of the former firehouse occupied by the Gay Activists Alliance in SoHo, which had served as a political and cultural center for lesbians and gays. "Gay Activists Alliance Firehouse," NYC LGBT Historic Sites Project, https://www.nyclgbtsites.org/site/gay-activists-alliance-firehouse/.

106. Wolfe, discussion.

107. Danzig, discussion.

108. Levine, discussion.

109. Shapiro, 2004 interview.

110. Shapiro, discussion, 2015.

111. Planned as an archives and museum, it was initiated by the Center's board and founded by Richard C. Wandel, a historian, photographer, and archivist.

112. The building had asbestos and was structurally at risk (Shapiro, discussion, 2015). A capital campaign began in 1995, and renovations started in 1998. The Center was relocated until 2001. "Center History," Lesbian, Gay, Bisexual and Transgender Community Center, https://gaycenter.org/about/history/.

113. Shapiro, discussion, 2015. The more effective HIV/AIDS treatment developed in 1995 and available in 1996 is known as the "AIDS cocktail." Combination therapy is also referred to as highly active antiretroviral therapy (HAART), combination antiretroviral therapy (cART), or antiretroviral therapy (ART).

114. Shapiro, discussion, 2015.

115. Shapiro, discussion, 2015.

116. Shapiro, 2004 interview.

117. Shapiro, 2004 interview.

118. Wolfe, discussion.

119. Danzig, discussion.

120. Thistlewaite, oral history interview, 44.

121. Shapiro, discussion, 2015.

122. Shapiro, discussion, 2015.

123. Shapiro, discussion, 2015.

124. Shapiro, 2017 e-mail.

125. Danzig, discussion.

126. Danzig, discussion.

127. Shapiro, discussion, 2015.

128. "About the Manuscripts and Archives Division," New York Public Library, https://www.nypl.org/about/divisions/manuscripts-division.

129. John Hammond and Bruce Eves' 1988 donation of their International Gay Information Center collection was, according to Bowling (discussion), the NYPL's first major LGBT collection.

130. Bowling, discussion.

131. Bowling, discussion.

132. Bowling, discussion.

133. Bowling, discussion.

134. Shapiro, discussion, 2015.

135. Shapiro, discussion, 2015.

136. Shapiro, discussion, 2015.

137. Shapiro, 2017 e-mail.

138. Shapiro, 2017 e-mail.

139. Finkelstein, discussion.

140. Shapiro, 2017 e-mail.

141. Shapiro, 2017 e-mail.

142. Shapiro, 2017 e-mail.

143. Shapiro, 2017 e-mail.

144. Shapiro, 2017 e-mail.

145. Shapiro, 2017 e-mail.

146. Shapiro, 2004 interview.

147. Shapiro, discussion, 2015.

148. Shapiro, discussion, 2015.

149. Shapiro, discussion, 2015.

150. Shapiro, discussion, 2015.

151. Bowling, discussion.

152. New York Public Library, "ACT UP/NY Archives Donated to The New York Public Library," news release, March 11, 1996, http://www.actupny.org/docu ments/nyplPR.html.

153. The NYPL received the ACT UP/NY records in 1995. Additional records, including from the workspace collection, were not initially donated. Some were held by Goldberg, who was planning to write a book; three years later, he gave up his plans and donated the materials to the NYPL (Shapiro, 2015 interview; Goldberg, oral history interview). The finding aid for the ACT UP/ NY Records notes additions from Jack Ben Levi, Conyers Thompson, and Shapiro between 1992 and 1997. ACT UP New York Records, 1969, 1982–97, n.d., Humanities and Social Sciences Library, Manuscripts and Archives Division, New York Public Library, May 2008, https://nyplorg-data-archives-produc tion.s3.amazonaws.com/uploads/collection/pdf_finding_aid/actupny.pdf.

154. Shapiro, 2004 interview.

155. Baumann, discussion, 2015.

156. Shapiro, discussion, 2015.

157. "Gay and Lesbian Collections & AIDS/HIV Collections," New York Public Library, https://www.nypl.org/lgbtqcollections.

158. Levine, discussion.

159. Shapiro, discussion, 2015.

160. New York Public Library, "ACT UP/NY Archives Donated."

161. New York Public Library, "ACT UP/NY Archives Donated."

162. Wolfe, discussion.

163. Thistlewaite, oral history interview, 48.

164. Wolfe, discussion.

165. Wolfe, discussion.

166. Wolfe, discussion.

167. Wolfe, discussion. Shapiro, in a 2017 e-mail to me, contested Wolfe's account of the timeline: "My recollection is that BEFORE NYPL came, not AFTER, Max[ine Wolfe] and Ron Goldberg went in and took materials out."

168. Wolfe, discussion.

169. "How to Use the Archives," Lesbian Herstory Archives, https://web.archive
.org/web/20190628064915/http://www.lesbianherstoryarchives.org/using
.html.

170. Shapiro, discussion, 2015.

171. Levine, discussion.

172. Goldberg, oral history interview, 23.

173. Thistlewaite, oral history interview, 34.

174. Julian de Mayo, in discussion with the author, New York City, August 27, 2016.

175. Finkelstein, discussion.

176. Danzig, discussion.

177. Baumann, discussion, 2015.

178. Jason Baumann, in discussion with the author, New York City, August 25,
2016.

179. Baumann, discussion, 2016.

180. Sellie et al., "Interference Archive," 456.

181. Sellie et al., "Interference Archive."

182. Baumann, discussion, 2016.

183. Baumann, discussion, 2016.

184. Poz Magazine, "Poz on Location: ACT UP 'Die-in' at NYPL," YouTube, October 9, 2013, video, 3:45, https://www.youtube.com/watch?v=pUcvehiXOJw.

185. Poz Magazine, "Poz on Location."

186. Winnie McCroy, "'AIDS Is Not History' Says Die-In at NYC Public Library,"
South Florida Gay News, October 8, 2013, https://southfloridagaynews.com/.

187. Nicholas Cimarusti, "ACT UP/NY Stages Die-In and Hackathon," *HIV Plus
Magazine,* October 25, 2013, http://www.hivplusmag.com/.

188. Cimarusti, "ACT UP/NY Stages Die-In and Hackathon."

189. Cimarusti, "ACT UP/NY Stages Die-In and Hackathon."

190. Foster, "Choreographies of Protest," 404. Strategically, the closeness of activists' bodies makes it difficult for police to surround and drag away any individual, thus providing communal care.

191. Milano, discussion.

192. Milano, discussion.

193. Milano, discussion.

194. Baumann, discussion, 2016.

195. New York Public Library, "How to ACT UP," January 15, 2014, https://www
.nypl.org/audiovideo/how-act.

196. Milano, discussion.

197. Baumann, discussion, 2016.

198. Baumann, discussion, 2016.

199. New York Public Library, "How to ACT UP: January 15, 2014."

200. Diedrich, *Indirect Action,* 199–216.

201. Baumann, discussion, 2016.

202. Baumann, discussion, 2015.

203. Baumann, discussion, 2015.

204. Baumann, discussion, 2015.

205. Baumann, discussion, 2015.

206. Baumann, discussion, 2015.

207. Baumann, discussion, 2015.

208. Baumann, discussion, 2015.

209. Baumann, discussion, 2015.

210. Morris, "ACT UP 25," 50.

211. Morris, "ACT UP 25," 50.

212. Marika Cifor and Jamie A. Lee, "Towards an Archival Critique: Opening Possibilities for Addressing Neoliberalism in the Archival Field," *Journal of Critical Library and Information Studies* 1, no. 1 (2017): 13, https://doi.org/10.24242/jclis.v1i1.10.

213. Cifor and Lee, "Towards an Archival Critique," 13.

214. In contrast, in 2015 the NYPL digitized 157 items from ACT UP/NY Records. On its Digital Collections website, these photographs, posters, and placards can be downloaded and reused without restriction.

215. Morris, "ACT UP 25," 50.

216. Morris, "ACT UP 25," 51.

217. Russo, "Why We Fight."

3. An Archival Cure

1. Kenyon Farrow, "What You Need to Know about the Second Person Likely Cured of HIV," Body Pro, March 6, 2019, https://www.thebodypro.com/article/need-to-know-second-person-likely-cured-hiv.

2. Kenyon Farrow, "No, Dr. Sebi Did Not Have the Cure for HIV—Despite Nipsey Hussle's Planned Documentary," Body, April 2, 2019, https://www.thebody.com/article/dr-sebi-did-not-cure-hiv-nipsey-hussle-documentary.

3. Farrow, "No, Dr. Sebi Did Not Have the Cure for HIV."

4. Nipsey Hussle, "Blue Laces 2," track 6 on *Victory Lap* (Atlantic Records, 2018).

5. Farrow, "No, Dr. Sebi Did Not Have the Cure for HIV."

6. Farrow, "No, Dr. Sebi Did Not Have the Cure for HIV."

7. Eunjung Kim, *Curative Violence: Rehabilitating Disability, Gender, and Sexuality in Modern Korea* (Durham, N.C.: Duke University Press, 2017), 4.

8. Eli Clare, *Brilliant Imperfection: Grappling with Cure* (Durham, N.C.: Duke University Press, 2017), 56.

9. Kim, *Curative Violence,* 14.

10. Joasia Krysa, "The Politics of Contemporary Curating: A Network Perspective," in *The Routledge Companion to Art and Politics,* ed. Randy Martin (New York: Routledge, 2015), 116.

11. Marika Cifor, "Towards an AIDS Archive," Gallery, Visual AIDS, June 2018, https://visualaids.org/gallery/detail/towards-an-aids-archive.

12. Clare, *Brilliant Imperfection*, xvi.

13. Flinn and Alexander, "Humanizing an Inevitably Political Craft." Whether social justice is an archival imperative is contested. See Mario H. Ramirez, "Being Assumed Not to Be: A Critique of Whiteness as an Archival Imperative," *American Archivist* 78, no. 2 (2015): 339–56, https://doi.org/10.17723/0360-9081.78.2.339.

14. Clare, *Brilliant Imperfection*, 6.

15. Kyle Croft, Tracy Fenix, David Hirsh, Eric Rhein, Sur Rodney (Sur), Nelson Santos, and Shirlene Cooper, "Activating the Archive Project" (event, Visual AIDS, Fales Library and Special Collections, Elmer Holmes Bobst Library, New York University, New York City [hereafter Fales], November 8, 2018), https://visualaids.org/events/detail/activating-the-archive-project.

16. Zidovudine (ZDV) or azidothymidine (AZT), brand name Retrovir (GlaxoSmithKline, original sponsor Burroughs-Wellcome), approved by the FDA in 1987, was the first antiretroviral HIV/AIDS treatment. Didanosine (ddI, DDI), sold as Videx (Bristol Myers-Squibb), was approved in 1991. Alcitabine (ddC), brand name Hivid (Hoffmann-La Roche), was approved in 1992. Lamivudine (3TC) sold as Epivir (GlaxoSmithKline), was approved in 1995. AZT, DDI, and 3TC are still used in combination therapies. Samuel Broder, "The Development of Antiretroviral Therapy and Its Impact on the HIV-1/AIDS Pandemic," *Antiviral Research* 85, no. 1 (2010): 1–18, https://doi.org/10.1016/j.antiviral.2009.10.002.

17. David Hirsh, in discussion with the author, telephone, December 5, 2018.

18. Hirsh, discussion, December 5, 2018.

19. Hirsh, discussion, December 5, 2018.

20. Hirsh, discussion, December 5, 2018.

21. Clare, *Brilliant Imperfection*, 15.

22. Clare, *Brilliant Imperfection*, 15.

23. Clare, *Brilliant Imperfection*, 15.

24. Clare, *Brilliant Imperfection*, 28.

25. Krysa, "Politics of Contemporary Curating," 116.

26. Walter Glannon, "Transcendence and Healing," *Journal of Medical Ethics* 30 (2004): 71, https://doi.org/10.1136/jmh.2002.000145; Krysa, "Politics of Contemporary Curating," 116; Carla Acevedo-Yates, "Curating Is a Double Game: *Curare* as an Alternative Model of Institutional Critique" (master's thesis, Bard College, 2014).

27. Hamid A. Abdulmumeen, Ahmed N. Risikat, and Agboola R. Sururah, "Food: Its Preservatives, Additives and Applications," *International Journal of Chemical and Biochemical Sciences* 1, no. 2012 (2012): 36–47.

28. Kim, *Curative Violence*, 6.

29. Kim, *Curative Violence*, 6.

30. Clare, *Brilliant Imperfection*, 106.

31. Clare, *Brilliant Imperfection*, 69.

32. Kim, *Curative Violence*, 7.

33. Robert McRuer, "Critical Investments: AIDS, Christopher Reeve, and Queer/Disabilities Studies," *Journal of Medical Humanities* 23, nos. 3–4 (2002): 230, https://doi.org/10.1023/A:1016846402426.

34. Katie Batza, *Before AIDS: Gay Health Politics in the 1970s* (Philadelphia: University of Pennsylvania Press, 2018), 133.

35. Batza (2018, 131) contests the dominant narrative placing AIDS activists in adversarial relationship to the state. From the 1970s, the state was enmeshed in the gay community's infrastructure of health services, research, and networks.

36. Diedrich, *Indirect Action*, 206–7.

37. Kim, *Curative Violence*, 8.

38. Clare, *Brilliant Imperfection*, 70.

39. Diedrich, *Indirect Action*, 131.

40. Martin Duberman, *Hold Tight Gently: Michael Callen, Essex Hemphill, and the Battlefield of AIDS* (New York: The New Press, 2014), 228.

41. Hirsh, discussion, December 5, 2018.

42. Hirsh, discussion, December 5, 2018.

43. Hirsh, discussion, December 5, 2018.

44. Hirsh, discussion, December 5, 2018.

45. Diedrich, *Indirect Action*, 16.

46. Diedrich, *Indirect Action*, 206.

47. Diedrich, *Indirect Action*, 2.

48. Jerry Friedland, "Still Here: Fighting HIV/AIDS in the Bronx" (panel presentation), September 10, 2016, Bronx Museum of the Arts, http://www.bronxmuseum.org/events/still-here-fighting-hiv-aids-in-the-bronx.

49. Clare, *Brilliant Imperfection*, 76.

50. Diedrich, *Indirect Action*, 131.

51. Jennifer Brier, *Infectious Ideas: U.S. Political Responses to the AIDS Crisis* (Chapel Hill: University of North Carolina Press, 2009), 168.

52. Diedrich, *Indirect Action*, 201; Brier, *Infectious Ideas*, 168; Gould, *Moving Politics*, 285–86; Duberman, *Hold Tight Gently*, 188; and Jan Huebenthal, "Injury and Resistance: Centering HIV/AIDS in Times of Queer Equality" (PhD diss., College of William and Mary, 2019) detail divisions within activist groups and their significance.

53. Diedrich, *Indirect Action*, 201.

54. Diedrich, *Indirect Action*, 16.

55. Clare, *Brilliant Imperfection*, 88.

56. Diedrich, *Indirect Action*, 200.

57. Hirsh, discussion, December 5, 2018.

58. Alexander McLelland and Jessica Whitbread, "PosterVirus: Claiming Sexual Autonomy for People with HIV through Collective Action," in *Mobilizing Metaphor: Art, Culture and Disability Activism in Canada,* ed. Christine Kelly and Michael Orsini (Vancouver: University of British Columbia Press, 2016), 86. On HIV/AIDS and disability, see Fink, *Forget Burial.*

59. McLelland and Whitbread, "PosterVirus," 86.

60. Kim, *Curative Violence,* 3.

61. Kim, *Curative Violence,* 11.

62. Alison Kafer, *Feminist, Queer, Crip* (Bloomington: Indiana University Press, 2013), 27.

63. Kim, *Curative Violence,* 8.

64. Kim, *Curative Violence,* 5.

65. Kafer, *Feminist, Queer, Crip,* 28.

66. Kim, *Curative Violence,* 11.

67. Kim, *Curative Violence,* 11.

68. David Hirsh, in discussion with the author, telephone, November 27, 2018.

69. Author's emphasis. Hirsh, discussion, November 27, 2018.

70. Nick Debs, "Essay," in *Arts' Communities, AIDS' Communities: Realizing the Archive Project* (New York: Visual AIDS, 1996), 20.

71. Sur Rodney (Sur), in discussion with the author, New York City, May 19, 2016.

72. Debs, "Essay," 20–21 (emphasis mine).

73. Debs, "Essay," 21.

74. Debs, "Essay," 21.

75. Debs, "Essay," 21.

76. Debs, "Essay," 21.

77. Frank Moore, "Frank Moore," in W. E. Scott Hoot, "Estate Planning for Artists: Will Your Art Survive?," *Columbia-VLA Journal of Law and the Arts* 1, no. 1 (1996): 21; David Hirsh, in discussion with the author, New York City, November 8, 2018.

78. Esther McGowan, in discussion with the author, New York City, May 27, 2016.

79. Diana K. Wakimoto, Chirstine Bruce, and Helen Partridge, "Archivist as Activist: Lessons from Three Queer Community Archives in California," *Archival Science* 13, no. 4 (2013): 293–316, https://doi.org/10.1007/s10502-013-9201-1; Marika Cifor, Michelle Caswell, Alda Allina Migoni, and Noah Geraci, "'What We Do Crosses Over to Activism': The Politics and Practice of Community Archives," *The Public Historian* 40, no. 2 (2018): 69–95, https://doi.org/10.1525/tph.2018.40.2.69.

80. "About Us," Visual AIDS, https://www.visualaids.org/about.

81. "About Us," Visual AIDS.

82. "The Archive Project," Visual AIDS, https://www.visualaids.org/projects/detail/the-archive-project.

83. Moore, "Frank Moore," 19.

84. Moore, "Frank Moore," 19.

85. Moore, "Frank Moore," 19.

86. Hirsh, discussion, November 8, 2018.

87. Hirsh, discussion, November 8, 2018.

88. Lisa Duggan and José Esteban Muñoz, "Hope and Hopelessness: A Dialogue," *Women and Performance* 19, no. 2 (July 2009): 278, https://doi.org/10.1080/07407700903064946.

89. Visual AIDS Staff, "The Multitudes of Frank Moore," "Gallery," Visual AIDS, November 2012, https://www.visualaids.org/gallery/detail/104.

90. W. E. Scott Hoot, "Estate Planning for Artists: Will Your Art Survive?" *Columbia-VLA Journal of Law and the Arts* 21, no. 1 (1996): 15.

91. "FM Notebook #82, 1993–1995," Frank Moore Papers, MSS 135, Box 5, Folder 138, Fales.

92. "FM Notebook #82, 1993–1995."

93. Douglas Crimp, "Right On, Girlfriend!" *Social Text* no. 33 (1992): 2, https://doi.org/10.2307/466431.

94. Daniel C. Brouwer, "Communication as Counterpublic," in *Communication as . . . Perspectives on Theory,* ed. T. G. Striphas, Gregory J. Shepherd, and Jeffery St. John (Thousand Oaks, Calif.: Sage, 2006), 199.

95. Gould, *Moving Politics,* 349, 392.

96. "FM Notebook #82, 1993–1995."

97. "FM Notebook #82, 1993–1995."

98. "FM Notebook #82, 1993–1995."

99. Hirsh, discussion, November 8, 2018.

100. Hirsh, discussion, December 5, 2018.

101. Hirsh, discussion, November 27, 2018.

102. Hirsh, discussion, November 8, 2018.

103. Hirsh, discussion, December 5, 2018.

104. Hirsh, discussion, November 8, 2018.

105. Hirsh, discussion, December 5, 2018.

106. Hirsh, discussion, December 5, 2018. For Moore, the archive committee was a practical fulfillment of the Estate Project for Artists with AIDS's estate-planning services, which addressed archiving only on "a theoretical level." Moore, "Frank Moore," 21.

107. Hirsh, discussion, November 8, 2018.

108. Honorary members Hirsh selected were people formative to the archives' vision, but who were unable to participate day to day. Hirsh, discussion, December 5, 2018.

109. It is difficult to establish a leadership roster. Worn down from loved ones "continuously dying" and facing financial challenges, of his decision to step back in the late 1990s, Hirsh said, "I had to take care of myself. It was as simple

as that." Moore was involved until his 2002 death. Others were involved briefly, such as Richardson. Because there was no secretary, few documents chart the archives' early development. Hirsh, discussion, November 27 and December 5, 2018.

110. Hirsh, discussion, November 27, 2018.

111. Hirsh, discussion, November 27, 2018.

112. Hirsh, discussion, November 27, 2018.

113. Hirsh, discussion, November 27, 2018.

114. Sur, discussion.

115. Eric Rhein, in discussion with the author, Jersey City, N.J., May 26, 2016.

116. Rhein, discussion.

117. Visual AIDS Staff, "The Multitudes of Frank Moore."

118. Hirsh, discussion, November 27, 2018.

119. Rhein, discussion.

120. Rhein, discussion.

121. Michelle Caswell, "Toward a Survivor-Centered Approach to Records Documenting Human Rights Abuse: Lessons from Community Archives," *Archival Science* 14, nos. 3–4 (2014): 313, https://doi.org/10.1007/s10502-014-9220-6.

122. Hirsh, discussion, November 8, 2018.

123. Roberto Juarez, in discussion with the author, New York City, May 23, 2016.

124. Ralph Blumenthal, "Artists with AIDS Race Time to Preserve Work for All Time," *New York Times,* June 20, 1995, https://www.nytimes.com/.

125. Blumenthal, "Artists with AIDS Race Time."

126. Lisa Pines, "Forward," in *Arts' Communities, AIDS' Communities: Realizing the Archive Project* (New York: Visual AIDS, 1996), 6.

127. Juarez, discussion.

128. Rhein, discussion.

129. Rhein, discussion.

130. Hirsh, discussion, November 27, 2018.

131. David Hirsh, in discussion with the author, telephone, April 25, 2019.

132. Hirsh, discussion, April 25, 2019.

133. Blumenthal, "Artists with AIDS Race Time."

134. Juarez, discussion.

135. Hirsh, discussion, April 25, 2019.

136. Hirsh, discussion, April 25, 2019.

137. Hirsh, discussion, April 25, 2019.

138. Joseph Stegenga, *Care and Cure: An Introduction to the Philosophy of Medicine* (Chicago: University of Chicago Press, 2018), 1.

139. Glannon, "Transcendence and Healing," 71; Krysa, "Politics of Contemporary Curating," 116.

140. Frank Moore, "Frank Moore"; Rhein, discussion.

141. Frank Moore, "Frank Moore," 21.

142. Marlon M. Bailey, "'Dear Audre': Black Gay and Lesbian Caregiving as HIV/AIDS Activism in the '80s," National Women's Studies Association, San Francisco, November 15, 2019.

143. Bailey, "Dear Audre."

144. Michelle Caswell and Marika Cifor, "From Human Rights to Feminist Ethics: Radical Empathy in the Archives," *Archivaria* 81 (2016): 24. On the Artist+ Registry as manifestation of a feminist ethics of care approach, see Michelle Caswell and Marika Cifor, "Neither a Beginning Nor an End: Applying an Ethics of Care to Digital Archival Collections," in *The Routledge International Handbook of New Digital Practices in Galleries, Libraries, Archives, Museums and Heritage Sites,* ed. Hannah Lewi, Wally Smith, Steven Cooke, and Dirk vom Lehn (London: Routledge, 2019).

145. Caswell and Cifor, "From Human Rights to Feminist Ethics," 31.

146. Hirsh, discussion, November 27, 2018.

147. Sur, discussion.

148. Paul Ashmore, Ruth Craggs, and Hannah Neate, "Working-With: Talking and Sorting in Personal Archives," *Journal of Historical Geography* 38, no. 1 (2012): 81, https://doi.org/10.1016/j.jhg.2011.06.002.

149. Geoffrey Hendricks and Sur Rodney (Sur), "A Dialogue," in *Arts' Communities, AIDS' Communities: Realizing the Archive Project* (New York: Visual AIDS, 1996), 56–57. Buczak died in 1987. Bill Olander (1950–89) was at the time a curator at the New Museum and Visual AIDS cofounder with whom Hendricks discussed the Buczak exhibition. He got Hendricks involved with Visual AIDS.

150. Hendricks and Sur, "Dialogue," 56.

151. Hendricks and Sur, "Dialogue," 56.

152. Hendricks and Sur, "Dialogue," 56.

153. Juarez, discussion.

154. Juarez, discussion.

155. Hendricks and Sur, "Dialogue," 57.

156. Sur, discussion.

157. Nelson Santos, in discussion with the author, New York City, May 25, 2016.

158. Debs, "Essay," 21.

159. Debs, "Essay," 21.

160. "FM Notebook #82, 1993–1995."

161. Debs, "Essay," 21.

162. Debs, "Essay," 21.

163. Sur, discussion.

164. Juarez, discussion.

165. Hirsh, discussion, November 27, 2018.

166. Hirsh, discussion, November 8, 2018.

167. "FM Notebook #82, 1993–1995," 22.

168. "The First 10," March 1995, Visual AIDS Organizational Files, Visual AIDS.

169. "First 10."

170. José Luis Cortés, in discussion with the author, Skype, January 18, 2019.

171. "FM Notebook #82, 1993–1995," 22.

172. Santos, discussion.

173. Santos, discussion.

174. Alex Fialho, in discussion with the author, New York City, May 25, 2016.

175. Rhein, discussion.

176. McGowan, discussion.

177. McGowan, discussion.

178. Hirsh, discussion, November 27, 2018.

179. Alexander R. Galloway and Eugene Thacker, "On Misanthropy," in *Curating Immateriality: The Work of the Curator in the Age of Network Systems,* DATA Browser 3, ed. Josaia Krysa (New York: Autonomedia, 2006), 176.

180. Hirsh, discussion, November 27, 2018.

181. Cortés, discussion.

182. Cortés, discussion.

183. Santos, discussion.

184. McGowan, discussion.

185. Hirsh, discussion, November 8, 2018.

186. McGowan, discussion.

187. Kerr, discussion.

188. Kerr, discussion.

189. McGowan, discussion.

190. McGowan, discussion.

191. McGowan, discussion.

192. McGowan, discussion.

193. Frank Moore, "The Archive Project: A Larger Vision," in *Arts' Communities, AIDS' Communities: Realizing the Archive Project* (New York: Visual AIDS, 1996), 23.

194. "FM Notebook #82, 1993–1995."

195. "Archive Project," Visual AIDS.

196. "Archive Project," Visual AIDS.

197. "FM Notebook #82, 1993–1995."

198. "FM Notebook #82, 1993–1995."

199. "FM Notebook #82, 1993–1995."

200. See Ryan Conrad, "Revisiting AIDS and Its Metaphors," *Drain Magazine* 13, no. 2 (2016), http://drainmag.com/revisiting-aids-and-its-metaphors/.

201. Conrad, "Revisiting AIDS and Its Metaphors."

202. "First 10."

203. "FM Notebook #82, 1993–1995."

204. "FM Notebook #82, 1993–1995."

205. "First 10."

206. Croft et al., "Activating the Archive Project."

207. "First 10."

208. Nelson Santos, "On Digitizing the Archive Project and Launching the Artist+ Registry," presentation, Visual AIDS, Fales, November 8, 2018.

209. "History," Visual AIDS, https://www.visualaids.org/history.

210. Visual AIDS was awarded a 2020–22 Andrew W. Mellon community-based archives grant to support collection development, digitization, and an oral history project with BIPOC artist members. It includes funding for a project archivist, Kailee Faber, hired in 2021.

211. The Joan Mitchell Foundation (2019) from 2005 to 2017 provided direct funding to community-based arts organizations, including Visual AIDS.

212. Sur, discussion.

213. Santos, "On Digitizing the Archive Project."

214. Santos, discussion. The term "registry" was potentially problematic in an AIDS context, where fears of mandatory registration and possible quarantine were justified. However, "registry" was selected for its arts legibility.

215. Santos, "On Digitizing the Archive Project."

216. Kerr, discussion.

217. McGowan, discussion.

218. McGowan, discussion.

219. Fialho, discussion.

220. Fialho, discussion.

221. Santos, discussion.

222. Fialho, discussion.

223. Fialho, discussion.

224. Fialho, discussion.

225. Rodney G. S. Carter, "Of Things Said and Unsaid: Power, Archival Silences, and Power in Silence," *Archivaria* 61 (2006): 227.

226. David Caron, *The Nearness of Others: Searching for Tact and Contact in the Age of HIV* (Minneapolis: University of Minnesota Press, 2014); Trevor Hoppe, *Punishing Disease: HIV and the Criminalization of Sickness* (Berkeley: University of California Press, 2017).

227. Santos, discussion.

228. Santos, discussion.

229. Santos, discussion.

230. McGowan, discussion.

231. Trevor Owens, *The Theory and Craft of Digital Preservation* (Baltimore, Md.: John Hopkins University Press, 2018), 5.

232. Owens, *Theory and Craft*, 4.

233. Croft et al., "Activating the Archive Project."

234. When I wrote this chapter in 2019–20, the web page was gone. However, I returned in October 2021, it was to a revamped Estate Project for Artists with AIDS web page.

235. Flinn, Stevens, and Shepherd, "Whose Memories, Whose Archives?," 79.

236. Moore, "Archive Project," 23.

237. Fialho, discussion.

238. Santos, discussion.

239. From 2003 to 2006, Visual AIDS collected Robert Blanchon's papers in creating his catalogue raisonné. Fales director Marvin J. Taylor acquired Blanchon's papers for the Downtown Collection. In 2011, after Chloe Dzubilo's death, Visual AIDS initially processed her papers before Fales acquired them. Santos, in his 2016 discussion with me, noted that he hoped that depositing their organizational records at Fales would provide context for the organization and make its records more accessible.

240. McGowan, discussion.

241. McGowan, discussion.

242. Fialho, discussion.

243. Rhein, discussion.

244. Claire Norton and Mark Donnelly, *Liberating Histories* (New York: Routledge, 2019), 110.

245. Kerr, discussion.

246. Fialho, discussion.

247. Well Project, "Long Term Survivors of HIV," submitted on October 30, 2018, https://www.thewellproject.org/hiv-information/long-term-survivors-hiv.

248. Rhein, discussion.

249. McGowan, discussion.

250. McGowan, discussion.

251. Fialho, discussion.

252. Since 2012, Visual AIDS has partnered with Residency Unlimited on a one-month residency focused on visual art and HIV/AIDS. X was the fourth curatorial resident.

253. "Introducing 2016 Visual AIDS Curatorial Resident Ajamu," Visual AIDS Blog, Visual AIDS, February 4, 2016, https://visualaids.org/blog/video-interviews -from-ajamus-archiving-activists-project.

254. Ajamu X, in discussion with the author, Skype, August 1, 2016.

255. X, discussion.

256. "Video Interviews from Ajamu's 'Archiving Activists Portrait Project,'" Visual AIDS Blog, Visual AIDS, April 11, 2016, https://visualaids.org/blog/video -interviews-from-ajamus-archiving-activists-project.

257. X, discussion.

258. X, discussion.

259. X, discussion.

260. Norton and Donnelly, *Liberating Histories,* 202.

261. Norton and Donnelly, *Liberating Histories,* 8.

262. Fialho, discussion.

263. Fialho, discussion.

264. Fialho, discussion.

265. Fialho, discussion.

266. Fialho, discussion.

267. Laws about HIV-specific criminal exposure were codified during the 1980s (Hoppe, *Punishing Disease*). As of 2019, thirty-four states and two territories have laws that criminalize alleged potential HIV exposure, nondisclosure, or potential transmission. Some laws criminalize behavior that cannot transmit HIV and apply regardless of actual transmission. Positive Women's Network, "Ending HIV Criminalization Factsheet," 2019, https://www.pwn-usa .org/issues/policy-agenda/ending-criminalization/ending-hiv-criminal ization/.

268. Fialho, discussion.

269. Hayden White, "The Burden of History," in *Tropics of Discourse: Essays in Cultural Criticism,* ed. Hayden White (Baltimore, Md.: John Hopkins University Press, 1978), 49.

270. Rhein, discussion.

271. Rhein, discussion.

272. Rhein, discussion.

273. The title of this section is a quote from my 2016 Skype discussion with X.

274. In January 2020, Fenix organized "the archive committee," a new initiative "to collectively develop and re-envision the strategic planning, BIPOC racial justice frameworks, and collections development policies and management of the Archive Project & Registry," "Archive Committee," Visual AIDS, 2020, https://visualaids.org/projects/archive-committee.

275. Clare, *Brilliant Imperfection,* 95.

276. Kim, *Curative Violence,* 11.

277. Shan Kelley, *With Curators Like These Who Needs a Cure,* 2015, oil paint, semen, resin on wood, 5 × 7 inches.

278. Debs, "Essay," 21.

279. Debs, "Essay," 21.

280. Rhein, discussion.

4. Status = Undetectable

1. Sara Ahmed, *The Cultural Politics of Emotion* (London: Routledge, 2004).

2. Undetectable Flash Collective, *What Is Undetectable?,* 2014, lenticular print, New York City, New York Public Library.

3. Solomon, "What Does It Mean to Remember AIDS?"

4. Steven W. Thrasher, "An Uprising Comes from the Viral Underclass," *Slate*, June 12, 2020, https://slate.com/.

5. Nathan Lee, "With the Aim of Making It Snap," in *Undetectable,* ed. Nathan Lee and Rachel Cook (New York: Visual AIDS, 2012), 9.

6. "HIV/AIDS Historical Time Line, 1981–1990," U.S. Food and Drug Administration, updated January 5, 2018, https://web.archive.org/web/201807261125 14/http://www.fda.gov/ForPatients/Illness/HIVAIDS/History/ucm151074 .htm.

7. Lee, "With the Aim," 2.

8. David Caron, *The Nearness of Others: Searching for Tact and Contact in the Age of HIV* (Minneapolis: University of Minnesota Press, 2014), 124.

9. Octavio R. González, "Resisting Erasure: AIDS and Modalities of Dissent," paper presented at the American Studies Association Conference, Chicago, November 12, 2017.

10. Liz Hunt, "'Cocktail' Opens New Chapter on AIDS," *Independent,* July 12, 1996, http://www.independent.co.uk/news/cocktail-opens-new-chapter-on -aids-1328432.html. The year 1996 was the first in which American AIDS-related deaths decreased.

11. Jan Huebenthal, "Injury and Resistance: Centering HIV/AIDS Histories in Times of Queer Equality" (PhD diss., College of William and Mary, 2019).

12. Susan Sontag, *AIDS and Its Metaphors* (New York: Farrar, Straus & Giroux, 1989).

13. Lee, "With the Aim," 10.

14. Debra Levine, in discussion with the author, Skype, October 28, 2016.

15. Sturken, "AIDS Activist Legacies."

16. Patricia Keller and Jonathan Snyder, "Encounters with the Unsightly: Reading (AIDS) History, Photography, and the Obscene," *Hispanic Issues On Line* 3 (2011): 97.

17. Gill-Peterson, "Haunting the Queer Spaces of AIDS," 279–300.

18. Katrin Köppert and Todd Sekuler, "Sick Memory: On the Un-dectable in Archiving AIDS," *Drain* 13, no. 2 (2016), http://drainmag.com/sick-memory -on-the-un-detectable-in-archiving-aids/.

19. Pietro Vernazza, Bernard Hirschel, Enos Bernasconi, and Markus Flepp, "HIV-Positive Individuals without Additional Sexually Transmitted Diseases (STD) and on Effective Anti-retroviral Therapy Are Sexually Non-infectious," *Bulletin des médecins suisses* 89 (2008): 165–69.

20. Halima Dao, Lynne M. Mofenson, Rene Ekpini, Charles F. Gilks, Matthew Barnhart, Omotayo Bolu, et al., "International Recommendations on Anti-retroviral Drugs for Treatment of HIV-Infected Women and Prevention of Mother-to-Child HIV Transmission in Resource-Limited Settings: 2006 Update," *American Journal of Obstetrics and Gynecology* 197, no. 3 (2007): S42–S55, https://doi.org/10.1016/j.ajog.2007.03.001.

21. "U = U Taking Off in 2017," *Lancet HIV* 4, no. 11 (2017): e475, https://doi .org/10.1016/S2352-3018(17)30183-2.

22. "U = U Taking Off in 2017."

23. Alice Park, "Are Some HIV Patients Non-infectious?," *Time*, February 4, 2008, http://content.time.com/time/health/article/0,8599,1709841,00.html.

24. NAM, "Does Undetectable Really Mean Uninfectious," *HIV Treatment Update* 175 (2008): 11, https://web.archive.org/web/20100103105303/http://www .aidsmap.com/files/file1002752.pdf.

25. Jan Huebenthal, "Un/detectability in Times of 'Equality': HIV, Queer Health, and Homonormativity," *European Journal of American Studies* 11, no. 3 (2017): 2, https://doi.org/10.4000/ejas.11729.

26. Köppert and Sekuler, "Sick Memory."

27. Douglas Crimp, "Introduction," *October* 43 (1987): 3, https://doi.org/10.23 07/3397562.

28. Paula A. Treichler, *How to Have Theory in an Epidemic: Cultural Chronicles of AIDS* (Durham, N.C.: Duke University Press, 1999), 1.

29. González, "Resisting Erasure."

30. UNAIDS, *90–90–90—An Ambitious Treatment Target to Help End the AIDS Epidemic,* Joint United Nations Programme on HIV/AIDS (UNAIDS), October 2014, http://www.unaids.org/en/resources/documents/2014/90-90-90.

31. Alison Howell, "Resilience as Enhancement: Governmentality and Political Economy beyond 'Responsibilisation,'" *Politics* 35, no. 1 (2015): 67–71, https://doi.org/10.1111/1467-9256.12080.

32. Roderic Crooks, "Accesso Libre: Equity of Access to Information through the Lens of Neoliberal Responsiblization," *Journal of Critical Library and Information Studies* 8, https://doi.org/10.24242/jclis.v2i1.91.

33. Thrasher, "Uprising Comes."

34. Judith Butler, *Frames of War: When Is Life Grievable?* (New York: Verso, 2009), 38.

35. Thrasher, "Uprising Comes."

36. Warren Buckingham, "HIV/AIDS in Maine and Beyond," paper presented at "The Local and the Global: Discussing HIV/AIDS in Maine and Beyond," Bowdoin College, Brunswick, Maine, November 29, 2017.

37. Eli Manning, "HAART in Art: Temporal Reflections on Artistic Representations of HIV Medication," Gallery, Visual AIDS, June 2018, https://visualaids .org/gallery/detail/743.

38. Andy Campbell, "Sister Undetectable . . . for Claudette," in *Undetectable,* ed. Nathan Lee and Rachel Cook (New York: Visual AIDS, 2012), 15.

39. Lee, "With the Aim," 10.

40. Campbell, "Sister Undetectable," 15.

41. "Undetectable: Curator Nathan Lee and Assistant Curator Rachel Cook," event, Visual AIDS, La MaMa La Galleria, New York City, May 31–June 30, 2012, https://visualaids.org/events/detail/undetectable.

42. Campbell, "Sister Undetectable," 15.

43. The curator's checklist also shows borrowed items from the Keith Haring Foundation and Fales's Downtown Collection.

44. González, "Resisting Erasure."

45. Jason Baumann, in discussion with the author, New York City, August 25, 2016.

46. Baumann, discussion, 2016.

47. AIDS activist videotapes were included within the NYPL's mid-2000s mass AV digitization.

48. Baumann, discussion, 2016.

49. Baumann, discussion, 2015.

50. Baumann, discussion, 2015.

51. Designed by graphic design firm DresserJohnson.

52. Burk, "From the Streets to the Gallery," 35.

53. Baumann, discussion, 2015.

54. Baumann, discussion, 2016.

55. Baumann, discussion, 2016.

56. Baumann, discussion, 2016.

57. Gill-Peterson, "Haunting the Queer Spaces of AIDS."

58. Emily Colucci, "More Demonstrations and Less Memorials in 'Why We Fight: Remembering AIDS Activism,'" Filthy Dreams (blog), October 19, 2013, https:// filthydreams.wordpress.com/2013/10/19/more-demonstrations-and-less -memorials-in-why-we-fight-remembering-aids-activism/.

59. Colucci, "More Demonstrations and Less Memorials."

60. Gill-Peterson, "Haunting the Queer Spaces of AIDS."

61. Colucci, "More Demonstrations and Less Memorials."

62. Baumann, discussion, 2015.

63. Baumann, discussion, 2015.

64. Baumann, discussion, 2016.

65. Undetectable Flash Collective, What Is Undetectable?, 2014, GIF, https://what isundetectable.tumblr.com/.

66. James Ash, "Sensation, Networks, and the GIF: Toward an Allotropic Account of Affect," in Networked Affect, ed. Ken Hillis, Susanna Paasonen, and Michael Petit (Cambridge, Mass.: MIT Press, 2015), 199.

67. Avram Finkelstein qtd. in Alex Fialho, "'The Collective Is Indeed a Flash: It Is a Sudden Rush of Energy that Occurs When All Points Touch,'" Visual AIDS Blog, Visual AIDS, May 29, 2015, https://www.visualaids.org/blog/detail/ the-collective-is-indeed-a-flash-it-is-a-sudden-rush-of-energy-that-occurs.

68. Finkelstein qtd. in Fialho, "Collective."

69. Finkelstein qtd. in Fialho, "Collective."

70. Finkelstein, discussion.

71. Kleist qtd. in Fialho, "Collective."

72. Finkelstein qtd. in Fialho, "Collective"

73. Baumann, discussion, 2016.

74. Avram Finkelstein qtd. in Larry Buhl, "Undetectable, Not Invisible: A Flash Collective Workshop Mounts an 'Art Intervention' at New York Public Library," *A&U Magazine*, December 14, 2014, https://web.archive.org/web/20170526160327/http://aumag.org/2014/12/18/undetectable-flash-collective/.

75. Undetectable Flash Collective members were Avram Finkelstein, Alex Fialho, Alina Oswald, Brendan Mahoney, Conrad Ventur, Filip Condeescu, Gerald Mocarsky, Hucklefaery Ken, Jano Cortijo, Jorge Sanchez, Kenneth Pietrobono, Lanai Daniels, Mark Blane, Nick Kleist, Pablo Herrera, and Spear Minteh.

76. Finkelstein, discussion.

77. Baumann, discussion, 2016.

78. Finkelstein, discussion.

79. Buhl, "Undetectable, Not Invisible."

80. Finkelstein, discussion.

81. Kleist qtd. in Fialho, "Collective."

82. Finkelstein, discussion.

83. Finkelstein, discussion.

84. Buhl, "Undetectable, Not Invisible."

85. Jano Cortijo qtd. in Fialho, "Collective."

86. Finkelstein, discussion.

87. Alina Oswald qtd. in Fialho, "Collective."

88. Oswald qtd. in Fialho, "Collective."

89. Oswald qtd. in Fialho, "Collective."

90. Rhein, discussion.

91. Rhein, discussion.

92. Rhein, discussion.

93. Fialho, discussion.

94. Alexandra Schwartz, "New York's Necessary New AIDS Memorial," *New Yorker*, December 8, 2016, www.newyorker.com/culture/cultural-comment/new-yorks-necessary-new-aids-memorial.

95. Schulman, *Gentrification of the Mind*.

96. *New York City HIV/AIDS Annual Surveillance Statistics* (New York: New York City Department of Health and Mental Hygiene, 2017), http://www1.nyc.gov/site/doh/data/data-sets/hiv-aids-annual-surveillance-statistics.page.

97. Finkelstein, discussion.

98. "What Is Undetectable?," event sponsored by Undetectable Flash Collective and Visual AIDS, Ideas City Festival, New Museum, Roosevelt Park, New York, May 30, 2015, https://www.visualaids.org/events/detail/undetectable-ideas-city.

99. Fialho, discussion.

100. Fialho, discussion.

101. Keller and Snyder, "Encounters with the Unsightly," 97.

102. Kerr, discussion.

103. Gilad Padva, *Queer Nostalgia in Cinema and Pop Culture* (New York: Palgrave Macmillan, 2014), 58–71.

104. Sasha Archibald and Robert Blanchon, *Robert Blanchon* (New York: Visual AIDS, 2006), 26.

105. Jason Foumberg, "Eye Exam: Queer Spirits," New City Art, May 30, 2011, http://art.newcity.com/2011/05/30/eye-exam-queer-spirits/.

106. Archibald and Blanchon, *Robert Blanchon*, 31.

107. "Guide to the Robert Blanchon Papers and Collection," March 13, 2019, Robert Blanchon Papers and Collection, Fales, http://dlib.nyu.edu/finding aids/html/fales/blanchon/.

108. Marvin J. Taylor, in discussion with the author, New York City, August 30, 2016.

109. Andrew Blackley, in discussion with the author, New York City, May 28, 2016.

110. Foumberg, "Eye Exam."

111. John Neff, in discussion with the author, Skype, July 26, 2016.

112. Golden Gallery, "John Neff Prints Robert Blanchon," news release, 2011, http://johnneff.org/neffprintsblanchon/wp-content/uploads/John-Neff -Prints-Robert-Blanchon.pdf.

113. "Guide to the Robert Blanchon Papers and Collection."

114. Blackley, discussion.

115. "Not Over: Part of the *Not Over* Exhibition Series," event sponsored by Visual AIDS, La MaMa La Galleria, New York, June 2013, https://visualaids.org/ events/detail/not-over-25-years-of-visual-aids.

116. Blackley, discussion.

117. For images, see Forrest Olivo, "'Not Only This, but 'New Language Beckons Us,' at Fales," *Office Notebook,* March 22, 2016, https://notebook.cagrp.org/ not-only-this-but-new-language-beckons-us-at-fales-library-and-special -collections-64fdb7a3f9af#.748iqfjbj.

118. Blackley, discussion.

119. Blackley, discussion.

120. Neff, discussion.

121. "Neff, John: Text," 2013, Box 1, Folder 35, *Not Only This, but "New Language Beckons Us"* Exhibition Archive, Fales.

122. "Neff, John: Text."

123. Blackley, discussion.

124. Blackley, discussion.

125. Blackley, discussion.

126. Blackley, discussion.

127. Blackley, discussion.

128. Blackley, discussion.

129. Julie Ault, Dodie Bellamy, Gregg Bordowitz, Nancy Brooks Brody, Elijah Burgher, Kathe Burkhart, Sean Carrillo, Peter Cramer, Matthias Herrmann, Jim Hubbard, Doug Ischar, William E. Jones, John Keene, Kevin Killian, Nathanaël, John Neff, Uzi Parnes, Mary Patten, Nina Sobell, Ela Troyano, Ultra-red, Jack Waters, Joe Westmoreland, and Danh Vo made contemporary works.

130. Blackley, discussion. Records from Kathy Acker, Robert Blanchon, Valerie Caris, Dennis Cooper, Lou Maletta, the MIX Collection, Frank Moore, Cookie Mueller, Polysexuality, Hunter Reynolds, Stuart Sherman, Jack Smith, James Wentzy, David Wojnarowicz, and Martin Wong's collections were included.

131. Julie Ault, in discussion with the author, telephone, September 14, 2016.

132. Ault, discussion.

133. Neff, discussion.

134. Neff, discussion.

135. "Neff, John: Text."

136. Blackley, discussion.

137. "Westmoreland, Joe: Dennis Cooper Documents," 2013, Box 1, Folder 49, *Not Only This, but "New Language Beckons Us"* Exhibition Archive, Fales.

138. "Westmoreland, Joe: Dennis Cooper Documents."

139. Ault, discussion.

140. Blackley, discussion.

141. Blackley, discussion.

142. Blackley, discussion.

143. Ault, discussion.

144. "Ault, Julie: Martin Wong Document," 2013, Box 1, Folder 4, *Not Only This, but "New Language Beckons Us"* Exhibition Archive, Fales.

145. "Ault, Julie: Martin Wong Document."

146. "Ault, Julie: Martin Wong Document."

147. Ault, discussion.

148. Ault, discussion.

149. Piepmeier qtd. in Jenna Brager and Jami Sailor, "Archiving the Underground," in *Make Your Own History: Documenting Feminist and Queer Activism in the 21st Century,* ed. Liz Bly and Kelly Wooten (Los Angeles: Litwin Books, 2012), 47.

150. Taylor, discussion.

151. Taylor, discussion.

152. Blackley, discussion.

153. Blackley, discussion.

154. Elizabeth Yakel, "Hidden Collections in Archives and Libraries," *OCLC Systems and Services: International Digital Library Perspectives* 21, no. 2 (2005): 95, https://doi.org/10.1108/10650750510598675.

155. Yakel, "Hidden Collections," 95.

156. Blackley, discussion.

157. Taylor, discussion.

158. Blackley, discussion.

159. Blackley, discussion.

160. Blackley, discussion.

161. González, "Resisting Erasure."

162. Ault, discussion.

163. Brothman, "Perfect Present, Perfect Gift."

5. Going Viral

1. Elizabeth Losh, *Hashtag* (New York: Bloomsbury, 2019).

2. Schulman, "Art of Protesting," 41.

3. Bradley-Perrin, discussion; Vincent Chevalier, in discussion with the author, Skype, August 2, 2016.

4. Gill-Peterson, "Haunting the Queer Spaces of AIDS," 279–300.

5. José Esteban Muñoz, *Disidentifications: Queers of Color and the Performance of Politics* (Minneapolis: University of Minnesota Press, 1999).

6. Muñoz, *Disidentifications,* 200, 31.

7. Muñoz, *Disidentifications,* 200.

8. Thrasher, "Uprising Comes."

9. Thrasher, "Uprising Comes."

10. Muñoz, *Disidentifications,* 200.

11. Marika Cifor and Cait McKinney, "Reclaiming HIV/AIDS in Digital Media Studies," *First Monday* 25, no. 10 (2020), https://doi.org/10.5210/fm.v25i10.10517; Cait McKinney, "Printing the Network: AIDS Activism and Online Access in the 1980s," *Continuum* 32, no. 1 (2018): 7–17.

12. Cifor and McKinney, "Reclaiming HIV/AIDS."

13. Michelle Caswell, "Dusting for Fingerprints: Introducing Feminist Standpoint Appraisal," *Journal of Critical Library and Information Studies* 3 (2020), https://journals.litwinbooks.com/index.php/jclis/article/view/113.

14. Jennifer Prybus, "Accumulating Affect: Social Networks and Their Archives of Feelings," in Hillis, Paasonen, and Petit, *Networked Affect,* 235–50, 240.

15. See Cifor and McKinney, "Reclaiming HIV/AIDS."

16. Marika Cifor, "'What Is Remembered Lives': Time and the Disruptive Animacy of Archiving AIDS on Instagram," *Convergence* 27, no. 2 (2021): 371–94, https://doi.org/10.1177/1354856520979961.

17. Hito Steyerl, "In Defense of the Poor Image," *e-flux* 10 (2009), https://www.e-flux.com/journal/10/61362/in-defense-of-the-poor-image/.

18. Steyerl, "In Defense of the Poor Image."

19. Steyerl, "In Defense of the Poor Image."

20. Jussi Parikka, *Digital Contagions: A Media Archaeology of Computer Viruses* (New York: Peter Lang, 2007), 120.

21. Parikka, *Digital Contagions,* 149.

22. Cait McKinney and Dylan Mulvin, "Bugs: Rethinking the History of Computing," *Communication, Culture, and Critique* 12, no. 4 (2019): 476.

23. Douglas Rushkoff, *Media Virus! Hidden Agendas in Popular Culture* (New York: Random House Digital, 1996).

24. Parikka, *Digital Contagions,* 131.

25. For example, a September 1989 *PC User* article describes the "viral marketing" of Macintosh computers. Now entire companies—viral agencies—generate and replicate hits.

26. Jeff D'Onofrio, "A Better, More Positive Tumblr," Tumblr Staff, 2018, https://staff.tumblr.com/post/180758987165/a-better-more-positive-tumblr.

27. Mason Sands, "Tumblocalypse: Where Tumblr and Its Users Are Headed after the Ban," *Forbes,* 2018, https://www.forbes.com/sites/masonsands/2018/12/20/tumblocalypse-where-tumblr-and-its-users-are-headed-after-the-ban/#70e7042d7020.

28. Oliver L. Haimson, Avery Dame-Griff, Elias Capello, and Zahari Richter, "Tumblr Was a Trans Technology: The Meaning, Importance, History, and Future of Trans Technologies," *Feminist Media Studies* 3 (2019): 1–17, https://doi.org/10.1080/14680777.2019.1678505.

29. Julia Craven, "Tumblr Is Betraying the Sex Workers and NSFW Artists Who Relied on the Platform," Huffington Post, 2018, https://www.huffpost.com/entry/tumblr-sex-workers-nsfw-artists-lose_n_5c0714fbe4b0fc236111037e.

30. Casey Fiesler and Brianna Dym, "Fandom's Fate Is Not Tied to Tumblr's: If Tumblr Doesn't Learn from History, It Will Be Headed for the Same Fate as LiveJournal," Slate, 2018, https://slate.com/.

31. Craven, "Tumblr Is Betraying the Sex Workers."

32. Alexander Cho, "Queer Reverb: Tumblr, Affect, Time," in Hillis, Paasonen, and Petit, *Networked Affect,* 43–57.

33. Jay D. Bolter, Blair MacIntyre, Michael Nitsche, and Kathryn T. Farley, "Liveness, Presence, and Performance in Contemporary Digital Media," in *Throughout: Art and Culture Emerging with Ubiquitous Computing,* ed. Ulrik Ekman (Cambridge, Mass.: MIT Press, 2012), 323–26; Carolin Gerlitz, "Acting on Data. Temporality and Self-Evaluation in Social Media," *tbc* (2012): 1–18.

34. Siân Lindley, "Making Time," in *Proceedings of the 18th ACM Conference on Computer Supported Cooperative Work and Social Computing* (2015), 1442–52.

35. Jess MacCormack, "A Cruising Ground of Aesthetics, Porn, Politics and Selfies: An Interview with Jess Mac," conducted by Mikhel Proulx, *No More Potlucks* 50 (2018), https://web.archive.org/web/20180709110820/http://nomorepotlucks.org/site/a-cruising-ground-of-aesthetics-porn-politics-and-selfies-an-interview-with-jess-mac-mikhel-proulx/.

36. Haimson, Dame-Griff, Capello, and Richter, "Tumblr Was a Trans Technology"; Andre Cavalcante, "Tumbling into Queer Utopias and Vortexes: Experiences of LGBTQ Social Media Users on Tumblr," *Journal of Homosexuality* 66, no. 12 (2018): 1715–35; Marty Fink and Quinn Miller, "Trans Media Moments Tumblr, 2011–2013," *Television and New Media* 15, no. 7 (2014): 611–26, https://doi.org/10.1177/1527476413505002; Avery Dame, "Making a Name for Yourself: Tagging as Transgender Ontological Practice on Tumblr," *Critical Studies in Media Communication* 33, no. 1 (2016): 23–37, https://doi.org/10.1080/15295036.2015.1130846.

37. MacCormack, "Cruising Ground."

38. Cho, "Queer Reverb."

39. Alexander Cho, "Acceleration, Extraction, Evasion: Social Media Sentiment Analysis and Queer of Color Resistance," paper presented at the Society for Cinema and Media Studies, Seattle, Washington, March 13, 2019.

40. MacCormack, "Cruising Ground."

41. Jess MacCormack, "My Social Network Swallowed Me Whole: A Conversation with Montreal Artist Jessica MacCormack," interview by Claire Paquet, *.dpi* 29 (2013), https://dpi.studioxx.org/en/no/29-The-Montreal-Issue/my-social-network-swallowed-me-whole-conversation-montreal-artist-jessica.

42. MacCormack, "My Social Network."

43. MacCormack, "Cruising Ground."

44. Kathryn Brewster and Bonnie Ruberg, "SURVIVORS: Archiving the History of Bulletin Board Systems and the AIDS Crisis," *First Monday* 25, no. 10 (2020).

45. Jess MacCormack, "David Wojnarowicz AIDS GIF," Tumblr blog, 2015, https://jessicamaccormackrmack.tumblr.com/post/104080011538.

46. Mac's GIF is also tied to Emily Roysdon's photographic series *Untitled*, a queer-feminist homage to Wojnarowicz's *Arthur Rimbaud in New York*. Mac brings this project into a digital milieu. Cait McKinney, e-mail message to author, September 28, 2020.

47. Rosa von Praunheim, dir. *Silence = Death* (First Run Features, 1990).

48. *A Fire in My Belly* is known for the 2010 controversy over its inclusion in the National Portrait Gallery's *Hide/Seek* exhibition. Begun in 1986–87, it was never completed by Wojnarowicz. The film is a thirteen-minute segment with a seven-minute section from a separate reel that Wojnarowicz labeled "Prostitution" on the cutting script. David Ng, "Getting the Facts Straight about Wojnarowicz's 'A Fire in My Belly,'" *Los Angeles Times*, February 2, 2011, https://latimesblogs.latimes.com/.

49. Olivia Laing, "A Stitch in Time," *frieze* 177 (February 13, 2016), https://frieze.com/article/stitch-time-0.

50. MacCormack, "Cruising Ground."

51. Jules Rosskam, "Making Trans Cinema: A Roundtable Discussion with Felix Endara, Reina Gossett, Chase Joynt, Jess Mac, and Madsen Minax," *Somatechnics* 8, no. 1 (2018): 14–26, 20.

52. MacCormack, "My Social Network."

53. MacCormack, "Cruising Ground."

54. MacCormack, "My Social Network."

55. MacCormack, "Cruising Ground."

56. MacCormack, "Cruising Ground."

57. Greg Elmer, *Profiling Machines: Mapping the Personal Information Economy* (Cambridge, Mass.: MIT Press, 2003).

58. Mark Andrejevic, *Infoglut: How Too Much Information Is Changing the Way We Think and Know* (New York: Routledge, 2013); John Cheney-Lippold, "A New Algorithmic Identity: Soft Biopolitics and the Modulation of Control," *Theory, Culture, and Society* 28, no. 6 (2011): 164–81, https://doi.org/10.1177%2F0263276411424420.

59. MacCormack, "My Social Network."

60. James Ash, "Sensation, Networks, and the GIF: Toward an Allotropic Account of Affect," in Hillis, Paasonen, and Petit, *Networked Affect,* 199.

61. Gil Bartholeyns, "The Instant Past: Nostalgia and Digital Retro Photography," in Niemeyer, *Media and Nostalgia,* 60.

62. Erik N. Jensen, "The Pink Triangle and Political Consciousness: Gays, Lesbians, and the Memory of Nazi Persecution," *Journal of the History of Sexuality* 11, no. 1 (2002): 331.

63. Conrad, "Revisiting AIDS and Its Metaphors."

64. MacCormack, "My Social Network."

65. Studio XX, "Jessica MacCormack," https://studioxx.org/en/participants/jessica-maccormack-2/.

66. Jess MacCormack, "Visual AIDS Interviews Jessica MacCormack, an Artist and Ally from Canada," interview by Visual AIDS, Visual AIDS Blog, Visual AIDS, July 20, 2013, https://visualaids.org/blog/visual-aids-interviews-jessica-maccormack-an-artist-and-ally-from-canada.

67. MacCormack, "Visual AIDS Interviews Jessica MacCormack."

68. MacCormack, "Visual AIDS Interviews Jessica MacCormack."

69. MacCormack, "Visual AIDS Interviews Jessica MacCormack."

70. Visual AIDS, "Kia LaBeija," Artist+ Registry, https://visualaids.org/artists/kia-labeija.

71. Kia LaBeija, "Artist Statement," Visual AIDS blog, January 5, 2018, https://visualaids.org/blog/alternate-endings-radical-beginnings-video-artist-statement-kia-labeija.

72. LaBeija, "Artist Statement."

73. Jareh Das, "The Multi-faceted Narrative of Illness," Visual AIDS Gallery, November 2018, https://visualaids.org/gallery/the-multi-faceted-narrative-of-illness.

74. Emily Colucci, "Queeroes 2019: How Kia LaBeija and Lyle Ashton Harris Use Art to Persevere," *Them,* June 24, 2019, https://www.them.us/story/queeroes-2019-kia-labeija-lyle-ashton-harris.

75. LaBeija, "Artist Statement."

76. Colucci, "Queeroes 2019."

77. LaBeija, "Artist Statement."

78. Kia LaBeija and Julie Tolentino, *Duets: Kia LaBeija and Julie Tolentino in Conversation* (New York: Visual AIDS, 2018), 35.

79. In the mid-twentieth century, Black and Latinx queer/trans people organized themselves into houses and created balls. Events started in Harlem and now happen worldwide. In 1977, Crystal LaBeija announced an event hosted by the "House of LaBeija," a phrase still used. House members can choose to take the name. Hugh Ryan, "Power in the Crisis: Kia LaBeija's Radical Art as a 25 Year Old, HIV Positive Woman of Color," Vice, June 6, 2015, https://www.vice.com/.

80. LaBeija and Tolentino, *Duets,* 60.

81. Will Rawls, "Bittersweet Kinetic," Visual AIDS blog, March 29, 2018 https://visualaids.org/blog/bittersweet-kinetic.

82. LaBeija and Tolentino, *Duets,* 58.

83. LaBeija and Tolentino, *Duets,* 58.

84. Rawls, "Bittersweet Kinetic."

85. Kia LaBeija, "#Undetectable," PosterVirus, 2016, https://postervirus.tumblr.com/post/153565653152/kia-labeija-undetectable.

86. See Cifor and McKinney, "Reclaiming HIV/AIDS."

87. Aria Dean, "Closing the Loop," *New Inquiry,* March 1, 2019, https://thenewinquiry.com/closing-the-loop/.

88. Ryan, "Power in the Crisis."

89. Ryan, "Power in the Crisis."

90. Sean Black, "Kwan's Song and the Allure of Immortality," *A&U Magazine,* May 1, 2015, https://web.archive.org/web/20160209084405/https://aumag.org/2015/05/01/kia-labeija/.

91. Black, "Kwan's Song."

92. LaBeija, "Artist Statement."

93. Laura Stamm, "Sustaining Life During the AIDS Crisis: New Queer Cinema and the Biopic" (PhD diss., University of Pittsburgh, 2018).

94. Julia S. Jordan-Zachery, *Shadow Bodies: Black Women, Ideology, Representation, and Politics* (New Brunswick, N.J.: Rutgers University Press, 2017), 98.

95. Jordan-Zachery, *Shadow Bodies,* 98.

96. Colucci, "Queeroes 2019."

97. Ryan, "Power in the Crisis."

98. LaBeija and Tolentino, *Duets,* 35.

99. Colucci, "Queeroes 2019."

100. Printmaker and graphic designer Deagle was involved in art-action collective Gran Fury's well-funded, professionally produced early campaigns. However, he left because "the working methods of Gran Fury just really didn't work for me." Deagle's works were produced quickly in response to specific events and

were targeted to queers. Kate Eichhorn, *Adjusted Margin: Xerography, Art, and Activism in the Late Twentieth Century* (Cambridge, Mass.: MIT Press, 2016), 125.

101. Thomas L. Long, *AIDS and American Apocalypticism: The Cultural Semiotics of an Epidemic* (New York: SUNY Press, 2005).

102. The 2015 digitization metadata attributes the poster to ACT UP/NY and does not include a creation date. ACT UP/NY, "American Flag [Our government continues to ignore the lives, deaths, and suffering of people with HIV infection . . .]," New York Public Library Digital Collections, https://digitalcollec tions.nypl.org/items/510d47e3-5f5e-a3d9-e040-e00a18064a99.

103. Visual AIDS and Demian DinéYazhi´, "HIV/AIDS Is Quiet at Times in Native Communities," Visual AIDS blog, December 3, 2014, https://visualaids.org/ blog/hiv-aids-is-quiet-at-times-in-native-communities.

104. National Indian Health Board, "HIV and Sexually Transmitted Infections (STI) in American Indian and Alaska Native Communities," https://www.nihb.org/ behavioral_health/hiv_indian_country.php.

105. David Titterington, "Indigenous American Flags," *Medium*, May 17, 2019, https://medium.com/@davidtitterington/indigenous-american-flags-41 9396a28df6.

106. Bertha Harvey, *Flag Rug*, 1991, wool, Portland (Ore.) Art Museum, 2001.72, http://portlandartmuseum.us/mwebcgi/mweb.exe?request=record;id=4534 ;type=101.

107. Titterington, "Indigenous American Flags."

108. Demian DinéYazhi´ and R.I.S.E., "High Resolution Poster," Bury My Art at Wounded Knee (Tumblr blog), December 1, 2015, https://burymyart.tumblr .com/post/134368863223/high-resolution-poster-based-on-hivaids-related.

109. manuel arturo abreu, "Embodying Survivance," *Art in America*, September 25, 2017, https://www.artnews.com/art-in-america/features/embodying-surviv ance-63297/.

110. abreu, "Embodying Survivance."

111. Visual AIDS and Demian DinéYazhi´, "HIV/AIDS Is Quiet at Times in Native Communities," Visual AIDS blog, December 3, 2014, https://visualaids.org/ blog/hiv-aids-is-quiet-at-times-in-native-communities.

112. Demian DinéYazhi´, "Make Native America Great Again," *Offing*, May 26, 2017, https://theoffingmag.com/art/make-native-america-great/.

113. Demian DinéYazhi´, Demian DinéYazhi´: Hallie Ford Fellow in the Visual Arts 2018, https://www.tfff.org/gallery/demian-din%C3%A9yazhi%E2%80%99.

114. Anishinaabe scholar Gerald Vizenor explains: "Survivance is an active sense of presence, the continuance of native stories, not a mere reaction, or a surviv-able name. Native survivance stories are renunciations of dominance, tragedy and victimry." Gerald Vizenor, *Manifest Manners: Narratives on Postindian Survivance* (Lincoln: University of Nebraska Press, 1999), vii.

115. Visual AIDS and DinéYazhi´, "HIV/AIDS Is Quiet at Times."

116. Visual AIDS and DinéYazhi´, "HIV/AIDS Is Quiet at Times."

117. The slogan was used on a screen print in the 2017 exhibition *One Day This Kid Will Get Larger,* curated by Danny Orendorff at the DePaul Art Museum. Trenton Straube, "AIDS Art in America That's Youthful, Even Joyous," *Poz,* February 10, 2017, https://www.poz.com/article/aids-art-america-youthful-even-joyous-depaul-slideshow.

118. Theodore Kerr, "Framing the Issue," *On Curating* 42 (2019), https://www.on-curating.org/issue-42-reader/framing-the-issue.html#.Xh3_FRdKjs0.

119. Demian DinéYazhi´ and R.I.S.E., "HIV Affects Indigenous Communities," *On Curating* 42 (2019), https://www.on-curating.org/issue-42-reader/hiv-affects-indigenous-communities.html#.Xh3_rxdKjs0.

120. DinéYazhi´ and R.I.S.E., "High Resolution Poster."

121. Kaitlyn Tiffany, "Tumblr's First Year without Porn," *Atlantic,* December 3, 2019, https://www.theatlantic.com/.

122. Cristina Criddle, "Transgender Users Accuse TikTok of Censorship," BBC News, February 12, 2020, https://www.bbc.com/news/technology-51474114.

123. (RED), "Turn Your TikTok Videos into a Force that Fights AIDS with #MakeItRed," press release, December 2, 2019, https://www.red.org/reditorial/makeitred-with-tiktok.

124. Haimson, Dame-Griff, Capello, and Richter. "Tumblr Was a Trans Technology."

Epilogue

1. Jordan-Zachery, *Shadow Bodies,* 98.

2. Cheng, Juhasz, and Shahani, introduction to *AIDS and the Distribution of Crises,* 2.

3. Villarosa, "America's Hidden HIV Epidemic."

4. Jallicia A. Jolly, "What HIV/AIDS Teaches Us about Covid-19," *Medium,* June 19, 2020, https://medium.com/national-center-for-institutional-diversity/what-hiv-aids-teaches-us-about-covid-19-7d80766f748b.

5. Laurie Marhoefer, "Coronavirus: Three Lessons from the AIDS Crisis," *Conversation,* March 16, 2020, https://theconversation.com/coronavirus-three-lessons-from-the-aids-crisis-133575.

6. Steven W. Thrasher, "I Study Prisons and AIDS History. Here's Why Self-Isolation Really Scares Me," Slate, March 20, 2020, https://slate.com/.

7. Edmund White, "Fear, Bigotry and Misinformation—This Reminds Me of the 1980s AIDS Pandemic," *Guardian,* April 6, 2020, https://www.theguardian.com/.

8. Tawana Petty, "Watched and Still Dying," Our Data Bodies (blog), April 26, 2020, https://www.odbproject.org/2020/04/26/watched-and-still-dying/.

9. Thrasher, "I Study Prisons and AIDS History."

10. Zack Beauchamp, "Trump Is Mishandling Coronavirus the Way Reagan Botched the AIDS Epidemic," *Vox*, March 30, 2020, https://www.vox.com/.

11. Marhoefer, "Coronavirus."

12. Michael J. O'Loughlin, "Facing the Fear: How Covid-19 and HIV/AIDS Responses Compare," *America Magazine*, March 16, 2020, https://www.americamagazine.org/.

13. Scott Shafer, "Could Lessons from the Early Fight against AIDS Inform the Coronavirus Response?," *NPR*, April 10, 2020, https://www.npr.org/.

14. Thrasher, "I Study Prisons and AIDS History."

15. Mark S. King, "Stop Comparing Coronavirus to Early HIV/AIDS. Just Stop," My Fabulous Disease (blog), March 14, 2020, https://marksking.com/my-fabulous-disease/stop-comparing-coronavirus-to-early-hiv-aids-just-stop/.

16. Theodore (Ted) Kerr, "How to Live with a Virus," *Poz*, March 23, 2020, https://www.poz.com/article/live-virus.

17. Abdul-Aliy A. Muhammad, "Our Covid-19 Response Is Living in the House HIV Activists Built," *Body*, April 1, 2020, https://www.thebody.com/article/covid-19-and-aids-epidemic.

18. Anne Price, "Normal Is What Got Us Here," *Medium*, May 5, 2020, https://insightcced.medium.com/normal-is-what-got-us-here-5f9c39f56d19.

19. Roxane Gay, "Remember, No One Is Coming to Save Us," *New York Times*, May 30, 2020, https://www.nytimes.com/.

20. "What Would an HIV Doula Do?," in *What Does a Covid-19 Doula Do?* (Los Angeles: ONE Archives Foundation, 2020), 6–7, https://www.onearchives.org/what-does-a-covid19-doula-do-zine/.

21. GLBT Historical Society, "Fighting Back: Lessons from AIDS for Covid-19," July 8, 2020, https://web.archive.org/web/20200805225722/https://www.glbthistory.org/fighting-back.

22. Yvette Ramírez, "Extending Affective Care in the Digital Realm," Visual AIDS Web Gallery, August 2020, https://visualaids.org/gallery/mapping-nyc-hyper-surveillance-during-covid-19.

23. June Lei, "Stages of Grief: A Dream within a Dream," Visual AIDS Web Gallery, May 2020, https://visualaids.org/gallery/stages-of-grief-a-dream-within-a-dream; Abdul-Aliy A. Muhammad, "Blesséd Are Those Who Remember: A Call to Cry, Feel and Mourn," Visual AIDS Web Gallery, July 2020, https://visualaids.org/gallery/blesse%CC%81d-are-those-who-remember-a-call-to-cry-feel-remember.

24. Ezra Benus and Noah Benus, "An Army of the Sick Can't Be Defeated: Reflections on Care Work in Perpetual Sick Times," Visual AIDS Web Gallery, April 2020, https://visualaids.org/gallery/caretaking-web-gallery; Journey Streams, "Ampler than Loneliness: Documenting Collective Resilience through HIV/AIDS and Covid-19," Visual AIDS Web Gallery, September 2020, https://

visualaids.org/gallery/documenting-collective-resilience-covid-hiv-2020 -web-gallery.

25. Jolly, "What HIV/AIDS Teaches Us about Covid-19."

26. My reflections on information and upheaval, aftermath, and aftercare are informed by the collaborative framing of AfterLab. Marika Cifor, Megan Finn, Anna Lauren Hoffmann, and Tonia Sutherland, "AfterLab: About Our Lab," https://www.afterlab.ischool.uw.edu/about-our-lab/.

27. Kerr, "How to Live with a Virus."

28. Juana María Rodríguez, *Sexual Futures, Queer Gestures, and Other Latina Longings* (New York: NYU Press, 2014); Marlon M. Bailey, "Nine Black Gay Men's Sexual Health and the Means of Pleasure in the Age of AIDS," in Cheng et al., *AIDS and the Distribution of Crises,* 217–35.

29. Shannon Faulkhead, "Connecting through Records: Narratives of Koorie Victoria," *Archives and Manuscripts* 37, no. 2 (2009): 60–88; Jamie A. Lee, *Producing the Archival Body* (New York: Routledge, 2020).

30. Hil Malatino, *Trans Care* (Minneapolis: University of Minnesota Press, 2020); Fink, *Forget Burial.*

31. Cifor et al., "AfterLab."

32. Cifor et al., "AfterLab."

33. Cifor et al., "AfterLab."

34. Roxane Gay, "Notes on Power in a Pandemic," *Medium,* April 3, 2020, https:// gay.medium.com/notes-on-power-in-a-pandemic-b43996c3e03.

35. Cifor et al., "AfterLab."

36. Crimp, "The Spectacle of Mourning," in *Melancholia and Moralism,* 201.

37. Gay, "Notes on Power in a Pandemic."

38. Visual AIDS, "Alternate Endings, Radical Beginnings," video curated by Erin Christovale and Vivian Crockett, 2017.

MARIKA CIFOR is assistant professor in the Information School and adjunct faculty in gender, women, and sexuality studies at the University of Washington.

NOT BILLS BUT BILLIONS

Power of Dreaming big et do it now Decret:

NOW I AM RICH!

I AM Rich, then I AM born then I forget.

Reading this book, you will be born again,

and your eyes will see your wealth.

$6000.000 in 3 Months

Small Book

By

Edje Bouka